THIRD EDITION

HUMAN RESOURCES

IN HEALTHCARE

Managing for Success

THIRD EDITION

HUMAN RESOURCES
IN HEALTHCARE

Managing for Success

**Bruce J. Fried and
Myron D. Fottler, Editors**

Health Administration Press, Chicago
Association of University Programs in Health Administration, Arlington, Virginia

12   11   10   09   5   4   3   2

Library of Congress Cataloging-in-Publication Data

Human resources in healthcare: managing for success / Bruce J. Fried
and Myron D. Fottler, editors.—3rd ed.
        p. cm.
Includes bibliographical references and index.
ISBN 978-1-56793-299-7 (alk. paper)
1. Health facilities—Personnel management. I. Fried, Bruce, 1952-
II. Fottler, Myron D.
[DNLM: 1. Personnel Management—methods. WX 159 H91807 2008]
RA971.35.H864 2008
362.1068'3—dc22

                                                                2008013657

The paper used in this publication meets the minimum requirements of American National Standard for Information Sciences—Permanence of Paper for Printed Library Materials, ANSI Z39.48-1984. ∞ ™

Project manager: Jane Calayag; Acquisitions editor: Audrey Kaufman; Cover designer: Anne LoCascio; Composition: Putman Productions, LLC

Health Administration Press
A division of the Foundation
   of the American College of
   Healthcare Executives
One North Franklin Street
Suite 1700
Chicago, IL 60606
(312) 424-2800

Association of University Programs
   in Health Administration
2000 14th Street North
Suite 780
Arlington, VA 22201
(703) 894-0940

BRIEF CONTENTS

DETAILED CONTENTS

FOREWORD

Human resources management is one of the most dynamic and rewarding responsibilities in healthcare delivery. Because a healthcare organization cannot exist without the people who provide care, both directly and indirectly, recruitment and retention of staff are critical. A healthcare organization can only be as competent and quality-focused as its employees, physicians, leaders, and volunteers. To ensure the delivery of safe patient care, recruitment and retention of a highly skilled and qualified workforce are essential and must be a top priority.

Today's healthcare organizations face many challenges, including significant shortages of physicians; nurses; respiratory therapists; radiologic, cardiovascular, and medical technologists; physical and occupational therapists; physician assistants; and nurse practitioners. Making recruitment particularly imperative is the fact that the population is aging and will be leaving the workforce in large numbers; consequently, more healthcare services will be demanded in the years ahead. Never before has it been so important for healthcare leaders and managers to understand employee satisfiers.

"Workforce development" is a relatively new term that refers to the continuing education and training of employees for current, new, and/or changing jobs. Such a program also aims to recruit and prepare students for the jobs of the future. Healthcare organizations that do not have a strong, committed workforce development program and/or a partnership with local high schools, colleges, and universities will find themselves grossly understaffed in the coming years. In addition, healthcare organizations must help the educational institutions in their communities to solve problems such as limited classroom capacity, inability to fill instructor vacancies, aging instructors, and long waiting lists of qualified students for allied health and nursing programs.

For the first time ever, people from four different generations are working together. Traditionalists, baby boomers, generation Xers, and millennials have differing work needs and expectations, challenging those who manage them to find appropriate ways to motivate, satisfy, reward, and recognize each group. The core values of one generation are also different from the other, so no longer will a one-size-fits-all approach to employee programs suffice. One theme that is common among members of these generations is the pursuit of work–life balance. No longer are employees interested in devoting their lives to their jobs. Time for friends, family, and self has become a significant worker value, making flexible work scheduling a must in contemporary organizations.

Workforce diversity and inclusion is another area of great challenge. There is fierce competition for talent with diverse backgrounds, and putting together a workforce that is diverse in culture, knowledge, perspective, and style is not easy. Many advances toward greater inclusion have been made, but major distances still need to be covered before the healthcare workforce can truly reflect the U.S. society as a whole.

Competitive compensation and benefit programs are especially essential in this tight labor market. Of even greater importance is ensuring that these programs motivate or provide an incentive to employees to achieve optimal performance. Performance management systems must be designed to clearly articulate expectations and to appropriately reward performance.

A recent addition to human resources challenges is disaster preparedness, and nowhere is this more important than in a healthcare organization. In the midst of a disaster, healthcare providers must be able to continue, and even expand, operations and services for their communities. At the same time, they must recognize and respond to the personal needs of their own staff, many of whom will be required to work during catastrophic events. Successful healthcare organizations are ready, willing, and able to respond when unforeseen circumstances occur, and they will occur.

Healthcare organizations have tremendous opportunities to recruit, retain, develop, and coach their workforce when reimbursement and other financial pressures are high. That is the time to be strategic and to make solid cost–benefit human resources decisions that support the organization's financial goals as well as the long-term ability to staff with highly qualified individuals. Although getting caught up in day-to-day problem solving is easy, quick fixes cannot address long-term issues.

Human resources management and strategic planning should mirror the strategic priorities and goals of the organization. Positive outcomes in human resources metrics are essential to financial health, patient satisfaction, and the ability to achieve goals each year.

This book provides a comprehensive discussion of these and other topics related to strategic human resources management. Whether you work in human resources specifically or management in general, you must understand and appreciate the connection between a positive workforce culture and outstanding patient care delivery. Human resources issues are complex, and the answers are not simple. Therefore, human resources thinking, planning, and execution must be strategic.

William K. Atkinson, PhD,
president and chief executive officer, WakeMed Health & Hospitals,
Raleigh, North Carolina

PREFACE

Change has become a staple of the healthcare system. It is omnipresent in our discussions about healthcare: A Google search for "healthcare change" yields more than 17 million results.

In the previous edition of this book, we made the observation that healthcare has undergone major transformations as a result of advances in technology, availability of information, and new forms of organizations and financing mechanisms. To this list we add the emerging impact of globalization not just on healthcare but also on the healthcare workforce, greater awareness of natural and man-made threats, and increased recognition of possible severe labor shortages because of the aging of the population and aging of the healthcare workforce.

An oft-repeated maxim is that "change creates opportunity." In the present healthcare environment, change inspires feelings of uncertainty. However, it does offer opportunities for honest people who seek solutions to healthcare problems, some of which have little precedent in terms of type or scope. This environment also creates opportunities for opportunists who, like snake-oil salesmen of days past, tempt us with quick fixes. Some of these fixes are merely repackaged and relabeled old strategies that are marketed effectively to a public desperate for new answers. Many of these fixes have little or no empirical support, but they are strongly promoted by "heroes of management." Simply turn your attention to the business section of any bookstore to see the array of fixes for sale.

Pfeffer and Sutton's (2006) book, *Hard Facts, Dangerous Half-Truths, and Total Nonsense,* provides an enlightening and amusing picture of the frivolous, trendy nature of the management book market. Even the titles of these books read like fads, even contradictory: *Love Is the Killer App: How to Win Business and Influence Friends* and *Business Is Combat: A Fighter Pilot's Guide to Winning in Modern Business Warfare.* With a few exceptions, the half-life of this genre of management "literature" is overall short but sufficiently long for its authors and publishers to reap a handsome profit and for business followers to jump on the next "revolutionary" method.

This new edition of *Human Resources in Healthcare* takes the approach supported by Pfeffer and Sutton and by responsible leaders in the healthcare industry who advocate the use of evidence in management and clinical work. In a recent *JAMA* article, Shortell, Rundall, and Hsu make an eloquent case for linking evidence-based medicine (EBM) and evidence-based management (EBMgt) to improve quality of care:

> Until both components are in place—identifying the best content (i.e., EBM) and applying it within effective organizational contexts (i.e., EBMgt)—consistent, sustainable improvement in the quality of care received by US residents is unlikely to occur (Shortell, Rundall, and Hsu 2007, 673).

Evidence-based management practices do not always have the shelf appeal of popular business methods contained in books sold at mall shops. However, such practices are robust and long-standing, owing to the fact that they have empirical support, have led to a sustained record of success, and have been designated as best practices. This edition, like the last two editions, is filled with concepts and strategies that have, over the years, been repeatedly tested and refined by practicing leaders and managers in actual organizations.

A word about the general concept of management is in order, however. The success of management practices is considerably less certain than, for example, the well-proven effectiveness of the measles vaccine. After all, clinical trials are hard to come by in management. What works in management and human resources management often depends on a myriad of factors, codified in organizational contingency theories. This fact does not make our management theories, research findings, and practices invalid, however. In medicine, we know that patients with the same disease respond very differently to the same medication, but we do not yet fully understand why that is the case and we cannot yet personalize medications to the unique characteristics of the individual. The same idea applies to management.

In light of this, our humble advice is for managers at all organizational levels to be aware of the unique contingent factors that may have an impact on the effectiveness of any recommended practice or strategy. We accept the fact that many people in our impatient society will be less than satisfied with strategies that do not work in every circumstance, every time. But then again, those people are more likely to purchase books at their local mall.

While we hope that this book imparts evidence-based knowledge, we also realize that having this knowledge alone does not guarantee that even the most studious reader will become an effective manager. We certainly would not expect someone who only carefully read and absorbed medical textbooks, but who never actually performed the procedures and obtained feedback, to perform any type of surgery, let alone a successful one. The point is that effectiveness takes a considerable amount of learning, practice, and time. Being an expert manager means getting to the point where book knowledge becomes intuitive and decisions are guided by this intuition. It is no wonder that the archetype of the wise old man or woman can be found across cultures.

Having said this, we encourage readers to supplement the empirical strategies and tools presented in this book with competency-building activities.

Book Overview

We have substantially revised the content of this book in our continuing efforts to impart, and keep up with, the knowledge base required to be competent in healthcare human resources management. This edition includes three new chapters:

- Chapter 3
- Chapter 9
- Chapter 12

In addition, the book contains three extensive cases that emphasize that human resources management goes beyond its own function and extends to other aspects of the organization.

Without exception, all other chapters have been expanded, updated, and improved. The new authors and coauthors in this edition not only further enrich the content but also add to the healthy mix of educators and practitioners who contributed to this book.

Chapters

Chapter 1, by Myron Fottler, explores strategic human resources management. For many years, the human resources function was synonymous with handling "personnel" and had a reputation for being passive and at times obstructionist in its relationship with internal customers. This chapter presents a progressive approach to human resources management that links human resources practices with organizational mission, strategies, and goals.

Chapter 2, by Tom Ricketts, offers an overview of human resources planning from a societal or national perspective. The chapter provides the reader with an appreciation of the regional, national, and global context of human resources planning and management.

Chapter 3, by Leah Masselink, discusses the increasing global mobility of healthcare professionals and its effects on the workforce and healthcare quality in this country and abroad. The chapter helps the reader consider the logistical and ethical challenges of this issue.

Chapter 4, by Kenneth White, Dolores Clement, and Kristie Stover, takes the reader through the world of various healthcare professions. This chapter lays out the functions, educational preparation, licensure requirements, changing roles, and management implications of those who directly provide and those who support the delivery of healthcare.

Chapter 5, by Beverly Rubin and Bruce Fried, is a guide in the vast legal environment surrounding healthcare human resources. Among other topics, the chapter addresses employee rights, discipline and privacy, sexual harassment, and equal employment opportunity.

Chapter 6, by Rupert Evans, focuses on the subject of societal and workforce diversity. This chapter gives a much-needed clarification on the meaning and application of diversity in healthcare organizations, pointing out that the term involves considerably more than a person's race and ethnicity.

Chapter 7, by Myron Fottler, brings us into, perhaps, the most critical foundational concept in human resources management: job analysis. The chapter explains the processes of and useful approaches to conducting a job analysis, creating job descriptions, and writing job specifications. Fottler contends that the deliberate structuring of work can lead to improved individual, group, and organizational performance.

Chapter 8, by Bruce Fried and Michael Gates, deals with recruitment, selection, and retention. In this edition, the chapter expands its coverage of retention, presenting recent evidence on the effectiveness of alternative retention strategies and discussing the costs of turnover.

Chapter 9, by Rita Quinton, offers useful, practical advice on designing and evaluating employee-training activities. The chapter is a comprehensive treatment of the many aspects of developing a training program that works.

Chapter 10, by Bruce Fried, describes a variety of approaches for managing employee performance, including providing feedback and building strategies for improvement. Fried emphasizes that for performance management to be effective, it needs to be viewed as positive rather than punitive and likely requires a change in organizational mind-set.

Chapter 11, by Howard Smith, Bruce Fried, Derek van Amerongen, and John Laughlin, is a comprehensive treatment of the issue of compensation, including balancing internal equity and external competitiveness and the conflicts that can arise within different compensation models.

Chapter 12, by Dolores Clement, Maria Curran, and Sharon Jahn, attends to a critical topic that was sorely missing in earlier editions: employee benefits. In this chapter, the authors dissect the aspects of employee benefits, including the history, current practices and challenges, budgetary implications, and benefits administration.

Chapter 13, by William Gentry, explores the issues of health and safety in the healthcare workplace. This chapter has been expanded to include disaster preparedness and disaster management.

Chapter 14, by Donna Malvey, covers labor relations and unionization. The chapter presents new information, including recent rulings that have direct relevance to healthcare. Malvey notes that the healthcare field and the public sector remain the two major targets for unionization in the United States.

Chapter 15, by Cheryl Jones and George Pink, is a broad discussion of nurse workload and measurement. The chapter addresses topics such as patient classification systems, evidence on the relationship between nurse workload and the quality of care, and nurse workload and nurse shortages. New exercises are included as well to stimulate thinking and discussion.

Chapter 16, by Eileen Hamby, concentrates on human resources budgeting and employee productivity. This chapter is particularly relevant today given the increased attention to using metrics in human resources management. Elements of a labor budget are described, and the controversial question of outsourcing is broken down and analyzed.

Chapter 17, by Myron Fottler and Robert Ford, emphasizes customer focus and the role of human resources in creating and maintaining a customer-focused organization. The chapter defines practical strategies to more closely align human resources systems with a customer-focused vision.

Chapter 18, by Bruce Fried and Myron Fottler, examines current and future societal and healthcare trends that have (and will have) implications for the healthcare workforce and human resources management. The authors posit that, in the face of challenges, human resources managers will need not only to play an active role as a strategic partner to the organization but also to be inquisitive, creative, and communicative about how human resources can best respond to these issues.

Cases

This edition also includes three integrative cases. Taking the perspective that human resources management is not confined to the "human resources silo," these cases challenge the reader to consider the larger environment of the organization when addressing human resources issues. Based on real situations, these cases analyze three different levels: the organization, the department, and the individual.

Case 1, by Sarah Huth and Sara Hofstetter, surrounds a downsizing effort at a VA facility and raises important questions about the many pitfalls of organizational reorganization.

Case 2, by Andy Garrard and Heather Grant, discusses a radiology department's struggle with its customer service role. The case involves the complex interplay among organizational trust, process improvement, organizational conflict, and technological change.

Case 3, by Lee Ellis, Dawn Morrow, and Adia Bradley, addresses the complex process of performance feedback and the difficult human issues that arise in providing feedback to employees.

Acknowledgments

Bruce Fried
First and foremost, I thank all of the authors who contributed to this book. All of them willingly and generously shared their knowledge and time. Thanks to staff at Health Administration Press—to Audrey Kaufman for humanely keeping us on schedule, and to Jane Calayag for her thoughtful and very helpful editing. I always appreciate the leadership of Peggy Leatt and Laurel Files in the Department of Health Policy and Administration at UNC. Together, Peggy and Laurel sustain a culture that encourages and nurtures innovation while challenging us always to look at the evidence.

I thank my children—Noah, Shoshana, and Aaron—who allow me to live vicariously through their growth. I also thank my parents, who have always supported my efforts, even when they are not quite certain how exactly I spend my time. Of course, I extend my gratitude to my wife, Nancy, who consistently provides me with tremendous emotional and intellectual support whether I think I need it or not.

Myron Fottler
Thanks to Megan McLendon, a student assistant and MHA student at the University of Central Florida. Her assistance and patience with typing various versions of my chapters, facilitating communications with editorial colleagues and other authors, and finding appropriate and relevant materials for updating chapters were invaluable and very much appreciated. My gratitude also goes to my wife, Carol, for her support on this and other projects over the years. Finally, I thank Aaron Liberman, chair of the Department of Health Administration and Informatics at the University of Central Florida, for his support of this project.

Bruce J. Fried, PhD
University of North Carolina at Chapel Hill

Myron D. Fottler, PhD
University of Central Florida

References

Pfeffer, J., and R. I. Sutton. 2006. *Hard Facts, Dangerous Half-Truths, and Total Nonsense: Profiting from Evidence-Based Management.* Boston: Harvard Business School Press.
Shortell, S. M., T. G. Rundall, and J. Hsu. 2007. "Improving Patient Care by Linking Evidence-Based Medicine and Evidence-Based Management." *JAMA* 298 (6): 673–76.

STRATEGIC HUMAN RESOURCES MANAGEMENT

Myron D. Fottler, PhD

Learning Objectives

After completing this chapter, the reader should be able to

- define strategic human resources management,
- outline key human resources functions,
- discuss the significance of human resources management to present and future healthcare executives, and
- describe the organizational and human resources systems that affect organizational outcomes.

Introduction

Like most other service industries, the healthcare industry is very labor intensive. One reason for healthcare's reliance on an extensive workforce is that it is not possible to produce a "service" and then store it for later consumption. In healthcare, the production of the service that is purchased and the consumption of that service occur simultaneously. Thus, the interaction between healthcare consumers and healthcare providers is an integral part of the delivery of health services. Given the dependence on healthcare professionals to deliver service, the possibility of heterogeneity of service quality must be recognized within an employee (as skills and competencies change over time) and among employees (as different individuals or representatives of various professions provide a service).

The intensive use of labor for service delivery and the possibility of variability in professional practice require that the attention of leaders in the industry be directed toward managing the performance of the persons involved in the delivery of services. The effective management of people requires that healthcare executives understand the factors that influence the performance of individuals employed in their organizations. These factors include not only the traditional *human resources management* (HRM) activities (i.e., recruitment and selection, training and development, appraisal, compensation, and employee relations) but also the environmental and other organizational aspects that impinge on human resources (HR) activities.

Strategic human resources management (SHRM) refers to the comprehensive set of managerial activities and tasks related to developing and maintaining a qualified workforce. This workforce, in turn, contributes to organizational effectiveness, as defined by the organization's strategic goals. SHRM occurs in a complex and dynamic milieu of forces within the organizational context. A significant trend that started within the last decade is for HR managers to adopt a strategic perspective of their job and to recognize critical linkages between organizational strategy and HR strategies (Fottler et al. 1990; Greer 2001).

This book explains and illustrates the methods and practices for increasing the probability that competent personnel will be available to provide the services delivered by the organization and that these employees will appropriately perform the necessary tasks. Implementing these methods and practices means that requirements for positions must be determined, qualified persons must be recruited and selected, employees must be trained and developed to meet future organizational needs, and adequate rewards must be provided to attract and retain top performers. All of these functions must be managed within the legal constraints imposed by society (i.e., legislation, regulation, and court decisions). This chapter emphasizes that HR functions are performed within the context of the overall activities of the organization. These functions are influenced or constrained by the environment, the organizational mission and strategies that are being pursued, and the systems indigenous to the institution.

Why study SHRM? How does this topic relate to the career interests or aspirations of present or future healthcare executives? Staffing the organization, designing jobs, building teams, developing employee skills, identifying approaches to improve performance and customer service, and rewarding employee success are as relevant to line managers as they are to HR managers. A successful healthcare executive needs to understand human behavior, work with employees effectively, and be knowledgeable about numerous systems and practices available to put together a skilled and motivated workforce. The executive also has to be aware of economic, technological, social, and legal issues that facilitate or constrain efforts to attain strategic objectives.

Healthcare executives do not want to hire the wrong person, to experience high turnover, to manage unmotivated employees, to be taken to court for discrimination actions, to be cited for unsafe practices, to have poorly trained staff undermine patient satisfaction, or to commit unfair labor practices. Despite their best efforts, executives often fail at HRM because they hire the wrong people or they do not motivate or develop their staff. The material in this book can help executives avoid mistakes and achieve great results with their workforce.

Healthcare organizations can gain a competitive advantage over competitors by effectively managing their human resources. This competitive advantage may include cost leadership (i.e., being a low-cost provider) and product differentiation (i.e., having high levels of service quality). A 1994 study examined the HRM practices and productivity levels of 968 organizations across 35 industries (Huselid 1994). The effectiveness of each organization's HRM practices was rated based on the presence of such benefits as incentive plans, employee grievance systems, formal performance appraisal systems, and employee participation in decision making. The study found that organizations with high HRM effectiveness ratings clearly outperformed those with low HRM rankings. A similar study of 293 publicly held companies reported that productivity was highly correlated with effective HRM practices (Huselid, Jackson, and Schuler 1997).

Based on "extensive reading of both popular and academic literature, talking with numerous executives in a variety of industries, and an application of common sense," Jeffrey Pfeffer (1998) identifies in his book, *The Human Equation*, the seven HRM practices that enhance an organization's competitive advantage. These practices seem to be present in organizations that are effective in managing their human resources, and they occur repeatedly in studies of high performing organizations. In addition, these themes are interrelated and mutually reinforcing; it is difficult to achieve positive results by implementing just one practice on its own. See Figure 1.1 for a list of the seven HRM themes relevant to healthcare. While these HR practices generally have a positive impact on organizational performance, their relative effectiveness may also vary depending on their alignment (or lack thereof) with each other and with the organizational mission, values, culture, strategies, goals, and objectives (Ford et al. 2006).

The bad news about achieving competitive advantage through the workforce is that it inevitably takes time to accomplish (Pfeffer 1998). The good news is that, once achieved, this type of competitive advantage is likely to be more enduring and more difficult for competitors to duplicate. Measurement is a crucial component for implementing the seven HR practices listed in Figure 1.1. Failure to evaluate the impact of HR practices dooms these practices to second-class status, neglect, and potential breakdown. Feedback from such measurement is essential in further development of or changes to practices as well as in monitoring how each practice is achieving its intended purpose.

Most of these HR practices are described in more detail throughout the book. Although the evidence presented in the literature shows that effective

1. *Provide employment security.* Employees can be fired if they do not perform, but they should not be put on the street quickly because of economic downturns or strategic errors by senior management over which employees have no control. An example that Pfeffer frequently cites is Southwest Airlines, which sees job security as a vital tool for building employee partnership and argues that short-term layoffs would "put our best assets, our people, in the arms of the competition."

2. *Use different criteria to select personnel.* Companies should screen for cultural fit and attitude, among other things, rather than just for skills that new employees can easily acquire through training.

3. *Use self-managed teams and decentralization as basic elements of organizational design.* Pfeffer is particularly keen on the way teams can substitute peer-based control of work for hierarchical control, thereby allowing for the elimination of management layers.

4. *Offer high compensation contingent on organizational performance.* High pay can produce economic success, as illustrated by the story of Pathmark. This large grocery store chain in the eastern United States had three months to turn the company around or go bust. The new boss increased the salaries of his store managers by 40 percent to 50 percent, enabling managers to concentrate on improving performance rather than complain about their pay.

5. *Train extensively.* Pfeffer notes that this activity "begs for some sort of return-on-investment calculations" but concludes that such analyses are difficult, if not impossible, to carry out. Successful companies that emphasize training do so almost as a matter of faith.

6. *Reduce status distinctions and barriers.* These include dress, language, office arrangements, parking, and wage differentials.

7. *Share financial and performance information.* The chief executive officer of Whole Foods Market has said that a high-trust organization "can't have secrets." His company shares salary information with every employee who is interested.

SOURCE: Pfeffer (1998)

HRM practices can strongly enhance an organization's competitive advantage, it fails to indicate why these practices have such an influence. In this chapter, we describe a model—the SHRM—that attempts to explain this phenomenon. First, however, a discussion of environmental trends is in order.

Environmental Trends

Among the major environmental trends that affect healthcare institutions are changing financing arrangements, emergence of new competitors, advent of new technology, low or declining inpatient occupancy rates, changes in physician–organization relationships, transformation of the demography and increase in diversity of the workforce, shortage of capital, increasing market penetration by managed care, heightened pressures to contain costs, and greater expectations of patients. The results of these trends have been increased competition, the need for higher levels of performance, and concern for institutional survival. Many healthcare organizations are closing facilities; undergoing corporate reorganization; instituting staffing freezes and/or reductions in workforce; allowing greater flexibility in work scheduling; providing services despite fewer resources; restructuring and/or redesigning jobs; outsourcing many functions; and developing leaner management structures, with fewer levels and wider spans of control.

Organizations are pursuing various major competitive strategies to respond to the current turbulent healthcare environment, including offering low-cost health services, providing superior patient service through high-quality technical capability and customer service, specializing in key clinical areas (e.g., becoming centers of excellence), and diversifying within or outside healthcare (Coddington and Moore 1987). In addition, organizations are entering into strategic alliances (Kaluzny, Zuckerman, and Ricketts 1995) and restructuring their organizations in various ways. Regardless of which strategies are being pursued, all healthcare organizations are experiencing a decrease in staffing levels in many traditional service areas and an increase in staffing in new ventures, specialized clinical areas, and related support services (Wilson 1986).

Staffing profiles in healthcare today are characterized by a limited number of highly skilled and well-compensated professionals. Healthcare organizations are no longer "employers of last resort" for the unskilled. At the same time, however, most organizations are experiencing shortages of various nursing and allied health personnel.

The development of appropriate responses to the ever-changing healthcare environment has received so much attention that HRM planning is now well accepted in healthcare organizations. However, implementation of such plans has often been problematic. The process often ends with the development of goals and objectives and does not include strategies or methods of implementation and ways to monitor results. Implementation appears to be the major difficulty in the overall management process (Porter 1980).

A major reason for this lack of implementation has been failure of healthcare executives to assess and manage the various external, interface, and internal stakeholders whose cooperation and support are necessary to successfully implement any business strategy (i.e., corporate, business, or functional) (Blair and Fottler 1990). A stakeholder is any individual or group with a "stake" in the organization. *External stakeholders* include patients and their families, public and private regulatory agencies, and third-party payers. *Interface stakeholders* are those who operate on the "interface" of the organization in both the internal and external environments; these stakeholders may include members of the medical staff who have admitting privileges or who are board members at several institutions. *Internal stakeholders* are those who operate within the organization, such as managers, professionals, and nonprofessional employees.

Involving supportive stakeholders, such as employees and HR managers, is crucial to the success of any HRM plan. If HR executives are not actively involved, then employee planning, recruitment, selection, development, appraisal, and compensation necessary for successful plan implementation are not likely to occur. McManis (1987, 19) notes that "[w]hile many hospitals have elegant and elaborate strategic plans, they often do not have supporting human resource strategies to ensure that the overall corporate plan can be implemented. But strategies don't fail, people do." Despite this fact, the healthcare industry as a whole spends less than one-half the amount that other industries are spending on human resources management (*Hospitals* 1989).

The SHRM Model

A strategic approach to human resources management includes the following (Fottler et al. 1990):

- Assessing the organization's environment and mission
- Formulating the organization's business strategy
- Identifying HR requirements based on the business strategy
- Comparing the current HR inventory—in terms of numbers, characteristics, and practices—with future strategic requirements
- Developing an HR strategy based on the differences between the current inventory and future requirements
- Implementing the appropriate HR practices to reinforce the business strategy and to attain competitive advantage

Figure 1.2 provides some examples of possible linkages between strategic decisions and HRM practices.

SHRM has not been given as high a priority in healthcare as it has received in many other industries. This neglect is particularly surprising in a labor-intensive industry that requires the right people in the right jobs at the right times and that often undergoes shortages in various occupations (Cerne 1988). In addition, the literature in the field offers fairly strong evidence that organizations that use more progressive HR approaches achieve significantly better financial results than comparable, although less progressive, organizations do (Gomez-Mejia 1988; Huselid 1994; Huselid, Jackson, and Schuler 1997; Kravetz 1988).

Strategic Decision	Implications on HR Practices
Pursue low-cost competitive strategy	→ Provide lower compensation Negotiate give-backs in labor relations Provide training to improve efficiency
Pursue service-quality differentiation competitive strategy	→ Provide high compensation Recruit top-quality candidates Evaluate performance on the basis of patient satisfaction Provide training in guest relations
Pursue growth through acquisition	→ Adjust compensation Select candidates from acquired organization Outplace redundant workers Provide training to new employees
Pursue growth through development of new markets	→ Promote existing employees on the basis of an objective performance-appraisal system
Purchase new technology	→ Provide training in using and maintaining the technology
Offer new service/product line	→ Recruit and select physicians and other personnel
Increase productivity and cost effectiveness through process improvement	→ Encourage work teams to be innovative Take risks Assume a long-term perspective

FIGURE 1.2

Implications of Strategic Decisions on HR Practices

Figure 1.3 illustrates some strategic HR trends that affect job analysis and planning, staffing, training and development, performance appraisal, compensation, employee rights and discipline, and employee and labor relations. These trends are discussed in more detail in later chapters in this book. The bottom line of Figure 1.3 is that organizations are moving to higher levels of flexibility, collaboration, decentralization, and team orientation. This transformation is driven by the environmental changes and the organizational responses to those changes discussed earlier.

FIGURE 1.3
Strategic
Human
Resources
Trends

Old HR Practices		*Current HR Practices*
Job Analysis/Planning		
Explicit job descriptions	⟶	Broad job classes
Detailed HR planning	⟶	Loose work planning
Detailed controls	⟶	Flexibility
Efficiency	⟶	Innovation
Staffing		
Supervisors make hiring decisions	⟶	Team makes hiring decisions
Emphasis on candidate's technical qualifications	⟶	Emphasis on "fit" of applicant within the culture
Layoffs	⟶	Voluntary incentives to retire
Letting laid-off workers fend for themselves	⟶	Providing continued support to terminated employees
Training and Development		
Individual training	⟶	Team-based training
Job-specific training	⟶	Generic training emphasizing flexibility
"Buy" skills by hiring experienced workers	⟶	"Make" skills by training less-skilled workers
Organization responsible for career development	⟶	Employee responsible for career development
Performance Appraisal		
Uniform appraisal procedures	⟶	Customized appraisals
Control-oriented appraisals	⟶	Developmental appraisals
Supervisor inputs only	⟶	Appraisals with multiple inputs
Compensation		
Seniority	⟶	Performance-based pay
Centralized pay decisions	⟶	Decentralized pay decisions
Fixed fringe benefits	⟶	Flexible fringe benefits (i.e., cafeteria approach)
Employee Rights and Discipline		
Emphasis on employer protection	⟶	Emphasis on employee protection
Informal ethical standards	⟶	Explicit ethical codes and enforcement procedures
Emphasis on discipline to reduce mistakes	⟶	Emphasis on prevention to reduce mistakes
Employee and Labor Relations		
Top-down communication	⟶	Bottom-up communication and feedback
Adversarial approach	⟶	Collaboration approach
Preventive labor relations	⟶	Employee freedom of choice

The SHRM Process

As illustrated in Figure 1.4, a healthcare organization is made up of systems that require constant interaction within the environment. To remain viable, an organization must adapt its strategic planning and thinking to extend to external changes. The internal components of the organization are affected by these changes, so the organization's plans may necessitate modifications in terms of the internal systems and HR process systems. There must be harmony among these systems.

The characteristics, performance levels, and amount of coherence in operating practices among these systems influence the outcomes achieved in terms of organizational and employee-level measures of performance. HR goals, objectives, process systems, culture, technology, and workforce must be aligned with each other (i.e., internal alignment) and with various levels of organizational strategies (i.e., external alignment) (Ford et al. 2006).

Internal and External Environmental Assessment

Environmental assessment is a crucial element of SHRM. As a result of changes in the legal/regulatory climate, economic conditions, and labor-market realities, healthcare organizations face constantly changing opportunities and threats. These opportunities and threats make particular services or markets more or less attractive in the organization's perspective.

Among the trends currently affecting the healthcare environment are increasing diversity of the workforce, aging of the workforce, labor shortages, changing worker values and attitudes, and advances in technology. Healthcare executives have responded to these external environmental pressures through various internal, structural changes, including developing network structures, joining healthcare systems, participating in mergers and acquisitions, forming work teams, implementing continuous quality improvement, allowing telecommuting, employee leasing, outsourcing, using more temporary or contingent workers, and globalization.

Healthcare executives need to assess not only their organizational strengths and weaknesses but also their internal systems; human resources' skills, knowledge, and abilities; and portfolio of service markets. Management of human resources involves paying attention to the effect of environmental and internal components on the HR process. Because of the critical role of healthcare professionals in delivering services, managers should develop HR policies and practices that are closely related to, influenced by, and supportive of the strategic goals and plans of their organization.

Organizations, either explicitly or implicitly, pursue a strategy in their operations. Deciding on a strategy means determining the products or services that will be created and the markets to which the chosen services will be offered. Once the selection is made, the methods to be used to compete in the

FIGURE 1.4
SHRM
Model

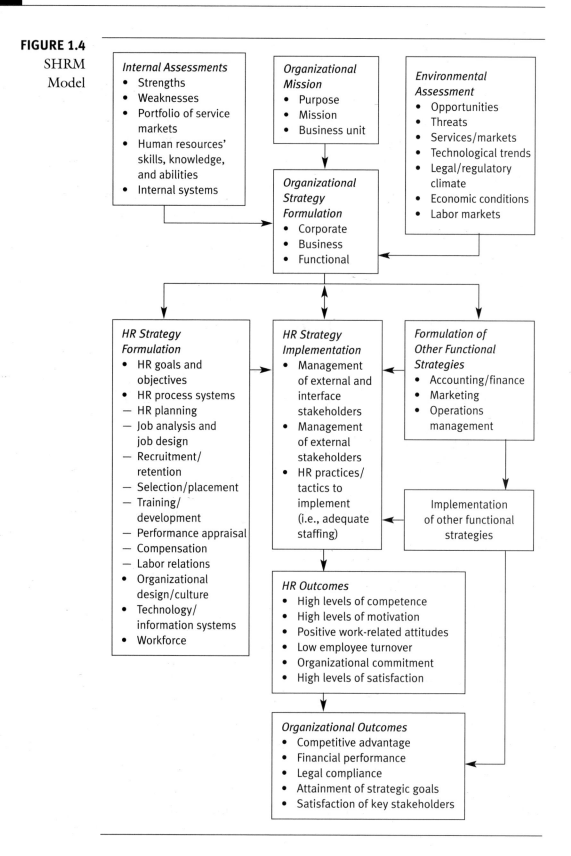

chosen market must be identified. The methods adopted are based on internal resources available, or potentially available, for use by managers. As shown in Figure 1.4, strategies should consider environmental conditions and organizational capabilities. To be in a position to take advantage of opportunities that are anticipated to occur, as well as to parry potential threats from changed conditions or competitor initiatives, managers must have detailed knowledge of the current and future operating environment. Cognizance of internal strengths and weaknesses allows managers to develop plans based on an accurate assessment of the organization's ability to perform in the marketplace at the desired level.

SHRM does not occur in a vacuum; rather, it occurs in a complex and dynamic constellation of forces in the organizational context. One significant trend has been for HR managers to adopt a strategic perspective and to recognize the critical links between human resources and organizational goals. As seen in Figure 1.4, the SHRM process starts with the identification of the organization's purpose, mission, and business unit, as defined by the board of directors and the senior management team. The process ends with the HR function serving as a strategic partner to the operating departments. Under this new view of human resources management, the HR manager's job is to help operating managers achieve their strategic goals by serving as the expert in all employment-related activities and issues.

When HR is viewed as a strategic partner, talking about the single best way to do anything makes no sense. Instead, the organization must adopt HR practices that are consistent with its strategic mission, goals, and objectives. In addition, all healthcare executives are HR managers. Proper management of employees entails having effective supervisors and line managers throughout the organization.

Organizational Mission and Corporate Strategy

An organization's *purpose* is its basic reason for existence. The purpose of a hospital may be to deliver high-quality clinical care to the population in a given service area. An organization's *mission*, created by its board and senior managers, specifies how the organization intends to manage itself to most effectively fulfill its purpose. The mission statement often provides subtle clues on the importance the organization places on its human resources. The purpose and mission affect HR practices in obvious ways. A nursing home, for example, must employ nursing personnel, nurse aides, and food service workers to meet the needs of its patients.

The first step in formulating a corporate and business strategy is doing a *SWOT* (strengths, weaknesses, opportunities, and threats) *analysis*. The managers then attempt to use the organization's strengths to capitalize on environmental opportunities and to cope with environmental threats. Human resources play a fundamental role in SWOT analysis because the nature and type of people who work within an organization and the organization's ability to attract new talent represent significant strengths and weaknesses.

Most organizations formulate strategy at three basic levels: the corporate level, the business level, and various functional levels. *Corporate strategy* is a set of strategic alternatives that an organization chooses from as it manages its operations simultaneously across several industries and markets. *Business strategy* is a set of strategic alternatives that an organization chooses from to most effectively compete in a particular industry or market. *Functional strategies* consider how the organization will manage each of its major functions (i.e., marketing, finance, and human resources).

A key challenge for HR managers when the organization is using a corporate growth strategy is recruiting and training large numbers of qualified employees, who are needed to provide services in added operations. New-hire training programs may also be needed to orient and update the skills of incoming employees. In Figure 1.4, the two-way arrows connecting "Organizational Strategy Formulation" and "HR Strategy Formulation" indicate that the impact of the HR function should be considered in the initial development of organizational strategy. When HR is a true strategic partner, all organizational parties consult with and support one another.

HR Strategy Formulation and Implementation

Once the organization's corporate and business strategies have been determined, managers can then develop an HR strategy. This strategy commonly includes a staffing strategy (planning, recruitment, selection, placement), a developmental strategy (performance management, training, development, career planning), and a compensation strategy (salary structure, employee incentives).

A *staffing strategy* refers to a set of activities used by the organization to determine its future HR needs, recruit qualified applicants with an interest in the organization, and select the best of those applicants as new employees. This strategy should be undertaken only after a careful and systematic development of the corporate and business strategies so that staffing activities mesh with other strategic elements of the organization. For example, if retrenchment is part of the business strategy, the staffing strategy will focus on determining which employees to retain and what process to use in termination.

A *developmental strategy* helps the organization enhance the quality of its human resources. This strategy must also be consistent with the corporate and business strategies. For example, if the organization wishes to follow a strategy of differentiating itself from competitors through customer focus and service quality, then it will need to invest heavily in training its employees to provide the highest-quality service and to ensure that performance management focuses on measuring, recognizing, and rewarding performance—all of which lead to high levels of service quality. Alternatively, if the business strategy is to be a leader in providing low-cost services, the developmental strategy may focus on training to enhance productivity to keep overall costs low.

A *compensation strategy* must also complement the organization's other strategies. For example, if the organization is pursuing a strategy of related diversification, its compensation strategy must be geared toward rewarding employees whose skills allow them to move from the original business to related businesses (e.g., inpatient care to home health care). The organization may choose to pay a premium to highly talented individuals who have skills that are relevant to one of its new businesses. When formulating and implementing an HR strategy and the basic HR components discussed earlier, managers must account for other key parts of the organization, such as organizational design, corporate culture, technology, and the workforce (Bamberger and Fiegelbaum 1996).

Organizational design refers to the framework of jobs, positions, groups of positions, and reporting relationships among positions. Most healthcare organizations use a *functional design* whereby members of a specific occupation or role are grouped into functional departments such as OB-GYN, surgery, and emergency services. Management roles are also divided into functional areas such as marketing, finance, and human resources. The top of the organizational chart is likely to reflect positions such as chief executive officer (CEO) and vice presidents of marketing, finance, and human resources. To operate efficiently, and allow for seamless service, an organization with a functional design requires considerable coordination across its various departments.

Many healthcare organizations have been moving toward a flat organizational structure or *horizontal corporation*. Such an organization is created by eliminating levels of management, reducing bureaucracy, using wide spans of control, and relying heavily on teamwork and coordination to get work accomplished. These horizontal corporations are designed to be highly flexible, adaptable, streamlined, and empowered. The HR function in such organizations is typically diffused throughout the system so that operating managers take on more of the responsibility for HR activities and the HR staff play a consultative role.

Corporate culture refers to the set of values that help members of that culture understand what they stand for, how they do things, and what they consider important. Because culture is the foundation of the organization's internal environment, it plays a major role in shaping the management of human resources, determining how well organizational members will function together and how well the organization will be able to achieve its goals. There is no ideal culture for all organizations, but a strong and well-articulated culture enables employees to know what the organization stands for, what it values, and how to behave. A number of forces shape an organization's culture, including the founder or founders, institutional affiliations, shared experiences, symbols, stories, slogans, heroes, and ceremonies.

Managers must recognize the importance of culture and take appropriate care to transmit that culture to others in the organization. Culture can be transmitted through orientation, training, consistent behavior (i.e., walking the talk), corporate history, and telling and retelling of stories. Culture may facilitate the work of either HR managers or line managers. If the organization has a strong, well-understood, and attractive culture, recruiting and retaining qualified employees become easier. If the culture is perceived as weak or unattractive, recruitment and retention become problematic. Likewise, the HR function can reinforce an existing culture by selecting new employees who have values that are consistent with that culture.

Technology also plays a role in the formulation and implementation of an HR strategy. The HR activities of healthcare organizations are quite different from those in the manufacturing industry. In healthcare, different criteria for hiring and methods of training are used. In addition, healthcare organizations typically emphasize educational credentials. Many aspects of technology play a role in HR in all healthcare settings. For example, automation of certain routine functions may reduce demand for certain HR activities but may increase it for others. Computers and robotics are important technological elements that affect HRM, and rapid changes in technology affect employee selection, training, compensation, and other areas.

Appropriately designed management information systems provide data to support planning and management decision making. HR information is a crucial element of such a system, as such information can be used for both planning and operational purposes. For example, strategic planning efforts may require data on the number of professionals in various positions who will be available to fill future needs. Internal planning may require HR data in categories such as productivity trends, employee skills, work demands, and employee turnover rates. The use of an intranet (an internal internet that is available to all members of an organization) can improve service to all employees, help the HR department, and reduce many routine administrative costs (Gray 1997).

Finally, *workforce composition* and trends also affect HR strategy formulation and implementation. The American workforce has become increasingly diverse in numerous ways. It has seen growth in the number of older employees, women, Latinos, Asians, African Americans, foreign born, the disabled, single parents, gays, lesbians, and people with special dietary preferences. Previously, most employers observed a fairly predictable employee pattern: People entered the workforce at a young age, maintained stable employment for many years, and retired at the usual age—on or around age 65. This pattern has changed and continues to evolve as a result of demographic factors, improved health, and the abolition of mandatory retirement.

As mentioned earlier, the successful implementation of an HR strategy generally requires identifying and managing key stakeholders (Blair and Fottler 1990, 1998). The HR strategy, as all other strategies, can only be implemented through people; therefore, such implementation requires motivational and communication processes, goal setting, and leadership. Specific practices or tactics are also necessary to implement the HR strategy. For example, if a healthcare organization's business strategy is to differentiate itself from competitors through its high-level focus on meeting customer (patient) needs, then the organization may formulate an HR strategy to provide all employees with training in guest relations.

However, that training strategy alone will not accomplish the business objective. Methods for implementation also need to be decided; for example, should the training be provided in-house or externally through programs such as those run by the Disney Institute? How will each employee's success in applying the principles learned be measured and rewarded? The answers to such questions provide the specific tactics needed to implement the HR strategy associated with the business goal of differentiation through customer service. Obviously, the organization will also develop and implement other functional strategies in accounting/finance, marketing, operations management, and other areas. Positive or negative organizational outcomes are determined by how well all of these functional strategies are formulated, aligned, and implemented.

HR Outcomes and Performance

The outcomes achieved by a healthcare organization depend on its environment, its mission, its strategies, its HR process systems, its internal systems and the consistency with which the operating practices are followed across these systems, and its capability to execute all of the above factors. The appropriate methods for organizing and relating these factors are determined by the outcomes desired by managers and other major stakeholders, and numerous methods exist for conceptualizing organizational performance and outcomes (Cameron and Whetten 1983; Goodman and Pennings and Associates 1977). For this discussion, the specific outcomes are HR outcomes and organizational outcomes (see the two bottom boxes in Figure 1.4).

Numerous HR outcomes are associated with HR practices. An organization should provide its workforce with job security, meaningful work, safe conditions of employment, equitable financial compensation, and a satisfactory quality of work life. Organizations will not be able to attract and retain the number, type, and quality of professionals required to deliver quality health services if the internal work environment is unsuitable. In addition, employees are a valuable stakeholder group whose concerns are important because of the complexity of the service they provide. Job satisfaction (Starkweather and Steinbacher 1998), commitment to the organization (Porter et al. 1974), motivation (Fottler et al. 2006), levels of job stress (DeFrank and

Ivancevich 1998), and other constructs can be used as measures of employee attitude and psychological condition.

Measuring the HR Function

HR metrics are measures of HR outcomes and performance. Part of HR's role as a strategic business partner is to measure the effectiveness of the HR function as a whole as well as the various HR tasks. Today, HR is under some scrutiny, as management and other areas of the organization inquire how various HR activities contribute to performance outcomes (*HR Focus* 2005a). Specifically, the questions often focus on the return on investment (ROI) of HR activities.

Human capital metrics have been developed to determine how HR activities contribute to the organization's bottom line (*HR Focus* 2005b). Some employers now gather data on the ROI of various recruitment sources, such as print advertising, Internet advertising, college recruitment, internal transfers, and career fairs (Garvey 2005). Other employers track productivity using cost metrics, such as the time to fill positions, the percentage of diverse candidates hired, interview-to-offer ratios, offer-to-acceptance ratios, hiring manager satisfaction, new-hire satisfaction, cost per hire, headcount ratios, turnover costs, financial benefits of employee retention, and the ROI of training (Garvey 2005; Schneider 2006).

Such metrics relate to specific HR activities, but there is also a need to measure the overall contribution of the HR function to organizational performance and outcomes (Lawler, Levenson, and Boudreau 2004).

The HR Scorecard is one method to measure this contribution. This tool is basically a modified version of the balanced scorecard (BSC), which is a measurement and control system that looks at a mix of quantitative and qualitative factors to evaluate organizational performance (Kaplan and Norton 1996). The "balance" reflects the need for short-term and long-term objectives, financial and nonfinancial metrics, lagging and leading indicators, and internal and external performance perspectives. A book entitled *The Workforce Scorecard* extends research on the BSC to maximize workforce potential (Huselid, Becker, and Beatty 2005). The authors show that traditional financial performance measures are "lagging" performance indicators, which can be predicted by the way organizations manage their human resources. HR practices are the "leading" indicators, predicting subsequent financial performance.

The Mayo Clinic has developed its own HR balanced scorecard that allows the HR function to become more involved in the organization's strategic planning (Fottler, Erickson, and Rivers 2006). Based on the assumption "what gets measured gets managed," Mayo's HR balanced scorecard measures and monitors a large number of input and output HR indicators that are aligned with the organization's mission and strategic goals. This HR scorecard measures financial (i.e., staff retention savings), customer (i.e., employee retention, patient satisfaction), internal (i.e., time to fill positions), and learning (i.e., staff satisfaction, perceived training participation) areas.

Organizational Outcomes and Performance

For long-term survival, a healthcare organization must have a balanced, exchange relationship with the environment. This equitable relationship must exist because it is mutually beneficial to the organization and to the environment with which it interacts. A number of outcome measures can be used to determine how well the organization is performing in the marketplace and is producing a service that will be valued by consumers, such as growth, profitability, ROI, competitive advantage, legal compliance, strategic objectives attainment, and key stakeholder satisfaction. The latter may include such indexes as patient satisfaction, cost per patient day, and community perception.

The mission and objectives of the organization are reflected in the outcomes that are stressed by management and in the strategies, general tactics, and HR practices that are chosen. Management makes decisions that, combined with the level of fit achieved among the internal systems, determine the outcomes the institution can achieve. For example, almost all healthcare organizations need to earn some profit for continued viability. However, some organizations refrain from initiating new ventures that may be highly profitable if the ventures do not fit their overall mission of providing quality services needed by a defined population group. Conversely, some organizations may start some services that are acknowledged to be break-even propositions at best because those services are viewed as critical to their mission and the needs of their target market.

The concerns of such an organization are reflected not only in the choice of services it offers but also in the HR approaches it uses and the outcome measures it views as important. This organization likely places more emphasis on assessment criteria for employee performance and nursing unit operations that stress the provision of quality care than on criteria concerned with efficient use of supplies and the maintenance of staffing ratios. This selection of priorities does not mean that the organization is ignoring efficiency of operations; it just signals that the organization places greater weight on the former criteria. The outcome measures used to judge the institution should reflect its priorities.

Another institution may place greater emphasis on economic return, profitability, and efficiency of operations. Quality of care is also important to that organization, but the driving force for becoming a low-cost provider causes the organization to make decisions that reflect its business strategy; therefore, it stresses maintenance or reduction of staffing levels and strictly prohibits overtime. Its recruitment and selection criteria stress identification and selection of employees who will meet minimum job requirements and expectations and, possibly, will accept lower pay levels. In an organization that strives to be efficient, less energy may be spent on "social maintenance" activities designed to meet employee needs and to keep them from leaving or unionizing. The outcomes in this situation will reflect, at least in the short run, higher economic return and lower measures of quality of work life.

Regardless of their specific outcome objectives, most healthcare organizations seek competitive advantage over similar institutions. The ultimate goal of the HR function should be to develop a distinctive brand so that employees, potential employees, and the general public view that particular organization as the "choice" rather than as the "last resort."

The HR Brand   In HR, *branding* refers to the organization's corporate image or culture (Johnson and Roberts 2006). Because organizations are constantly competing for the best talent, developing an attractive HR brand is extremely important. A brand embodies the values and standards that guide employee behavior. It indicates the purpose of the organization, the types of people it hires, and the results it recognizes and rewards (Barker 2005). If an organization can convey that it is a great place to work for, it can attract the "right" people (*HR Focus* 2005c). Being acknowledged by an external source is a good way to create a recognized HR brand. Inclusion on national, published "best" lists, such as the following, helps an organization build a base of followers and enhances its recruitment and retention programs:

- *Fortune*'s 100 Best Companies to Work For
- *Working Mothers*'s 100 Best Companies for Working Mothers
- *Computerworld*'s Best Places to Work in IT
- Robert Levering and Milton Moskowitz's 100 Best Companies to Work for in America

Being selected for *Fortune*'s 100 Best Companies list is so desirable that some organizations try to change their culture, philosophy, and brand just to be included (Phillips 2005).

Cardinal Health in Dublin, Ohio, ranks 19th on *Fortune*'s list and is a major provider of healthcare products, services, and technologies (Schoeff 2006). Corporate leaders at Cardinal recently decided that the organization's competitive advantage lies with its people. As a result, the organization is concentrating its HR efforts on more strategic issues and outsourcing more administrative functions. Among its strategic activities are identifying and developing talent and more closely linking HR activities to strategic objectives. Cardinal's management believes that these changes will enable HR to become a strategic player and will greatly increase the organization's global HR capability.

The immediate goal of building a strong HR brand is to attract and retain the best employees. However, the ultimate goal is to enhance the organization's outcomes and performance—that is, to achieve competitive advantage.

Human Resources and the Joint Commission

The Joint Commission initiated a pilot project to assess the relationship between adequate staffing and clinical outcomes (Lovern 2001). The project was led by a 20-member national task force composed of hospital leaders, clinicians, and technical experts, among others (Joint Commission 2002). The task force submitted its recommendations, which became a standard—Standard HR 1.30—that was implemented in January 2004. This standard requires healthcare organizations to assess their *staffing effectiveness* by continually screening for issues that can potentially arise as a result of inadequate staffing. Staffing effectiveness is defined as the number, competency, and skill mix of staff related to the provision of needed care, treatment, and services. The Joint Commission's focus is on the link between HR strategy implementation (i.e., adequate staffing) and organizational outcomes (i.e., clinical outcomes)—see these two boxes in Figure 1.4.

Under Standard HR 1.30, a healthcare facility selects a minimum of four screening indicators—two for clinical/service and two for human resources. The idea behind using two sets of indicators is to understand their relationship with one another; it also emphasizes that no indicator, in and of itself, can directly demonstrate staffing effectiveness. An example of a clinical/service screening indicator is an adverse drug event, and examples of HR screening indicators are overtime and staff vacancy rates. Staffing inefficiencies may be revealed by examining multiple screening indicators related to patient outcomes.

A facility has to choose at least one indicator for each clinical/service and HR category from the Joint Commission's list, and additional screening indicators can be selected based on the facility's unique characteristics, specialties, and services. This selection also defines the expected impact that the absence of direct and indirect caregivers may have on patient outcomes. The data collected on these indicators are analyzed to identify potential staffing-effectiveness issues when performance varies from expected targets—that is, ranges of performance are evaluated, external comparisons are made, and improvement goals are assessed. The data are analyzed over time against the screening indicators to identify trends, patterns, or the stability of a process. At least once a year, managers report to the senior management team regarding the aggregation and analysis of data related to staffing effectiveness and regarding any actions taken to improve staffing.

HR screening indicators include the following:

- Overtime
- Staff vacancy rates
- Staff turnover rates

- Understaffing, as compared to the facility's staffing plan
- Nursing hours per patient day
- Staff injuries on the job
- On-call per diem use
- Sick time

Clinical/service screening indicators include the following:

- Patient readmission rates
- Patient infection rates
- Patient clinical outcomes by diagnostic category

    The healthcare organization is expected to drill down to determine the causes of variation when data vary from expectation. The organization then undertakes steps leading to appropriate actions that are likely to remedy identified problems. For example, analysis of the data may indicate the need for evaluation of the organization's staffing practices. If so, the organization takes specific actions to improve its performance. Examples of strategies that may be used to address identified staffing issues include the following:

- Staff recruitment
- Education/training
- Service curtailment
- Increased technology support
- Reorganization of work flow
- Provision of additional ancillary or support staff
- Adjustment of skill base

A Strategic Perspective on Human Resources

Managers at all levels are becoming increasingly aware that critical sources of competitive advantage include appropriate systems for attracting, motivating, and managing the organization's human resources. Adopting a strategic view of human resources involves considering employees as human "assets" and developing appropriate policies and programs to increase the value of these assets to the organization and the marketplace. Effective organizations realize that their employees have value, much as the organization's physical and capital assets have value.

    Viewing human resources from an investment perspective, rather than as variable costs of production, allows the organization to determine how to best invest in its people. This leads to a dilemma. An organization that does not invest in its employees may be less attractive to both current and prospective employees, which causes inefficiency and weakens the organization's competitive position. However, an organization that does invest in its people needs to ensure that these investments are not lost. Consequently, an organization needs to develop strategies to ensure that its employees stay on long enough so that it can realize an acceptable return on its investment in employee skills and knowledge.

Not all organizations realize that human assets can be strategically managed from an investment perspective. Management may or may not have an appreciation of the value of its human assets relative to its other assets such as brand names, distribution channels, real estate, and facilities and equipment. Organizations may be characterized as human-resources oriented or not based on their answers to the following:

- Does the organization see its people as central to its mission and strategy?
- Do the organization's mission statement and strategy objectives mention or espouse the value of human assets?
- Does the organization's management philosophy encourage the development of any strategy that prevents the depreciation of its human assets, or does the organization view its human assets as a cost to be minimized?

Often, an HR investment perspective is not adopted because it involves making a longer-term commitment to employees. Because employees can leave and most organizations are infused with short-term measures of performance, investments in human assets are often ignored. Organizations that are performing well may feel no need to change their HR strategies. Those that are not doing as well usually need a quick fix to turn things around and therefore ignore longer-term investments in people. However, although investment in human resources does not yield immediate results, it yields positive outcomes that are likely to last longer and are more difficult to duplicate by competitors.

Who Performs HR Tasks?

The person or unit that performs HR tasks has changed drastically in recent years. Today, the typical HR department does not exist, and no particular unit or individual is charged with performing HR tasks (*HR Focus* 2005b). Internal restructuring has often resulted in a shift as to who carries out HR tasks, but it has not eliminated those functions identified in Figure 1.4. In fact, in some healthcare organizations, the HR department continues to perform the majority of HR functions. However, questions are now being raised such as, Can some HR tasks be performed more efficiently by line managers or by outside vendors? Can some HR tasks be centralized or eliminated altogether? Can technology perform HR tasks that were once previously done by HR staff? (Rison and Tower 2005).

Over time, the number of HR staff has declined, and continues to decline, as others have begun to assume responsibility for certain HR functions

(*HR Magazine* 2005). Outsourcing, shared service centers, and line managers now assist in performing many HR functions and activities. While most organizations are expected to outsource more HR tasks in the future, the strategic components of HR will likely remain within the organization itself (Pomeroy 2005; *HR Focus* 2006a). HR managers will continue to be involved with strategic HR matters and other key functions, including performance management and compensation management (Davolt 2006; Pomeroy 2005).

The shift toward strategic HR is beginning to permit the HR function to shed its administrative image and to focus on more mission-oriented activities, as noted earlier (*HR Focus* 2006b). This shift also means that all healthcare executives need to become skilled managers of their human resources. More HR professionals are assuming a strategic perspective when it comes to managing HR-related issues (*HR Focus* 2005d; Meisinger 2005). As they do so, they are continually upgrading and enhancing their professional capabilities (Khatri 2006). This means that they must be given a seat at the board of director's table to help the chief officers, senior management, and board members make appropriate decisions concerning HR matters (*HR Focus* 2004; Fottler et al. 2006).

The three critical HR issues to which an HR professional can lend expertise and therefore help organizational governance include selecting the incoming CEO, tying the CEO's compensation to performance, and identifying and developing optimum business and HR strategies (Kenney 2005). In addition, the HR professional can also contribute to leveraging HR's role in major change strategies (e.g., mergers and acquisitions), developing and implementing HR metrics that are aligned with business strategies, and helping line managers achieve their unit goals (Pinola 2002).

In a study of HR leaders in more than 1,000 organizations, 67 percent of the respondents reported that they belonged to the executive team in their organization (*HR Focus* 2003). Similarly, a 2006 survey of 427 HR professionals revealed that of the respondents who oversaw the HR department, 63 percent directly reported to the CEO or president (*HR Focus* 2006c). Moreover, the same survey found that more than half of the respondents worked for an organization that had an established strategic HR plan, and most of the respondents worked directly with senior management in developing organizational strategies. Of course, these data are not necessarily representative of the healthcare industry. If such data were available for the healthcare industry, the results may indicate somewhat lower levels of HR function influence.

Summary

In healthcare, the intensive reliance on professionals to deliver high-quality services requires organizations and their leaders to focus attention on the strategic management of their human resources and to be aware of the factors that influence the performance of all their employees. To assist healthcare executives in understanding this dynamic, this chapter presents a model that explains the interrelationship among corporate strategy, selected organizational-design features, HRM activities, employee outcomes, and organizational outcomes.

The outcomes achieved by the organization are influenced by numerous HR and non-HR factors. The mission determines the direction that is being taken by the organization and the goals it desires to achieve. The amount of integration or alignment of mission, strategy, HR functions, behavioral components, and non-HR strategies defines the level of achievement that is possible.

Healthcare organizations are increasingly striving to impress a distinctive HR brand image upon employees, potential employees, and the general public. They are doing this by modifying their cultures and working hard to be included on various national lists of "best companies." Successful branding results in competitive advantage in both labor and service markets. Organizations are also increasing the volume and quality of HR metrics they collect and use in an effort to better align their HR strategies with their business strategies. Finally, the locus of HRM is shifting, as strategic functions are retained by HR professionals within the organization while administrative tasks are outsourced elsewhere or delegated to line managers.

Discussion Questions

1. Distinguish among corporate, business, and functional strategies. How does each strategy relate to human resources management? Why?

2. How may an organization's human resources be viewed as either a strength or a weakness when doing a SWOT analysis? What could be done to strengthen human resources in the event that it is seen as a weakness?

3. List factors under the control of healthcare managers that contribute to the decrease in the number of people applying to health professions schools. Describe the steps that healthcare organizations can take to improve this situation.

4. What are the organizational advantages of integrating strategic management and human resources management? What are the steps involved in such an integration?

5. One healthcare organization is pursuing a business strategy of differentiating its service product through providing excellent customer service. What HR metrics do you recommend to reinforce this business strategy? Why?

6. In what sense are all healthcare executives human resources managers? How can executives best prepare to perform well in this HR function?

Experiential Exercises

Exercise 1 Before class, obtain the annual report of any healthcare organization of your choice. Review the material presented and the language used. Write a one-page memo that assesses that organization's philosophy regarding its human resources. In class, form a group of four or five students. As a group, compare the similarities and differences among the organizations that each group member investigated. Discuss the following:

- How can you differentiate those organizations that merely "talk the talk" from those that also "walk the walk"?
- What factors influence how an organization perceives its human resources?
- How do "better" organizations perceive their human resources?
- What did you learn from this exercise?

Exercise 2 Before class, review the seven HR practices developed by Jeffrey Pfeffer and shown in Figure 1.1. Consider how your current/most recent employer follows any three of these seven practices. Write a 1–2 page summary that lists the three practices you selected and their compatibilities (or incompatibilities) with your employer's HRM practices. In class, form a group of four or five students and share your perceptions. Discuss the following:

- What similarities and differences arise among the practices in your organization and those in your group members' employers?
- Which of the seven practices seem to be least followed by these organizations, and why?

Exercise 3 Each year, *Fortune* magazine publishes a list of "The Best Companies to Work For in America." Editors of the magazine base their selection on an extensive review of the HR practices of many organizations as well as on surveys of those organizations' current and former employees.

Use the Internet to identify three healthcare organizations on the latest *Fortune* "best companies" list. Next, visit the websites of these organizations, and review the posted information from the perspective of a prospective job applicant. Then, as a potential employee, answer the following:

- What information on the websites most interested you, and why?
- Which organization's website scored best with you, and why?

Based on the information posted on these websites, what are the implications for you as a future healthcare executive who will be planning and implementing HRM practices? What information will you include on your organization's website that will attract and retain employees?

References

Bamberger, P., and A. Fiegelbaum. 1996. "The Role of Strategic Reference Points in Explaining the Nature and Consequences of Human Resource Strategy." *Academy of Management Review* 21 (4): 926–58.

Barker, J. 2005. "How to Pick the Best People (and Keep Them)." *Potentials* 38 (4): 33–36.

Blair, J. D., and M. D. Fottler. 1990. *Challenges in Healthcare Management: Strategic Perspectives for Managing Key Stakeholders.* San Francisco: Jossey-Bass.

———. 1998. *Strategic Leadership for Medical Groups.* San Francisco: Jossey-Bass.

Cameron, K. S., and D. A. Whetten. 1983. *Organizational Effectiveness: A Comparison of Multiple Models.* New York: Academic Press.

Cerne, F. 1988. "CEO Builds Employee Morale to Improve Finances." *Hospitals* 62 (11): 100.

Coddington, D. C., and K. D. Moore. 1987. *Market-Driven Strategies in Healthcare.* San Francisco: Jossey-Bass.

Davolt, S. 2006. "The Half-Truth of Total HRO." *Employee Benefit News* 20 (6): 26–27.

DeFrank, R. S., and J. M. Ivancevich. 1998. "Stress on the Job." *Academy of Management Executives* 12 (3): 55–65.

Ford, R. C., S. A. Sivo, M. D. Fottler, D. Dickson, K. Bradley, and L. Johnson. 2006. "Aligning Internal Organizational Factors with a Service Excellence Mission: An Exploratory Investigation in Healthcare." *Health Care Management Review* 31 (4): 259–69.

Fottler, M. D., J. D. Blair, R. L. Phillips, and C. A. Duran. 1990. "Achieving Competitive Advantage Through Strategic Human Resource Management." *Hospital & Health Services Administration* 35 (3): 341–63.

Fottler, M. D., S. J. O'Connor, T. D'Aunno, and M. Gilmartin. 2006. "Motivating People." In *Healthcare Management,* 5th Edition, edited by S. M. Shortell and A. D. Kaluzny, 78–124. Albany, NY: Delmar.

Fottler, M. D., E. Erickson, and P. A. Rivers. 2006. "Bringing Human Resources to the Table: Utilization of an HR Balanced Score Card at Mayo Clinic." *Healthcare Management Review* 31 (1): 64–72.

Garvey, C. 2005. "New Generation Hiring Metrics." *HR Magazine* 50 (4): 70–76.

Gomez-Mejia, L. R. 1988. "The Role of Human Resources Strategy in Expert Performance." *Strategic Management Journal* 9: 493–505.

Goodman, P. S., and J. M. Pennings and Associates. 1977. *New Perspectives on Organizational Effectiveness.* San Francisco: Jossey-Bass.

Gray, F. 1997. "How to Become Intranet Savvy." *HR Magazine* (4): 66–71.

Greer, C. R. 2001. *Strategic Human Resource Management.* Upper Saddle River, NJ: Prentice-Hall.

Hospitals. 1989. "Human Resources." *Hospitals* 63: 46–47.

HR Focus. 2003. "Survey Supports Link Between HR Strategies and Profitability." *HR Focus* 83 (12): 8.

———. 2004. "What Lies Ahead for HR?" *HR Focus* 81 (10): 1–15.

———. 2005a. "Getting Real and Specific with Measurement." *HR Focus* 82 (1): 11–13.

———. 2005b. "SHRM Predicts the Human Capital Metrics of the Future." *HR Focus* 82 (8): 7–10.

———. 2005c. "HR Brand Building in Today's Market." *HR Focus* 82 (2): 1–15.

———. 2005d. "HR's Growing Role in M&A." *HR Focus* 82 (8): 1–15.

———. 2006a. "HR Technology Is Fueling Profits, Cost Savings and Strategy." *HR Focus* 84 (1): 7–10.

———. 2006b. "HR Departments Struggle to Move Up from Administrative to Strategic Status." *HR Focus* 83 (3): 8.

———. 2006c. "How Strategic Is HR Now, the Latest Research Shows Progress." *HR Focus* 83 (12): 3–5.

HR Magazine. 2005. "Advice to HR: Simplify and Save." *HR Magazine* 50 (9): 18.

Huselid, M. A. 1994. "Documenting HR's Effect on Company Performance." *HR Magazine* 39 (1): 79–85.

Huselid, M. A., S. E. Jackson, and R. S. Schuler. 1997. "Technical and Strategic Human Resources Management Effectiveness as Determinants of Firm Performance." *Academy of Management Journal* 40 (1): 171–88.

Huselid, M. A., B. E. Becker, and R. W. Beatty. 2005. *The Workforce Scorecard.* Boston: Harvard Business School Press.

Johnson, M., and P. Roberts. 2006. "Rules of Attraction." *Marketing Health Services* 26 (1): 38–40.

Joint Commission. 2002. "Healthcare at the Crossroads: Strategies for Addressing the Evolving Nursing Crisis." [Online publication; accessed 7/12/05.] www.jcaho.org/about+us/public+policy+initatives/health+care+at+the+crossroads.pdf.

Kaluzny, A., H. Zuckerman, and T. Ricketts. 1995. *Partners for the Dance: Forming Strategic Alliances in Healthcare.* Chicago: Health Administration Press.

Kaplan, R. S., and D. P. Norton. 1996. *The Balanced Scorecard.* Boston: Harvard Business School Press.

Kenney, R. 2005. "The Boardroom Role of Human Resources." *Corporate Board* 26 (1): 12–16.

Khatri, N. 2006. "Building HR Capability in HR Organizations." *Healthcare Management Review* 31 (1): 45–54.

Kravetz, D. J. 1988. *The Human Resources Revolution: Implementing Progressive Management Practices for Bottom Line Success.* San Francisco: Jossey-Bass.

Lawler, E. E., A. Levenson, and J. W. Boudreau. 2004. "HR Metrics and Analytics: Use and Impact." *Human Resources Planning* 27 (1): 27–35.

Lovern, E. 2001. "JCAHO to Study Staffing Issues." *Modern Healthcare* 31 (3): 6–8.

McManis, G. L. 1987. "Managing Competitively: The Human Factor." *Healthcare Executive* 2 (6): 18–23.

Meisinger, S. 2005. "Fast Company: Do They Really Hate HR?" *HR Magazine* 50 (9): 12.

Pfeffer, J. 1998. *The Human Equation: Building Profits by Putting People First.* Boston: Harvard Business School Press

Phillips, J. J. 2005. "The Value of Human Capital: What Logic and Intuition Are Telling Us." *Chief Learning Officer* 4 (8): 50–52.

Pinola, R. 2002. "What CFOs Want from HR." *HR Focus* 79 (9): 1.

Pomeroy, A. 2005. "Outsourcing, One Step at a Time." *HR Magazine* 50 (6): 12.

Porter, L. W., R. M. Steers, R. T. Mowday, and P. V. Boulian. 1974. "Organizational Commitment, Job Satisfaction, and Turnover Among Psychiatric Technicians." *Journal of Applied Psychology* 59: 603–9.

Porter, M. E. 1980. *Competitive Strategy.* New York: The Free Press.

Rison, R. P., and J. Tower. 2005. "How to Reduce the Cost of HR and Continue to Provide Value." *Human Resource Planning* 28 (1): 14–19.

Schneider, C. 2006. "The New Human Capital Metrics." *CFO* 22 (2): 22–27.

Schoeff, M. 2006. "Cardinal Health HR to Take a More Strategic Role." *Workforce Management* (2): 7–8.

Starkweather, R. A., and C. L. Steinbacher. 1998. "Job Satisfaction Affects the Bottom Line." *HR Magazine* (9): 110–12.

Wilson, T. B. 1986. *A Guide to Strategic Human Resource Planning for the Healthcare Industry.* Chicago: American Society for Healthcare Human Resource Administration, American Hospital Association.

HEALTHCARE WORKFORCE PLANNING

Thomas C. Ricketts, III, PhD

Learning Objectives

After completing this chapter, the reader should be able to

- trace the history of human resources for health and workforce planning;
- learn why and when workforce planning is undertaken;
- briefly describe the five major methods used in workforce planning;
- understand the key concepts of benchmarking, adjusted needs, and demand as they apply to workforce planning;
- develop a simple estimate of the future supply of a profession for a population; and
- interpret the results of workforce planning reports as they relate to individual healthcare organizations and delivery systems.

Introduction

Most of this book views human resources management (HRM) from the perspective of the healthcare organization. Chapters focus on such topics as job design, recruitment and retention, and evaluation of individual performance. However, organizations are also affected by the larger external environment in which they are situated. In HRM, broad workforce policy and labor market factors, which are external aspects, affect an organization's ability to attract and retain employees. An organization may have a theoretically sound recruitment program for nurses, but if sufficient numbers of nurses are not being trained in the national healthcare system, the program will likely prove unsuccessful.

This chapter's focus is unique among the chapters in this book in that it addresses workforce planning for communities, regions, states, countries, and other jurisdictions. It devotes attention to the healthcare workforce needs throughout society rather than the needs of a particular organization.

Human resources for health (HRH) workforce planning deals with questions, including the following:

- How do we determine the number of surgeons needed in a particular geographic area?
- What factors help us to best anticipate future supply and need for various types of healthcare workers?
- What methods are used to project future workforce needs? What are the strengths and weaknesses of different approaches, and how may they be most effectively applied?

This chapter, therefore, takes a macro-level perspective on the healthcare workforce and examines concepts and methodologies that are useful in projecting workforce requirements for communities and larger regions. Much of the remainder of this book focuses on internal strategies for managing human resources, which we can view as micro-level approaches, and addresses workforce concerns from the perspective of a single organization.

Workforce planning is the assessment of needs for human resources. This process can be very formal and complex or depend on "back-of-the-envelope" estimates and can be applied to small organizations or practices as well as to national and international healthcare delivery systems. Workforce planning fits in with overall health systems planning and human resources development and management. One conceptualization sees workforce planning as one of three steps in workforce development (De Geyndt 2000):

1. Planning is the quantity concern.
2. Training is the quality concern.
3. Managing is the performance and output concern.

The Australian Medical Workforce Advisory Committee (2003) describes workforce planning succinctly: "ensuring that the right practitioners are in the right place at the right time with the right skills." However, the consensus remains that workforce planning is "not an exact science" (Fried 1997).

Workforce planning is used to support decision making and policy development for a wide range of concerns. For healthcare organizations to meet their clinical and operating goals and objectives, they must effectively deploy and support workers of all kinds. Doing so requires that the numbers and types of workers match the needs of the patients, regulators, and payers who make up the functional environment of the healthcare organization. For state, provincial, and regional or national systems, policymakers also require information from planning processes that include workforce projections and assessments. Functionally, workforce planning does several things:

- Interprets tasks and roles
- Establishes education and training needs

- Explains the dynamics of the workforce
- Describes and disseminates information about workforce and workplace change
- Defines and identifies shortages and surpluses

The History of Healthcare Workforce Planning

HRH planning dates back to the origins of organized medicine and healthcare. Military planners recognized the need to provide adequate numbers of caregivers for wounded and ill soldiers, and very rough assessments of the requirements for qualified medical workers were part of the preparation for military campaigns. The healthcare system in the Soviet Union, and later in socialized nations, made use of systemwide planning (which includes an estimate of the numbers and types of workers) in structuring healthcare. As European democracies moved toward national healthcare insurance systems, they recognized the need to balance their policies for training and preparing healthcare workers with the anticipated needs of the covered populations. Given the importance of human resources to healthcare systems and the examples of planning that were in existence, it was still possible for an expert group to observe that "only very recently has there been more of a substantive debate about this issue internationally" (Dubois, McKee, and Nolte 2006). While HRH planning has a fairly rich history within individual nations and among international bodies like the United Nations, it has received little reflection in most other countries. The United States offers an exception.

Daniel Fox (1996) describes healthcare workforce policy in the United States as "contentious and uncertain" and characterizes its history as a process that moved from "piety, to platitudes, to pork." His observations apply mostly to the ongoing debate over whether the government should directly support the education and preparation of physicians, or indirectly through some levy on social insurance, or not at all. Fox tracked the history of policies that were discussed and applied over time to support medical education. His analysis pertains to the development of policy that depends on workforce planning, but he did not speak specifically of that development process.

Fox's observations provide a useful context for understanding why we would or would not plan for a healthcare workforce in the United States. These reasons have implications for whether planning should be supported. By calling the initial stage of workforce policymaking the result of "pious" thinking, Fox implies that policymakers knew exactly the "right thing to do" and needed no or little specific guidance or planning to assist them. The subsequent dependence on "platitudes" about the reality of need and supply of physicians and nurses was made by using "accepted wisdom," which again meant that there was little need for either planning or research. The culmination of the policy stream with "pork" meant that resources were distributed according to political power with little regard for the "facts"—again, a situation that does not require the development of information and specific planning.

Healthcare workforce policy has traditionally been driven by a perception of a shortage of one or more of the healthcare professions. The history of concern over shortages may have started with physicians, but nurses were also considered a special part of the healthcare workforce and were subject to policy attention. The Nurse Training Act of 1941 attempted to expand nursing schools during wartime to provide nurses for the military. An apparent shortage of nurses in the late 1950s generated the first federal legislation to support training of healthcare professionals for the "market," not for some specific federal role. Subsidies for nursing education and public health traineeships were included in the Health Amendments Act of 1956, beginning an incremental expansion of federal government support for healthcare workforce training.

What followed were a series of healthcare professions laws that encouraged the creation of training programs, supported faculty, expanded schools, or provided special aid for programs to redistribute the workforce. The Health Professions Educational Assistance Act of 1963 (P.L. 88-129) provided construction money for healthcare professions schools—funds tied to increased enrollment requirements to assist with the school's operating expenses as well as loans and scholarship programs. The Act authorized support to medical schools for the first time and firmly established the presence of the federal government in health-related educational institutions. This was followed by an almost annual succession of laws that added support for nurses, created loan-repayment plans, and paid for construction. In 1970, the National Health Service Corps was created, which put the federal government in a role as a direct provider of healthcare professional service for the general population.

The precedent had been set for federal involvement in workforce policy in 1956, but early in the twentieth century many states took on healthcare professions education and regulation as an extension of their responsibility for public education and their implied "police powers" to protect the health, safety, and welfare of their citizens. Assuming a combination of power over both education and entry into the healthcare professions seems to suggest that the conditions were ripe for some form of planning on the part of the states that were investing substantial resources in medical and other health professions schools and that had ready policy levers to control the supply of practitioners. However, the politics of the healthcare professions were clearly dominated by the professions themselves, and the dominant culture was to support the market for a highly paid elite physician workforce assisted by less-well-paid nurses and other caregivers (Starr 1982). According to Weissert and Silberman (1998), not until the 1990s did the states begin to "send a message that the medical schools have a responsibility to the state and its citizens." For some reason, the states were not overly concerned with healthcare workforce supply and needs until the beginning of the twenty-first century.

Workforce planning can be considered a subtopic in the general area of HRH planning, but the two do not necessarily share a common history, and important differences exist in the way they are approached. Planning is usually initiated when a perception exists that limited resources are available to meet all possible needs and that the market will not adequately distribute the available benefits.

The Rationale for Healthcare Workforce Planning

History tells us that policy and political pressures are generated when either the market or the public signals a shortage of some type of basic good or service. In the case of healthcare workforce, the shortage is of healing practitioners and their supporting trades and professions. The case for formal planning, however, is often made in a more abstract and value-free context. Advocates for workforce planning sometimes appeal to a need for "rational policymaking," but often the stimulus for formal action is when people claim that they cannot get what they want, need, or deserve.

In the United States today, the perception of a nursing shortage and the concern over a potential physician shortage are stimulating the demand for workforce planning. In Canada and the United Kingdom, both of which provide national healthcare coverage, queues for certain types of care are long, drawing attention to the need for workforce planning. The World Health Organization (2000, 2006) recognizes that HRH planning has to be able to respond to changes in technology and global patterns of migration in both population and profession. The drivers of HRH planning have expanded to include the workforce's adaptation to technology as well as the match of needs to supply. Figure 2.1 describes an analytical framework for HRH planning that considers the emerging concerns over global markets; migration; and changes in technology, institutions, and populations. The figure emphasizes that the healthcare system is embedded in a complex web of very strong external forces that shape the inputs to the system, including the human resources necessary for the system to function.

FIGURE 2.1

The Contexts
for Planning in
HRH
Workforce
Planning

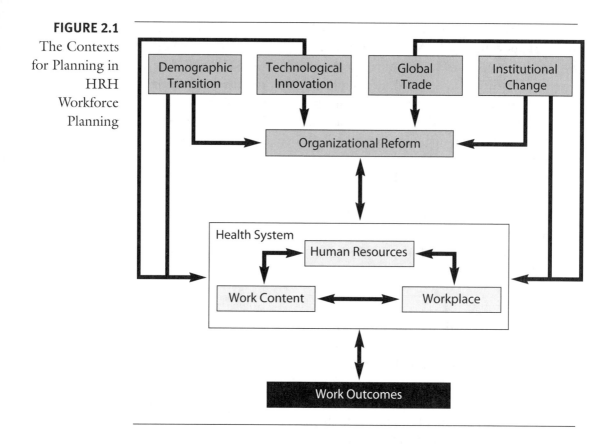

Overview of Workforce Planning Methodologies

Five basic strategies are used in workforce planning: (1) population-based estimating, (2) benchmarking, (3) needs-based assessment, (4) demand-based assessment, and (5) training-output estimating. Each approach has its strengths and weaknesses, depending on the goal of the planning exercise and the context in which it will be applied. These methods may be used separately or in combination, depending on the system at which the planning is targeted as well as the specific policy questions posed during planning.

For national health systems, *population-based estimating* combined with training-output estimating may be more applicable than the other methods. The goal of planning in such systems may be to balance investments in training with the healthcare needs of the overall population. For individual organizations, benchmarking with peer institutions may provide useful information on how to staff a hospital or clinic to achieve productivity. Demand-based assessment can allow managers to anticipate the effects of changes in requirements for staff after increased marketing efforts or proactive modifications to product mix (Schnelle et al. 2004). Needs-based assessment may be appropriate as systems and agencies try to cope with changes in disease prevalence or the availability of new technologies.

Population-Based Estimating

This method rests on presumed appropriate or normative ratios of personnel and professionals to population. These ratios are not always generated from epidemiological analysis or careful study of productivity and utilization, but they often come from rules of thumb or from the current state of balance of practitioners to population. In the United States, several proposals for the most appropriate ratio of physicians to population have been based on observations of current and past ratios. For example, in the United States, the Health Professional Shortage Area criterion views a ratio of 1 full-time equivalent primary care physician for every 3,500 people as an indicator of a severe level of need. A ratio of 1 physician to 3,000 people accompanied by elevated population-risk indicators, such as high infant mortality and a high proportion of people older than 65 years in a "rational service" area, also signals high need, making the area or population eligible for shortage designation.

In a description of the origins of the Health Professional Shortage Area (formerly Health Manpower Shortage Area) criterion, a federal report suggested that the 1:3,500 ratio was selected because it was 1.5 times the mean population-to-primary-care-physician ratio by county in 1974 and because it qualifies a quarter of all counties with the worst ratios (Bureau of Health Manpower 1977). That report indicated that the ratio of 1:2,500 was selected as a measure of relative adequacy, being close to the median ratio for all U.S. counties in 1974.

Many ratios have been suggested as indicative of adequate supply. Figure 2.2 summarizes 16 such "ideal" or "adequate" ratios. The ratios are drawn from work by David Kindig (1994) and the Council on Graduate Medical Education (1996, 1999). The wide variation in ratios points to the weaknesses inherent in population-based approaches. Variability can be the result of differences in assumptions concerning the productivity of practitioners, the needs for services in the population, and even miscalculations caused by poor data in surveys and practice lists. Nevertheless, analysts and planners persist in using ratios as standard indicators of desired staffing or as guides to their studies of professional supply.

Benchmarking

The *benchmarking* method takes into consideration existing ratios but adds a test of efficiency to the analysis. The most prominent example focuses on the physician workforce in the United States, where regional, population-based ratios have been estimated and compared to organizational ratios (Schroeder 1996; Goodman et al. 1996). In this case, regional ratios for hospital-referral areas generated for the *Dartmouth Atlas of Health Care* were compared to the ratio in a large managed care system and selected market-area ratios where there was intense or little managed care penetration. This approach to setting national standards is much more controversial than its use for organizations

(Malone 1997; Wholey, Burns, and Lavizzo-Mourey 1998). The ratios used in the Goodman analysis included an adjusted HMO (health maintenance organization) staffing ratio (1:1,908) and the actual generalist ratio for the Wichita (1:1,527) and Minneapolis (1:1,316) hospital-referral regions (see Figure 2.2). Across the United States, using the hospital-referral regions to calculate denominators, 96 percent of the population lived in areas with more generalist physicians than the HMO benchmark, 60 percent lived in areas that exceeded the Wichita standard, and 27 percent lived in areas that exceeded the Minneapolis standard.

Advocates of benchmarking view these ratios as achievable, optimal ratios and accept the implication that these ratios describe the most efficient supply of practitioners. Benchmarking has become a part of the workforce-analysis process, and the influence of the *Dartmouth Atlas of Health Care* in guiding policy debate may make this approach more important. However, there has been little acceptance of specific standards for setting policy targets or for setting standards for underservice. The development of a revised standard for underservice for primary medical care has been under discussion by the federal government since 1998 when a formal proposal was published but withdrawn (Ricketts et al. 2007).

Needs-Based Assessment

Perhaps the most obvious method of determining how many healthcare professionals should be supported in a system or an organization is to match the consensus healthcare needs of a population or client base with their biological need for care. Unfortunately, healthcare need is difficult to determine and is subject to much variation. The substantial differences in physician opinions over the indicators and conditions that signal need for various procedures—such as carotid endarterectomy and coronary bypass graft operations, among other costly and specialized interventions—have been well documented (Birkmeyer et al. 1998; Wennberg et al. 1998). That variation has been persistent, and even concerted efforts to develop consensus on the need for specialist care have not been altogether successful (Fink et al. 1984). Those consensus methods, however, can be applied to more localized situations, and useful guidance can be developed to determine how many individuals in a population are likely to require selected services.

The consensus process for *needs-based assessment* is iterative, where lists of indicators, signs, and conditions are presented in various combinations and where "expert" clinicians are asked to determine if these combinations are high-, medium-, or low-level reasons for hospitalization, for conducting a specific procedure, for course of therapy, or for prescribing a specific medication. The expert panel members rate these combinations, discuss the results, and re-rate them. These steps usually result in a mix of

FIGURE 2.2
Summary of
Population-to-
Physician
Ratios,
Suggested as
Standards

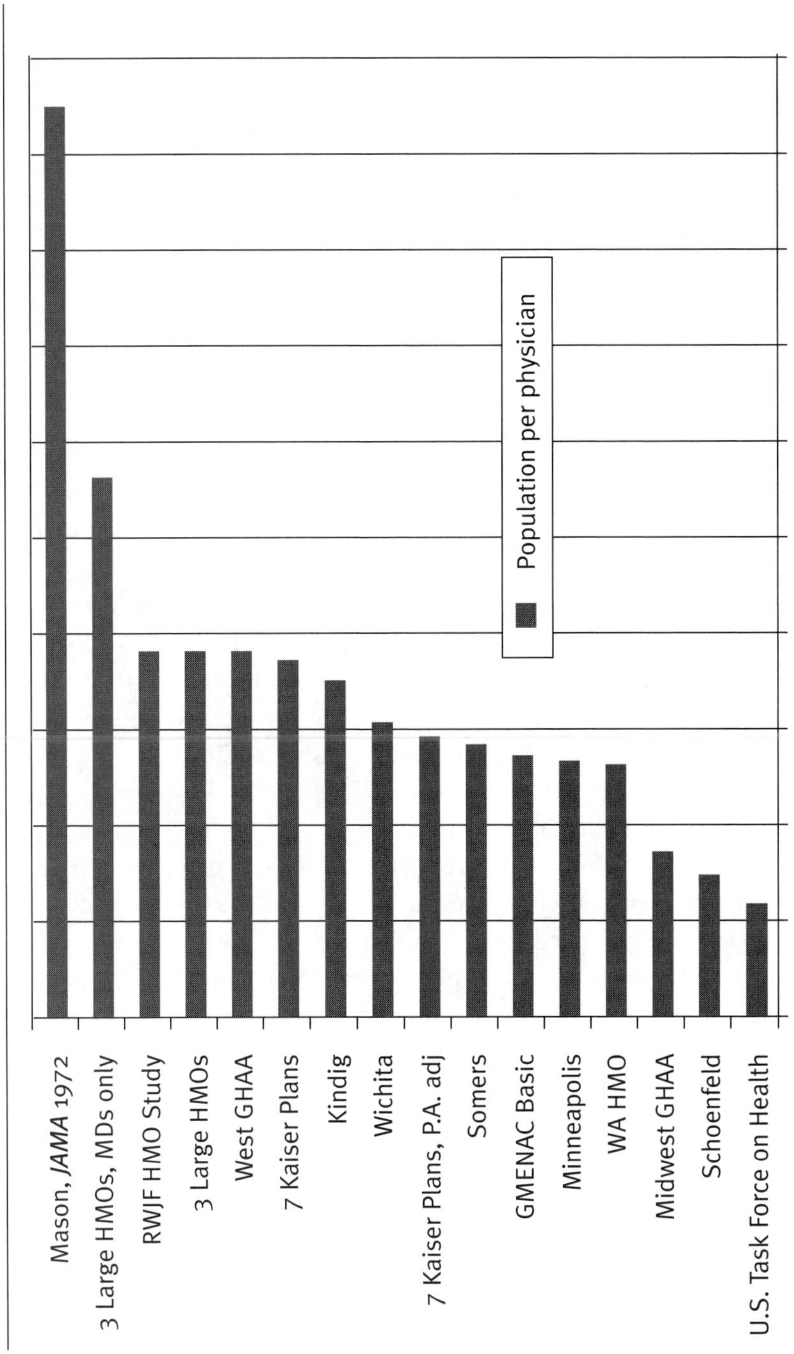

SOURCES: COGME (1996, 1999); Kindig (1994)

combinations—strong agreement on a particular care pathway is achieved, but agreement on other situations is not as high. However, the area of agreement is usually sufficiently large to allow for estimation of the total burden of care that certain groups of people are likely to require.

For national or other large populations, analysts can combine separate classes of diseases and their associated estimates of care to develop projections of staffing requirements. This was the approach taken by the Graduate Medical Education National Advisory Committee (1980) when it developed national projections of need and supply of physicians and primary care practitioners. That process was called "adjusted needs-based approach" to workforce planning, and it has been used since its development for specialty-specific estimates of requirements (Elisha, Levinson, and Grinshpoon 2004). For very specific specialties, the task of determining even supply is very difficult: "The actual number of FTE [full-time equivalent] neurosurgeons in practice is more difficult to determine, because the number is constantly changing as a result of death, retirement, modification of practice habits and mix of clinical practice versus other professional activities" (Popp and Toselli 1996).

The use of needs-based assessment to plan for staffing is supported in some sectors of the healthcare system by more carefully structured studies. An example includes the development of appropriate ratios of dental care practitioners (DeFriese and Barker 1982). Practical applications in healthcare organizations and bounded delivery systems require a focus on a particular type of need related to a specific type of organizational form—for example, the need in relation to staffing for outpatient mental health clinics that are managed centrally and that are located in areas where few alternative sources of this type of care exist (Elisha, Levinson, and Grinshpoon 2004).

Demand-Based Assessment

This workforce planning method is explicitly economic in nature and is based largely on past patterns of service utilization. Demand is considered to be somewhat independent of need for care in that some individuals may seek care when they are not ill, because they either misread their symptoms or desire to be treated regardless of medical need. In practice, need and demand are considered very closely tied. In an economic sense, demand is equal to utilization—what is consumed is what is demanded; that is, there is a balance in supply and demand in the market that is regulated by the price of the goods and services that are consumed. However, often the case is that demand and supply are not in balance in a sector such as healthcare because prices are not easily determined by either the purchaser or the supplier. Still, utilization can be a strong indicator of demand in a system in which the few barriers to care are caused by access restrictions. An open argument in the United States is whether or not the government restricts access by market rationing—a system that is opposite the explicit budget-rationing system in countries such as the United Kingdom and Canada.

A good example of the use of *demand-based assessment* is provided in studies commissioned by the American Medical Association (Marder et al. 1988). Any mathematical model that projects the supply or demand for healthcare professionals must include certain assumptions about the future. For example, knowing that a substantial growth is likely in the outdated number and population proportion allows the planner to anticipate much higher levels of utilization. These elevated levels of demand will be reflected in increased supplies of practitioners who are trained to care for the elderly, provided the training system is able to respond. In an application of this principle at a very macro level, a study by Cooper and colleagues (2002) demonstrates that overall economic activity is what determines the future supply of physicians in the United States. The authors' assumption is that the supply of medical practitioners is determined by the degree to which demand can be expressed in a relatively open market for care.

Training-Output Estimating

Training-output estimating is perhaps the most common method for anticipating supply of practitioners. Essentially, it draws on data from training programs, such as the number of enrollees, the number of anticipated graduates, and the trends in applications. This approach has been used to anticipate trends in the general supply of physicians (Cooper, Stoflet, and Wartman 2003), general surgeons (Jonasson, Kwakwa, and Sheldon 1995), internists (Andersen et al. 1990), pediatricians (Bazell and Salsberg 1998), and allied health professionals (DePoy, Wood, and Miller 1997).

Estimations of the supply of nurse practitioners and physician assistants rely heavily on trends in enrollment in training programs (Hooker and Cawley 2002; Buerhaus, Staiger, and Auerbach 2000). Anticipating the characteristics of the future workforce in relation to current training patterns is important to understand how well today's practitioners will meet clinical and social needs in the future. This issue has become critical in the United States, as the focus of national policy has shifted toward having a workforce that matches the racial and ethnic structure of the population (Fiscella et al. 2000).

Challenges and Difficulties of Workforce Planning

The fundamental challenge to HRH planning is that any credible analysis that points to an impending shortage or surplus of practitioners is likely to result in a policy or an organizational response that precludes that scenario from occurring. Retrospective analyses of "how well we did" often emphasize how poorly the projections performed rather than how much reaction these projections generated (Cooper et al. 2002). Disappointingly, such retrospective analyses are applied only to national estimates of the state of the workforce at some unspecified future time. In planning for physician supply, rarely are organizational or delivery system analyses discussed and critiqued, except when making them the basis of national estimates (Weiner 2004, 1994, 1987; Hart et al. 1997).

Planning for nursing staffing includes much more organizational emphasis because such planning is considered a "staffing" problem subject to management, rather than a need to anticipate a market response (Seago et al. 2001). Nursing staffing, however, is also subject to broad-scale analyses to anticipate local conditions (Cooper and Aiken 2001).

International Perspectives

National-level HRH workforce planning is practiced more often in other countries. This is a function of the political economy of these countries' healthcare systems, in which central direction and planning is the norm. In other countries, most ministries or departments of health include a human resources division or section that is responsible for the planning function. The planning that goes on is applicable to the overall system, where decisions are made concerning the number of practitioners and support staff to be trained or allowed into the country. Planning for specific staffing needs of institutions often takes place within the same part of the bureaucracy, but sometimes delineation is made between strategic planning for national needs and strategic planning for policy and institutional planning for staffing and management decision making.

Canada, for example, developed the Pan-Canadian Health Human Resources (HHR) Planning Initiative intended to bring more evidence-based methods to the work of Health Canada. This consortium effort relies on external research and analysis groups as well as on internal staff. The task of the Canadian HHR planning group is focused on assessing the future staffing and contracting needs of Health Canada and the provincial ministries and departments, as that nation attempts to reform the Canadian healthcare system in response to the 2003 First Ministers' Accord on Health Care Renewal. The 2003 Canadian federal budget allocated $90 million over five years to strengthen healthcare human resources planning and coordination. The national work and interprovincial planning activities are coordinated through the Advisory Committee on Health Delivery and Human Resources, which has assigned a planning subcommittee to develop evidence-based recommendations on education strategies, especially interprofessional education, and on establishing a workforce that can respond to a patient-centered healthcare system.

In 1995, Australia developed formal structures in its Department of Health to oversee planning activities for its healthcare workforce. For political and practical reasons, the oversight of planning functions was divided between two committees—one for medical positions (Australian Medical Workforce Advisory Committee) and one for all other professions and occupations (Australian Health Workforce Advisory Committee). The central technical task of these committees is to estimate the "required health workforce to meet future health service requirements and the development of strategies to meet that need" (Australian Medical Workforce Advisory Committee 2003).

The World Health Organization supports the Human Resources for Health program, which has invested heavily in developing skills of personnel who can do workforce planning for national and regional healthcare systems (see www.wpro.who.int/sites/whd for an example of work done in the western Pacific). Australia, for example, has committed substantial resources and energy in the development of plans for its rural and remote workforce, and it has developed a national public health workforce program (see www.nphp.gov.au/workprog/workforce).

Barriers to healthcare workforce development in all countries include a failure to specify health goals, limited liaison between the health and education sectors, and resource constraints. Other factors that have complicated a strategic approach to healthcare workforce development include the diversity and rapid evolution of health services, the long training period for most healthcare professions, and the increasing mobility of the healthcare workforce. Political ideology can also be a major player. In New Zealand, the market-oriented health reforms of the 1990s created a competitive rather than a collaborative environment in which workforce development was not a priority (Hornblow 2002). That has changed to some extent in recent years, but the Health Workforce Advisory Committee that was established to direct policy was disbanded in 2006 (see www.hwac.govt.nz).

One international development that is beginning to have widespread effects on workforce planning and planning in a management context is the European Union's Working Time Directive (WTD) (Roche-Nagle 2004; Paice and Reid 2004). This rule applies to a wide range of healthcare professionals and sets limits on the amount of time an individual is allowed to work in a day and over a work week. The initial implementation of the WTD began in August 2007. In August 2009, the directive will restrict the hours that trainees can work from 58 hours to 48 hours per week. The response to the restrictions has been to increase the intake of trainees in some systems, such as the National Health Service in the United Kingdom, and to restructure some training program schedules.

Workforce Supply Metrics

Measuring the supply of healthcare professionals is not as straightforward as it seems. A doctor is what a doctor does, but when considering the overall professional supply needed for a specific area or organization, the distinction between what a doctor is and what a doctor does is harder to make. For example, in counting primary care physicians, most experts and many explicit policies consider a family physician as dedicated to providing primary care, which is defined as healthcare that most people need most of the time. Under that description, a primary care practitioner, then, takes care of the most common complaints and coordinates the care needs of a patient—be it specialty or inpatient. However, is a psychiatrist or an OB-GYN a primary care physician? Each may be the patient's first contact with the medical system, and each may coordinate the care for many individuals, but the practice of a psychiatrist and an OB-GYN is limited to certain aspects of human health and illness.

To add more confusion, in many states and under certain federal regulations, these practitioners are considered primary care physicians. In other systems, the primary care physician's work is proscribed by certain rules to include only ambulatory care. These physicians are most often termed "GPs" or general practitioners. They may, however, have greater autonomy in the system and be able to control entry into hospitals. This kind of gatekeeping power may, in turn, influence the resulting demand or expressed need for surgery and, subsequently, for surgeons. The dynamics of the system, thus, become important to the estimation of the need for specialists and the staff who support them.

The extent of details involved in creating an inventory of primary care physicians is indicative of the complexity of any process that tries to ascertain how well the supply of healthcare professionals meets the needs of a population or an organization. This challenge often deters managers as well as planners from attempting to balance their anticipated needs for healthcare professionals with likely scenarios for supply. Sufficient models are available on how to approach HRH workforce planning that can make the effort well worthwhile in reducing overall costs of staffing or training and the costs associated with mismatches of needs and resources.

Summary

HRH workforce planning is the anticipation of how many practitioners and support workers an organization or a system will require to achieve its mission. The development of effective workforce plans depends on the use of accurate and reliable data that describe current supply, pattern of entry and exit from professions and positions, and the number of incoming workers from training programs and schools. At the national level, HRH planning requires an understanding of major economic and social trends as well as a keen sense of the politics involved in labor and professions.

Five basic methods are used in workforce planning: (1) population-based estimating, (2) benchmarking, (3) needs-based assessment, (4) demand-based assessment, and (5) training-output estimating. Each approach offers strengths and presents weaknesses, depending on the context in which it is applied. The institutional planner can use all or a combination of these approaches in developing staffing plans, preparing for turnover and transitions, and positioning the organization to compete effectively for resources.

Discussion Questions

1. What are the major types of healthcare workforce planning? Provide examples of situations where each strategy would be more appropriate than the others.
2. Healthcare workforce planning is often done after a shortage in a particular profession is recognized. How could planning help avert those shortages?
3. Counting healthcare professionals as part of healthcare workforce planning is not always straightforward. For a specific profession—nursing, dentistry, or medicine—describe how the practice patterns of the professionals may change the effective supply of that profession.

Experiential Exercise

Case   In 1999, California became the first state to pass a law that requires minimum staffing ratios for nurses in general acute care hospitals (Coffman, Seago, and Spetz 2002). California Assembly Bill 394 (AB 394) mandated the Department of Health Services to create "minimum, specific, and numerical nurse-to-patient ratios by licensed nurse classification and by hospital unit for the inpatient parts of general hospitals in the state." In January 2004, those regulations came into effect, translating into the following: In the emergency department, one nurse cannot care for more than four patients, while in postoperative surgical units, nurses cannot care for more than six patients.

Using the national nursing supply-and-demand model, the following table on page 42 shows the projected supply of registered nurses (RNs) and a trend for inpatient days in general acute care hospitals in North Carolina, from 2007 through 2023.

The North Carolina General Assembly is considering implementing a mandatory staffing ratio that matches the California rules for emergency departments and post-op

Year	Number of RNs	Trend of Inpatient Days
2007	67,712	4,024,336
2008	68,382	4,090,608
2009	69,049	4,156,880
2010	69,718	4,223,151
2011	74,387	4,289,423
2012	75,050	4,355,695
2013	75,536	4,421,967
2014	75,730	4,488,239
2015	75,890	4,554,511
2016	76,020	4,620,782
2017	76,160	4,687,054
2018	76,210	4,753,326
2019	76,208	4,819,598
2020	76,199	4,885,870
2021	76,165	4,952,141
2022	76,065	5,018,413
2023	75,800	5,084,685

surgical units in general acute care hospitals. The North Carolina Hospital Association found that in all of the hospitals in the state with emergency departments and post-op surgical units, emergency departments accounted for 8 percent of total inpatient days in 2007, and the post-op units accounted for 11 percent of inpatient days. Overall, hospital RNs accounted for 38 percent of all RNs practicing in North Carolina. Three percent of these hospital RNs worked in emergency departments, while 2.2 percent worked in post-op units. The available supply of RNs in 2007 allowed all hospitals in the state to fully staff their emergency departments and post-op units.

Exercise   If North Carolina implements a staffing law exactly like the one in California, and that law is put into effect on January 1, 2009, how would the numbers in the above table change? Estimate the change in the number of RNs required to staff the emergency departments and post-op units of acute care hospitals in North Carolina. The use of both units is expected to rise in direct proportion to the overall use of hospitals as measured by inpatient days.

References

Andersen, R. M., C. Lyttle, C. H. Kohrman, G. S. Levey, K. Neymarc, and C. Schmidt. 1990. "National Study of Internal Medicine Manpower: XVII. Changes in the Characteristics of Internal Medicine Residents and Their Training Programs, 1988–1989." *Annals of Internal Medicine* 113 (3): 243–49.

Australian Medical Workforce Advisory Committee. 2003. *Specialist Medical Workforce Planning in Australia.* North Sydney, Australia: Australian Medical Workforce Advisory Committee.

Bazell, C., and E. Salsberg. 1998. "The Impact of Graduate Medical Education Financing Policies on Pediatric Residency Training." *Pediatrics* 101 (4 Pt 2): 785–92; discussion 793–94.

Birkmeyer, J. D., S. M. Sharp, S. R. Finlayson, E. S. Fisher, and J. E. Wennberg. 1998. "Variation Profiles of Common Surgical Procedures." *Surgery* 124 (5): 917–23.

Buerhaus, P. I., D. O. Staiger, and D. I. Auerbach. 2000. "Implications of an Aging Registered Nurse Workforce." *JAMA* 283 (22): 2948–54.

Bureau of Health Manpower. 1977. *Report on Development of Criteria for Designation of Health Manpower Shortage Areas.* Rockville, MD: Health Resources Administration.

Coffman, J. M., J. A. Seago, and J. Spetz. 2002. "Minimum Nurse-to-Patient Ratios in Acute Care Hospitals in California." *Health Affairs (Millwood)* 21 (5): 53–64.

Cooper, R. A., and L. H. Aiken. 2001. "Human Inputs: The Healthcare Workforce and Medical Markets." *Journal of Health Politics, Policy & Law* 26 (5): 925–38.

Cooper, R. A., T. E. Getzen, H. J. McKee, and P. Laud. 2002. "Economic and Demographic Trends Signal an Impending Physician Shortage." *Health Affairs* 21 (1): 140–54.

Cooper, R. A., S. J. Stoflet, and S. A. Wartman. 2003. "Perceptions of Medical School Deans and State Medical Society Executives About Physician Supply." *JAMA* 290 (22): 2992–95.

Council on Graduate Medical Education (COGME). 1996. *Eighth Report: Patient Care Physician Supply and Requirements: Testing COGME Recommendations.* Washington, DC: Bureau of Health Professions, HRSA.

———. 1999. *Fourteenth Report: COGME Physician Workforce Policies: Recent Developments and Remaining Challenges in Meeting National Goals.* Washington, DC: Bureau of Health Professions, HRSA.

DeFriese, G. H., and B. D. Barker. 1982. *Assessing Dental Manpower Requirements: Alternative Approaches for State and Local Planning, Issues in Dental Health Policy.* Cambridge, MA: Ballinger.

De Geyndt, W. 2000. "Health Workforce Development in the NIS." In *NIS (New Independent States)/US Health Workforce Planning 2000,* edited by G. L. Filerman. Washington, DC: American International Health Alliance.

DePoy, E., C. Wood, and M. Miller. 1997. "Educating Rural Allied Health Professionals: An Interdisciplinary Effort." *Journal of Allied Health* 26 (3): 127–32.

Dubois, C. A., M. McKee, and E. Nolte (eds.). 2006. *Human Resources for Health in Europe.* Maidenhead, England: Open University Press.

Elisha, D., D. Levinson, and A. Grinshpoon. 2004. "A Need-Based Model for Determining Staffing Needs for the Public Sector Outpatient Mental Health Service System." *Journal of Behavioral Health Services Research* 31 (3): 324–33.

Fink, A., J. Kosecoff, M. Chassin, and R. H. Brook. 1984. "Consensus Methods: Characteristics and Guidelines for Use." *American Journal of Public Health* 74 (9): 979–83.

Fiscella, K., P. Franks, M. R. Gold, and C. M. Clancy. 2000. "Inequalities in Racial Access to Healthcare." *JAMA* 284 (16): 2053.

Fox, D. M. 1996. "From Piety to Platitudes to Pork: The Changing Politics of Health Workforce Policy." *Journal of Health Politics, Policy & Law* 21 (4): 825–44.

Fried, B. J. 1997. "Physician Resource Planning in an Era of Uncertainty and Change." *Canadian Medical Association Journal* 157 (9): 1227–28.

Goodman, D. C., E. S. Fisher, T. A. Bubolz, J. E. Mohr, J. F. Poage, and J. E. Wennberg. 1996. "Benchmarking the US Physician Workforce: An Alternative to Needs-Based or Demand-Based Planning." *JAMA* 276 (22): 1811–17.

Graduate Medical Education National Advisory Committee. 1980. *Report of the Graduate Medical Education National Advisory Committee to the Secretary, Department of Health and Human Services, Volume 1.* Washington, DC: Office of Graduate Medical Education.

Hart, L. G., E. Wagner, S. Pirzada, A. F. Nelson, and R. A. Rosenblatt. 1997. "Physician Staffing Ratios in Staff-Model HMOs: A Cautionary Tale." *Health Affairs (Millwood)* 16 (1): 55–70.

Hooker, R., and J. F. Cawley. 2002. *Physician Assistants in American Medicine*, 2nd ed. Philadelphia: W. B. Saunders.

Hornblow, A. 2002. Second NCETA Workforce Development Symposium, Adelaide, Australia, May 1.

Jonasson, O., F. Kwakwa, and G. F. Sheldon. 1995. "Calculating the Workforce in General Surgery." *JAMA* 274 (9): 731–34.

Kindig, D. A. 1994. "Counting Generalist Physicians." *JAMA* 271 (19): 1505–07.

Malone, S. 1997. "Staffing to Volume in Integrated Delivery Networks." *Journal of AHIMA* 68 (9): 42, 44, 46–48.

Marder, W. D., P. R. Kletke, A. B. Silberger, and R. J. Willke. 1988. *Physician Supply and Utilization by Specialty: Trends and Projections.* Chicago: American Medical Association.

Paice, E., and W. Reid. 2004. "Can Training and Service Survive the European Working Time Directive?" *Medical Education* 38 (4): 336–38.

Popp, A. J., and R. Toselli. 1996. "Workforce Requirements for Neurosurgery." *Surgery and Neurology* 46: 181–85.

Ricketts, T. C., L. J. Goldsmith, G. M. Holmes, R. M. Randolph, R. Lee, D. H. Taylor, and J. Ostermann. 2007. "Designating Places and Populations as Medically Underserved: A Proposal for a New Approach." *Journal of Health Care for the Poor and Underserved* 18 (3): 567–89.

Roche-Nagle, G. 2004. "The European Working Time Directive: A Survey of Surgical Specialist Registrars." *International Medical Journal* 97 (6): 175–78.

Schnelle, J. F., S. F. Simmons, C. Harrington, M. Cadogan, E. Garcia, and M. Bates-Jensen. 2004. "Relationship of Nursing Home Staffing to Quality of Care." *Health Services Research* 39 (2): 225–50.

Schroeder, S. A. 1996. "How Can We Tell Whether There Are Too Many or Too Few Physicians? The Case for Benchmarking" [editorial; comment]. *JAMA* 276 (22): 1841–34.

Seago, J. A., M. Ash, J. Spetz, J. Coffman, and K. Grumbach. 2001. "Hospital Registered Nurse Shortages: Environmental, Patient, and Institutional Predictors." *Health Services Research* 36 (5): 831–52.

Starr, P. 1982. *The Social Transformation of American Medicine.* New York: Basic Books.

Weiner, J. P. 1987. "Primary Care Delivery in the United States and Four Northwest European Countries: Comparing the 'Corporatized' with the 'Socialized'." *Milbank Quarterly* 65 (3): 426–61.

————. 1994. "Forecasting the Effects of Health Reform on U.S. Physician Workforce Requirement. Evidence from HMO Staffing Patterns." *JAMA* 272 (3): 222–30.

————. 2004. "Prepaid Group Practice Staffing and U.S. Physician Supply: Lessons for Workforce Policy." *Health Affairs (Millwood)* (Supplement Web Exclusives): W4, 43–59.

Weissert, C. S., and S. L. Silberman. 1998. "Sending a Policy Signal: State Legislatures, Medical Schools and Primary Care Mandates." *Journal of Health Politics, Policy & Law* 23 (5): 743–45.

Wennberg, D. E., F. L. Lucas, J. D. Birkmeyer, C. E. Bredenberg, and E. S. Fisher. 1998. "Variation in Carotid Endarterectomy Mortality in the Medicare Population: Trial Hospitals, Volume, and Patient Characteristics." *JAMA* 279 (16): 1278–81.

Wholey, D. R., L. R. Burns, and R. Lavizzo-Mourey. 1998. "Managed Care and the Delivery of Primary Care to the Elderly and the Chronically Ill." *Health Services Research* 33 (2 Pt II): 322–53.

World Health Organization. 2000. "What Resources Are Needed?" In *World Health Report 2000. Health Systems: Improving Performance.* Geneva, Switzerland: WHO.

————. 2006. "Working Together for Health." In *World Health Report 2006.* Geneva, Switzerland: WHO.

GLOBALIZATION AND THE HEALTHCARE WORKFORCE

Leah E. Masselink

Learning Objectives

After completing this chapter, the reader should be able to

- describe the history and current trends in international migration of physicians and nurses;
- enumerate the factors that motivate physicians and nurses to migrate to other countries;
- discuss the implications of physician and nurse migration for sending and receiving countries;
- understand the policy context and policy interventions that attempt to manage physician and nurse migration; and
- explain the issues of ethical recruitment, visa regulation, credentialing, and adaptation for managers of foreign-born and -trained physicians and nurses.

Introduction

In an increasingly interconnected world, the movement of people and information across international borders has become a phenomenon that is often taken for granted. As skilled healthcare providers, physicians and nurses have had opportunities to seek employment internationally for several decades, and foreign-trained professionals are important parts of the healthcare systems in many countries. In the United States alone, about 25 percent of physicians are foreign born and educated and about 4 percent of nurses were educated overseas (Cooper and Aiken 2006; Aiken et al. 2004).

The implications of *international migration* of physicians and nurses are complex, becoming a source of increasing debate in recent years. While physicians and nurses who migrate to other countries can benefit from better working conditions or salaries in their destinations, their movement can exacerbate inequalities in the worldwide distribution of healthcare workers. Migration of healthcare workers from developing countries has particularly far-reaching implications. These developing countries not only lose their investments in education and training, income tax revenue, and potential for national growth, buy they also see adverse health effects on their populations. In nations where healthcare workforce shortages are already severe, the need to replace healthcare professionals who have left for other countries only further depletes the health system's resources—funds that normally go toward fighting diseases and promoting public health. In addition, the lack of highly skilled care providers prevents these countries from meeting their own needs for healthcare innovation and problem solving. These factors exacerbate the existing inequalities in healthcare between developed and developing countries.

Given that foreign-trained physicians and nurses play an important role in many healthcare organizations in the United States, healthcare managers in this country must understand several issues related to the globalization of the healthcare workforce:

- In what areas do international migration of physicians and nurses occur? What can explain these patterns?
- What factors motivate the international migration of physicians and nurses?
- What are the ethical and logistical implications of physician and nurse migration for sending and receiving countries?

International migration of physicians and nurses is inherently difficult to manage because policies designed to direct and oversee it must balance two often competing objectives: (1) to protect the inherent right of people to migrate and (2) to ensure that quality healthcare services are available to all. This chapter describes past and current migration trends, causes, policy context, and responses. It also explores several international migration issues, such as ethical recruitment, visa regulation, credentialing, and adaptation. All of these topics are essential knowledge for U.S. healthcare managers.

History and Current Trends

Anecdotal accounts of international migration of physicians and nurses began to circulate in the 1960s. Initial reports mostly documented migration between developed countries, such as from Canada to the United States (*BMJ* 1968). In the 1970s, the World Health Organization (WHO) commissioned *The Multinational Study of the International Migration of Physicians*. This notable study found that, at the time, significant numbers of *international medical graduates* (IMGs) were practicing in the United States (about one in every five physicians), the United Kingdom (more than one in every four physicians), and Canada (one in every three physicians). Germany also had substantial numbers of migrant physicians, including many from Iran and the Middle East (Mejía 1978). In addition, the study reported that significant numbers of *international nursing graduates* (INGs) worked in the United States, European countries, and other developed nations. *Sending countries* (the countries from which healthcare professionals migrate) with particularly high proportions of nurses who go abroad to work include Haiti, Suriname, Hong Kong, Jordan, and the Philippines. In absolute numbers, more Filipino nurses were registered in the United States and Canada than in the Philippines in 1970 (Mejía 1978).

The characteristics of healthcare workforce migration have shifted since the WHO study was conducted in the 1970s. New sending countries have become significant sources of migrant physicians, including Egypt, Cuba, and nations in the Caribbean; sub-Saharan Africa; and the former Soviet Union. New *receiving countries* (the destinations of migrant healthcare professionals), such as the Persian Gulf states, have begun to draw physicians and nurses from all over the world, including Europe and India. Migration between the European Union and African countries has also increased (Martineau, Decker, and Bundred 2004). Some countries—particularly South Africa—have emerged as "holding grounds" for migrant workers who stay temporarily on their way to their final destination country (Vujicic et al. 2004).

According to Mullan (2005), the countries that send the largest numbers of physicians abroad are India, the Philippines, and Pakistan, while the countries that receive the greatest numbers of IMGs are the United States, the United Kingdom, Canada, and Australia. IMGs compose approximately 25 percent of the physician workforce in the United States, 28 percent in the United Kingdom, 23 percent in Canada, and 27 percent in Australia (Mullan 2005). In the United States, the three largest sending countries or regions for INGs are the Philippines, Canada, and Africa (especially South Africa and Nigeria). Between 1997 and 2000, 33 percent of foreign-born nursing-licensure applicants were Filipino, 22 percent were Canadian, and 7 percent were African (Buchan, Parkin, and Sochalski 2003).

Migration streams, particularly between English-speaking countries, appear to be well established: While IMGs make up more than 20 percent of the total physician workforces in the United States, the United Kingdom, Australia, and Canada, they represent only a tiny proportion of the physician workforces in France (3 percent) and Japan (1 percent) (Mullan 2005). In sub-Saharan Africa, rates of nurse migration are also markedly higher in Anglophone countries than in French- and Portuguese-speaking countries (Dovlo 2007). Many sending countries tend to have historical relationships with English-speaking receiving countries. For example, physicians from India and Pakistan make up the largest and third-largest groups, respectively, of IMGs in the United Kingdom, and doctors from the Philippines are the second-largest group of noncitizen IMGs in the United States (Mullan 2005).[1]

Many policymakers in both sending and receiving countries have expressed concern about the fact that the largest receiving countries draw significant proportions of their IMG workforces from lower-income countries. More than 75 percent of the IMGs in the United Kingdom come from lower-income countries, and other receiving countries have substantial proportions as well: Sixty percent of IMGs in the United States and about 40 percent of those in Canada and Australia are from developing nations (Mullan 2005).

Causes of International Migration

Determinants of physician and nurse migration are often discussed in terms of "push" and "pull" factors. *Push factors* motivate physicians and nurses to leave their home countries, while *pull factors* cause them to choose particular receiving countries. The reasons are chiefly discussed within an economic framework, considering a variety of factors as potential determinants. These include per capita gross domestic product, physician coverage, manpower production rates, rural/urban distribution of physicians and nurses, and workforce imbalances.

Push factors cited by the majority of studies include low pay, poor working conditions, political instability and insecurity, inadequate housing and social services, and lack of educational opportunities and professional development. Job dissatisfaction, lack of motivation, and weak professional leadership are also mentioned as contributing factors (Saravia and Miranda 2004). Pull factors, on the other hand, include opportunities for professional training, better job opportunities, and higher wages (Forcier, Simoens, and Giuffrida 2004). Other pull factors relate to workforce-supply issues that have created an imbalance between the demand for services and the supply of workers in receiving countries, such as aging of both the general population and the nursing workforce and the slowdowns in enrollment in training programs (Buchan and Sochalski 2004). The nursing workforces in receiving countries are vulnerable to such shortages, particularly with the opening of male-dominated careers to women (Marchal and Kegels 2003). IMGs and INGs are particularly needed in some receiving countries where domestically trained providers are reluctant to serve in certain capacities, such as in remote areas or in nursing homes.

Sending Country/Region Trends

Physician and nurse migration can be managed to varying degrees by sending countries. Some regions (such as sub-Saharan Africa and the Caribbean) continue to lose workers in the face of severe shortages, while other nations (such as Cuba, India, and the Philippines) purposely train surplus physicians and nurses for overseas employment. Still other countries (particularly China) are currently looking to shift into a training-for-export mode. This section sheds light on the diverse situations faced by sending countries and describes in detail the factors that contribute to each situation.

Brain Drain: Sub-Saharan Africa and the Caribbean

The situation in sub-Saharan Africa and the Caribbean is often referred to as *brain drain*—the widespread, uncontrolled departure of physicians and nurses from countries that already suffer healthcare worker shortages.

In sub-Saharan Africa, the largest sending countries are South Africa and Nigeria. In 2005, nearly 7,000 South African physicians and more than 4,000 Nigerian physicians were practicing in the United States, the United Kingdom, Canada, and Australia (Mullan 2005). Ghana has also experienced high rates of physician and nurse emigration: In 2000, that country lost more practicing nurses than the number of nursing graduates it produced (Dovlo 2007). As a relatively wealthy sub-Saharan African state, South Africa is unique in that it acts as both a sending and a receiving country for migrant physicians and nurses, many of whom come from other countries in the region.

In Africa, among the factors that influence health professionals' decisions to leave are low quality of life, high crime rates, conflict, political repression, and lack of educational opportunities for children. The HIV/AIDS epidemic has seriously depleted the healthcare workforce through death and attrition, and caring for growing numbers of patients with HIV/AIDS has overburdened the remaining providers. Nurses in this region are poorly paid, and this lack of adequate compensation also contributes to the workforce shortage. Sub-Saharan Africa suffers from a serious maldistribution of healthcare workers, with uneven supply between the public and private sectors, urban and rural areas, and tertiary and primary levels of care (Padarath et al. 2004).

A lack of higher education and career-development opportunities is another major push factor in this region. This dearth reflects a pattern of underinvestment in higher education by governments and outside donors. Health-professional education and training not only subsist on very limited material resources but are also plagued by a shortage of qualified teachers.

Similarly, countries in the Caribbean are overwhelmed by extremely high rates of HIV infection that are second only to the epidemic in sub-Saharan Africa. This region has also experienced crippling losses of nurses in recent years: 42 percent of all nursing positions across the Caribbean are vacant, and the lack of nursing educational capacity serves only to perpetuate the massive losses of nursing educators and experienced nurses. Jamaica is particularly affected, with a 58 percent average nursing vacancy rate in 2003. Many Jamaican nurses left to work in the United States, the United Kingdom, and Canada, and Jamaican healthcare leaders have begun to recruit from other countries in the Caribbean to make up for losses (Salmon et al. 2007).

Strategic Deployment: Cuba, the Philippines, and India

Some developing countries train surplus physicians and nurses for overseas employment, and both state and business interests promote and manage this practice. Cuba has a long-standing program of physician deployment, and the Philippine government has worked to manage nurse migration for many years. Recently, strategic deployment programs have also arisen in India.

For several decades now, Cuba has made the provision of healthcare workers to developing countries a part of its foreign policy, sending physicians to developing countries as participants in a Peace Corps–style international medical-aid program (Feinsilver 1989). These efforts are part of a larger effort by the Cuban government to promote its political agenda and to position itself as a "world medical power." Dozens of countries have received Cuban physicians over the years, including Algeria, South Africa (Lee 1996), and more recently Venezuela (Muntaner et al. 2006). Cuban physicians who participate in the program often provide services in isolated rural areas and are often involved in training their host countries' indigenous healthcare workers (Feinsilver 1989).

The Philippine government has been particularly active in establishing policies that aim to make the country the niche producer of nurses in the global economy (Ball 1996). The Philippines produces about 20,000 new nurses every year (Lorenzo et al. 2007), and the vast majority of these graduates eventually find work overseas: In 2004, 85 percent of all Filipino nurses practiced abroad (Aiken et al. 2004). A government agency regulates recruitment of Filipino overseas workers and processes documents for those bound to work in other countries. The emergence of nursing as a pathway to migration has led to unprecedented demand for nursing education in the Philippines. The number of nursing schools has grown exponentially in the past few decades, from 40 schools in the 1970s to 460 schools in 2006 (Lorenzo et al. 2007). This growth has led to concerns about the quality of nursing education, as schools compete with each other for faculty and hospital training space (Lorenzo et al. 2007).

Historically, India has been one of the largest sending countries of physicians to developed nations, including the United States and the United Kingdom (Mullan 2006). In recent years, it has also become a popular source country for nurses. Since the 1990s, it has moved from sixth to second position (after the Philippines) among countries that send nurses to the United States. Like the Philippines, India has a huge overall labor surplus, although it also has a very low nurse-to-population ratio. It has also become the site of increasing commercial activity around nursing education and migration. Indian hospitals have become involved in recruiting and training nurses for overseas markets, and local recruitment agencies that partner with U.S.-based recruiters have appeared in many urban areas. In recent years, some state governments have also begun to engage in international deployment of nurses (Khadria 2007).

The most frequently cited reason for the strategic deployment of physicians and nurses is the remittance income that migrant workers send to their home countries. Remittances can be a substantial source of revenue for sending countries. For example, Filipino migrant workers remitted $10.7 billion in 2005 (Lorenzo et al. 2007). Remittance income is often considered a potentially positive outcome of emigration. However, while such income may offset sending countries' financial losses, it may not make up for the staffing issues and poor outcomes associated with workforce migration.

Up-and-Coming Player: China

China is a relative newcomer to the global nursing market. It has sent nurses abroad for about 15 years, when the government began deploying groups of English-speaking nurses to Singapore and Saudi Arabia under temporary government-arranged contracts (Fang 2007). Since the early 2000s, this migration has shifted to countries such as Australia and the United Kingdom, where it is usually arranged by private agencies. U.S. healthcare organizations have begun to express interest in recruiting nurses from China.

For some Chinese nurses, the desire to seek employment abroad is influenced by several domestic factors. First, China has not invested enough in healthcare to employ all of its trained and educated nurses. Like the Philippines, China has a surplus of nurses based on the number of budgeted positions. Many nurses are unable to find work, or they are forced to retire early to make room for new graduates who are entering the workforce. Also, China has more physicians than nurses, contrary to recommendations by the WHO. In this context, overseas markets are becoming a desirable alternative for some Chinese nurses.

Consequences for Receiving Countries

The presence of IMGs and INGs has several important consequences for receiving countries. Some of the consequences of physician and nurse migration relate to larger issues of recruitment and retention. International recruitment is suggested to be a quick fix for recruitment and retention problems in receiving countries, allowing domestic supply lines to avoid developing their own solutions to unmet health-system needs. International migration may help receiving countries to fill positions in areas that are not as attractive to domestic workers. This leads to concerns that foreign-trained professionals may be subject to exploitation or may be forced to work in positions that are below their expertise—a phenomenon referred to as "brain waste" (Marchal and Kegels 2003).

The effects of having immigrant physicians and nurses on accessibility and quality of care are unclear: Some suggest that the quality and safety of care provided by internationally trained providers may be cause for concern, while others argue that the presence of these professionals may improve access to care, lower prices, and induce competition and higher quality (Forcier, Simoens, and Giuffrida 2004). The "safety net" use of immigrant healthcare workers has been demonstrated to be a real phenomenon (Forcier, Simoens, and Giuffrida 2004). The presence of immigrant health workers may prevent receiving healthcare systems from solving their own training and staffing problems. For example, while U.S. hospitals hire thousands of IMGs each year, thousands of domestic medical-school applicants are turned away (Martineau, Decker, and Bundred 2004).

The Policy Context

International migration occurs in the context of several important trade agreements. One such agreement that could affect future migration dynamics is the General Agreement on Trade in Services (GATS), which was implemented in 1995. GATS is an international treaty that governs the trade of services, including health services, among member countries of the World Trade Organization. GATS has three main objectives: (1) to liberalize trade in services, (2) to encourage economic growth through liberalizing trade in services, and (3) to increase the participation of developing countries in the world trade in services. The four modes of trade governed by GATS are (1) cross-border supply (services provided by workers in one country for organizations in another country), (2) consumption abroad (including medical tourism and education of foreign students), (3) commercial presence (investment of capital from one country into another), and (4) movement of natural persons (temporary cross-border migration of workers to provide services in another country [Kingma 2006]). While the GATS provision for temporary migration has caused concern that it would encourage further migration of health workers from developing countries to developed countries, this element is still being negotiated, and its final effects remain unclear (Kingma 2007).

Another agreement that particularly affects migration patterns in the United States is the North American Free Trade Agreement (NAFTA), which was implemented in 1994. NAFTA provides for the movement of workers between Canada, the United States, and Mexico, including special visa categories and mutual recognition of nurse licensure in the United States and Canada. This agreement has raised Canada's profile as a sending country of nurses in the United States, but movement between the two countries has been mostly unidirectional: About 15,000 Canadian nurses have moved to the United States under NAFTA, but relatively few U.S.-trained nurses have moved to Canada (Kingma 2006; Mautino 2003).

Policy Responses

A broad variety of policy initiatives have been proposed and implemented by sending and receiving countries to manage international migration of physicians and nurses. These include programs instituted by worldwide bodies such as the WHO and the International Council of Nurses (ICN), domestic policy changes in sending and receiving countries, government-to-government bilateral agreements, and proposed compensation schemes. Some countries or regions have adopted unique policies to manage the effects of physician and nurse migration: The Caribbean, as a sending region, has adopted a program called Managed Migration, and the United Kingdom, as a receiving country, has established the "Code of Practice on International Recruitment."

WHO Activities

The WHO (2007) has developed a variety of initiatives to manage the migration of healthcare workers. It is working with the Global Health Workforce Alliance Task Force to support efforts to scale up health-worker education, particularly in countries faced by workforce crises. It also provides technical support to countries and assists regional human resources for health observatories. Additionally, the WHO supports the Treat, Train, Retain (TTR) initiative, begun in 2006 to curb the effects of HIV/AIDS on the healthcare workforce and health systems in low- and middle-income countries. The goals of TTR are threefold: (1) to provide treatment, prevention, and support to health workers affected by HIV/AIDS; (2) to train providers (including community health workers) to maximize existing capacity to treat HIV/AIDS; and (3) to retain health workers in rural areas and the public sector in underresourced countries. The WHO will provide assistance to participating countries in developing TTR plans and budgeting for proposed changes, but TTR's implementation and financing will be managed by individual countries.

ICN Statement

The ICN—the federation of national nurses associations (e.g., American Nurses Association, Philippine Nurses Association)—has developed a position statement on ethical recruitment of nurses to guide the recruitment efforts between its member countries. While acknowledging nurses' inherent right to migrate, the statement also calls for receiving countries to work toward building self-sustainable, domestically trained nursing workforces. The statement also aims to protect migrant nurses, calling for several measures such as good-faith contracting, freedom of employment and association, and fair pay and working conditions (ICN 2007).

Domestic Policies in Sending Countries

Some sending countries have implemented domestic policy changes to reduce the effects of push factors that motivate physicians and nurses to seek overseas employment. These changes include improvement in pay, career opportunities, and working conditions; provision of incentives to induce overseas workers to return home; and the development of private-sector opportunities. Other measures focus more specifically on medical education, including pre-education screening of candidates likely to stay in-country, shortening of domestic training programs, and adaptations of curriculum to local conditions.

Still other policies aim to use financial disincentives to keep workers in-country, requiring emigrants to pay fees upon departure. For example, Eritrea has a bond program in which departing physicians are required to make up-front payments that guarantee their return from studies in South Africa (Marchal and Kegels 2003). This type of system could be particularly useful if revenues generated were used to fund human resources development in sending countries (Saravia and Miranda 2004).

Domestic Policies in Receiving Countries

Some receiving countries have adopted domestic policy changes to address the underlying human resources imbalances that contribute to the demand for foreign-trained workers. In many developed countries, nursing shortages are exacerbated by difficulties in retaining domestically trained nurses—difficulties that are often related to poor working conditions and low salaries (Janiszewski Goodin 2003). Turnover rates for nurses in U.S. hospitals were estimated at between 10 percent and 30 percent in 2000 (HSM Group 2002). To improve domestic retention, receiving countries, such as the United Kingdom and Australia, have implemented programs to recruit and retain domestic healthcare workers (Martineau, Decker, and Bundred 2004). Other countries have begun recruiting nonconventional workers, such as firefighters, to the healthcare field (Marchal and Kegels 2003).

In 2002, the U.S. Congress passed the Nurse Reinvestment Act, a piece of legislation that uses a combination of expanded eligibility for loan repayment, education vouchers, and other measures to improve retention of nurses (Andrews 2004). While this legislation represents a positive step in improving retention of domestically trained nurses, its funding stream has been subject to frequent cuts in the past few years, so its overall impact is unclear (Janiszewski Goodin 2003).

Government-to-Government Bilateral Agreements

Some sending and receiving countries have attempted to regulate the migration of healthcare workers between them by signing government-to-government *bilateral agreements.* Under this agreement, a receiving country pledges to underwrite the costs of training additional staff; to recruit staff for a fixed period (often providing training before staff return to the sending country); or to recruit surplus staff from a sending country (Buchan 2007). For example, the United Kingdom has bilateral agreements with the Philippines and Spain that allows the United Kingdom to recruit nurses from these two countries for temporary work in the National Health Service (Kline 2003). Bilateral agreements can help to manage the flow of physicians or nurses between sending and receiving countries by mandating short-term rather than permanent migration.

Another policy intervention that has been proposed requires receiving countries to compensate sending countries for the financial losses associated with worker migration. Various versions of this plan call for remuneration of the costs of educating migrant workers, for assistance with human resources development in sending countries, and for additional compensation for sending countries' lost tax revenue. Although well intended, these measures are difficult to implement because administrative costs would likely be high and because determining payment amounts, procedures, and enforcement would present further challenges to sending and receiving countries (Marchal and Kegels 2003).

Compensation Schemes

The Managed Migration program in the Caribbean is one of the most sophisticated policy responses to the issue of nurse migration in a sending country or region. Managed Migration aims to promote regional cooperation and strategic planning in six critical areas:

Managed Migration in the Caribbean

1. Terms and conditions of work
2. Recruitment, retention, and training
3. Value of nursing
4. Utilization and deployment
5. Management practices
6. Policy development

This program was developed by a partnership among national, regional, bilateral, and international stakeholders. Initiatives developed under the program include efforts to promote temporary or part-time migration of Caribbean-trained nurses to developed countries, agreements requiring receiving countries to invest in sending countries' health-professions education systems, and promotion of health tourism in Caribbean countries (Salmon et al. 2007).

The United Kingdom is one of the few major receiving countries to develop a specific policy to guide the recruitment of internationally trained physicians and nurses. Its National Health Service (NHS) has created the Code of Practice on International Recruitment, which includes the following provisions (Buchan 2007):

Code of Practice on International Recruitment in the United Kingdom

• Developing countries should not be targeted for active recruitment by the NHS unless the government of that country formally agrees.
• NHS employers should only use recruitment agencies that have agreed to comply with the Code.

- NHS employers should consider regional collaboration in international recruitment activities.
- Staff recruited from abroad have the same legal protection as other employees.
- Staff recruited from abroad should have the same access to further training as other employees.

While the Code has been touted as an example for other countries to follow, its effectiveness is somewhat limited by the fact that it only applies to the public sector (not to independent or private employers or recruitment agencies), and employers and migrant healthcare workers have found many ways to work around it. Nonetheless, the Code represents a deliberate effort by a receiving country to reduce the negative effects of healthcare worker recruitment from developing countries.

Issues for Managers

The movement of IMGs and INGs into the U.S. healthcare system raises several important issues for managers and leaders. In particular, managers must be aware of issues of ethical recruitment, regulation (visas), credentialing, and adaptation for internationally trained physicians and nurses. (For a summary of the elements in these issues, see Table 3.1.) Careful consideration of all of these areas is necessary to facilitate the successful recruitment and incorporation of internationally trained healthcare professionals into the U.S. healthcare system and to minimize the migration's negative effects on sending countries.

Recruitment

Healthcare organizations can recruit workers from overseas through several mechanisms. These include, but are not limited to, the following (Buchan and Perfilieva 2006):

- *Twinning.* Hospitals in sending and receiving countries develop links, based on staff exchanges, staff support, and flow of resources.
- *Staff exchange.* Healthcare workers temporarily move between organizations in sending and receiving countries for career and personal development opportunities or for organizational growth.
- *Educational support.* Educators and/or educational/funding resources temporarily move from receiving to sending organizations.
- *Bilateral agreement.* Employers in the receiving country develop an agreement with employers or educators in the sending country to help pay the costs of training additional staff or to recruit staff for training and development before returning staff to the sending country.

TABLE 3.1 Management Issues with Internationally Trained Physicians and Nurses

Issues	International Medical Graduate (IMG)	International Nursing Graduate (ING)
Regulation— Visas	*Temporary* J-1 • Category for trainees • Sponsored by ECFMG[1] for resident IMGs H-1B • Category for "specialty occupations" • 3-year length of stay, renewable for 3 additional years O • Category for "outstanding" researchers or specialists • Indefinite length of stay *Permanent* Labor Certification Process • Requires employer to demonstrate shortage of qualified workers in the geographic area • IMG is obligated to remain with employer for 18 months to 5 years after application is approved National Interest Waiver • No employer link • Requires demonstration of unique abilities that contribute to national quality of life	*Temporary* H-1B • Category for "specialty occupations" • 3-year length of stay, renewable for 3 additional years H-1C • Category for workers in underserved areas • Yearly cap of 500 nurses • 3-year length of stay TN • Linked to NAFTA[2] • Applies to nurses from Mexico and Canada • 1-year length of stay, renewable EB-3 • Employment-based visa • Released to India, the Philippines, and China for nurses and other health workers in 2005 *Permanent* Labor Certification Process • Requires employer to demonstrate shortage of qualified workers in the geographic area • ING is obligated to remain with employer for 18 months to 5 years after application is approved

(Continued)

TABLE 3.1   Continued

Credentialing	*Requirements* • Entry into residency programs certified by ECFMG • Verifiable medical school diploma • Passing scores on USMLE[3] Step 1 and Step 2 (clinical knowledge and clinical skills) • Acceptable scores on TOEFL[4]	*Requirements* • CGFNS[5] review of educational background and credentials • Passing score on NCLEX-RN[6] • Acceptable scores on TOEFL
Adaptation	*Training Needs* • Culture of medicine • Models of family relationships • Communication with patients • Communication with nursing and support staff	*Training Needs* • Nursing culture and communication • Supervision and delegation of care • Hospital systems, technology, and documentation • Clinical skills and drug administration

[1]ECFMG: Educational Commission for Foreign Medical Graduates; [2]NAFTA: North American Free Trade Agreement; [3]USMLE: U.S. Medical Licensing Examination; [4]TOEFL: Test of English as a Foreign Language; [5]CGFNS: Commission on Graduates of Foreign Nursing Schools; [6]NCLEX-RN: National Council Licensure Examination for Registered Nurses

SOURCES: ECFMG (2007); Mautino (2002, 2003); Bieski (2007); Kingma (2006); Arends-Kuenning (2006); Whelan et al. (2002); and Whelan (2006)

Additionally, IMGs and INGs also find jobs through informal mechanisms, such as personal and professional contacts (Bagchi 2001). In all of these models, the recruitment process can be conducted directly by the employer or mediated by either domestic or overseas recruitment agencies. A recruitment agency typically charges a hiring organization between $5,000 and $10,000 per nurse. In return, nurses agree to work for the hiring organization for a fixed period of time—usually two to three years. For-profit recruitment agencies represent an important and growing presence in overseas hiring of nurses in particular; many of them set up both domestic and sending-country offices to facilitate the process (Brush, Sochalski, and Berger 2004).

Employers in receiving countries must consider the implications of their recruiting practices for the countries and organizations from which they are recruiting. They must also be aware of the rights of the workers themselves. The United States has no overarching code of practice for international recruitment of healthcare workers, so the decisions about how to balance ethical concerns with domestic staffing needs are the responsibility of individual employers and the recruitment agencies with which they work. Recruitment agencies' behavior has improved since a rash of abuses was documented in the 1980s. Today, efforts toward better practice are fueled by market competition between agencies (Kingma 2006). Employers and recruiters must take responsibility for not recruiting from countries with severe shortages and for providing a safe and transparent recruitment process for migrant workers.

Regulation (Visas)

Because most IMGs enter the United States as residents, the first type of visa that they commonly obtain is the J-1 visa, a category for trainees. The Educational Commission for Foreign Medical Graduates (ECFMG 2007) is authorized by the U.S. Department of State to sponsor J-1 visas for IMGs. After completing their training, some physicians obtain permanent residency status, while others remain in the country on H-1B or O temporary visas.

Physicians

H-1B visas apply to immigrants in "specialty occupations," which usually require at least a bachelor's degree. These visas allow for a three-year length of stay, which can then be extended for three additional years. O visas can be obtained by physicians who have "outstanding" abilities in their field; these are usually researchers or specialists. O visas are more loosely tied to employers than H-1B visas and allow their holders to stay in the United States indefinitely (Mautino 2002).

IMGs who wish to work permanently in the United States can pursue permanent residency through one of two main avenues: going through a labor certification process or obtaining a national interest waiver. The *labor certification process* requires that an IMG's employer demonstrate a shortage of qualified workers to fill the position in the geographic area; if approved, the physician is obligated to remain with his or her employer for 18 months to

5 years after the application is approved. The *national interest waiver* requires the IMG to demonstrate that he or she has exceptional abilities in a field, such that his or her admission to the workforce is in the national interest of the United States. Physicians who seek a national interest waiver need not be linked to a specific employer, but they must demonstrate unique abilities that contribute to the country's quality of life, which may include service in a medically underserved area for five years or more (Mautino 2002).

Nurses   From 1990 to 1995, many INGs entered the United States under H-1A visas, which were aimed at encouraging the migration of overseas-educated nurses. This visa category was withdrawn after many U.S. healthcare organizations downsized in the mid-1990s. Since 1995, nurses have entered the country under one of four visa categories:

1. *H-1B:* See the provisions described in the physicians visa section earlier.
2. *H-1C:* Established under the Nursing Relief for Disadvantaged Areas Act of 1999, this visa allows INGs to work in underserved areas. It has a yearly cap of 500 nurses and permits a three-year length of stay (Bieski 2007).
3. *TN:* Linked to NAFTA, this visa applies to nurses from Mexico and Canada. It is good for a one-year stay in the United States and is renewable.
4. *EB-3:* A permanent employment-based visa, this was made available in 2005 to nurses and other healthcare workers from sending countries such as India, the Philippines, and China. Although the EB-3 visa quotas had been reached, the visa was extended to 50,000 more workers, enabling U.S. healthcare organizations to hire many overseas-trained nurses (Kingma 2006). Employers that hire nurses are not subject to the usual provision that requires them to prove that no U.S. workers are available to take jobs to be filled by visa recipients (Arends-Kuenning 2006).

Many of these visa categories either have very specific requirements or are difficult to obtain. Thus, many INGs apply for permanent residency permits (green cards) when coming to the United States (Kingma 2006). INGs can pursue permanent residency through the employer-dependent labor certification process, which is described earlier in the IMG visa section (Mautino 2003).

Credentialing

Physicians   IMGs who desire to work as physicians in the United States must complete their residency training in a U.S. healthcare organization before they can practice. Their entry into these training programs must be certified by the ECFMG, which has been managing the entry of IMGs into the U.S. workforce since 1958 (Whelan et al. 2002). Applicants must submit a verifiable diploma from a medical school listed in the *International Medical Education Directory* published by the Foundation for Advancement of International Medical Education and Research. They must also show a passing score on Step 1 and Step 2 (clinical knowledge and clinical skills) of the U.S. Medical Licensing Examination (USMLE), along with acceptable scores on the Test of English as a Foreign Language (TOEFL). The USMLE Step 1 and Step 2 examination and the TOEFL are given at test centers worldwide, while the USMLE Step 2 examination is given at regional test centers in the United States (ECFMG 2007).

IMGs must obtain a USMLE/ECFMG identification number to take the required examinations. They are certified by the ECFMG after completion of (and acceptable scores in) all examinations and meeting all other requirements, including school/diploma verification. Candidates may apply to residency programs before their certification is completed, but they must be fully certified before their programs begin. IMGs follow the same residency application and matching process as followed by U.S. medical graduates, although IMGs are also eligible to sign residency contracts outside of the matching system (ECFMG 2007).

Nurses

Credentialing of INGs in the United States is managed by the Commission on Graduates of Foreign Nursing Schools (CGFNS), which was established in 1977 to standardize the examination process for internationally trained nurses. The CGFNS conducts mandatory reviews of incoming nurses' educational backgrounds and credentials, documentation of English proficiency, and successful completion of the National Council Licensure Examination for Registered Nurses (NCLEX-RN) (Bieski 2007). The CGFNS credential review ensures that nurses have at least the minimum credentials required for licensure within the United States, although precise licensing requirements are still managed by state boards of nursing and may vary. The English-language proficiency requirement can be fulfilled through the submission of test scores on the TOEFL or another test of English proficiency.

The CGFNS offers a pre-immigration examination in more than 30 countries around the world. While the examination is not a substitute for the NCLEX-RN, it is an important predictor of success on the NCLEX-RN, which is required for employment in the United States. The NCLEX-RN is given at testing locations nationwide and in testing centers throughout Europe, Asia, and South America.

Adaptation

Physicians

IMGs in the United States face a variety of barriers that may inhibit their successful adaptation to working in the healthcare system. These barriers include the culture of medicine in this country—for example, patient-centered care and more accepting views of mental illness—that is most likely different from that in the IMG's homeland. The IMG will also need to adjust to various models of the American family—for example, single-parent and step families—that can influence physician–patient/family interactions (Whelan 2006). Also, some IMGs may encounter language difficulties when communicating with patients, some of whom may be suspicious of being treated by "foreign" physicians, and when working with nursing and support staff. IMGs' professional experiences, attitudes, and practices in their home countries may also cause misunderstanding or conflict with American staff members (Kuczkowski 2004).

Managers must take into account these and other potential adaptation issues when designing orientation and ongoing support programs to help foreign-trained physicians to adapt to their new roles within the U.S. healthcare system.

Nurses Once INGs, who have a broad variety of job experiences and expectations, arrive at their jobs in the United States, their organizations must provide adequate information and training to ensure that they can successfully perform their new roles within the American healthcare system. Managers who hire INGs have found the following areas in which training is especially useful:

- Culture (e.g., relative independence of nurses, work with professional care staff rather than with patients' family members) and communication
- Supervision and delegation of care
- Hospital systems, technology, and documentation
- Clinical skills and drug administration

Many healthcare organizations have found that INGs require additional orientation relative to U.S.-trained nurses, and to this end, organizations have initiated longer orientation programs that include elements such as those listed above. Nurse managers who supervise INGs will also benefit from educational programs that address many of the same areas. Such training will enable managers to facilitate the quick adaptation of their nurses and head off potential problems (Sherman 2007).

The Future of International Health Workforce Migration

The international migration of physicians and nurses is a long-standing phenomenon that is likely to continue for many years in the future. Healthcare organizations in many developed countries rely on these physicians and nurses to offset domestic staffing shortages. In some cases, this migration can exacerbate healthcare workforce shortages in sending countries. In other cases, however, this migration is anticipated, moving sending countries to educate and train surplus physicians and nurses for export.

While some receiving countries, such as the United Kingdom, have taken steps to minimize the negative effects of international recruitment on sending countries, the United States has not enacted similar policies. American healthcare workforce planners have made little effort to ensure that the supply of U.S.-trained physicians and nurses is self-sufficient. As a result, at least for the moment, this country will likely continue to need foreign-trained healthcare professionals to meet the demand. Although this reliance on international migration is unlikely to be a sustainable long-term strategy, it is and will be an essential part of the U.S. healthcare system for many years to come. Because the federal government has yet to develop a coherent workforce policy on this issue, the responsibility for managing the effects of international recruitment lies with leaders of individual healthcare organizations.

Issues of ethical recruitment will also continue to be important for healthcare workforce planners and organizational managers. These leaders must carefully consider how domestic needs place burdens on other countries' healthcare systems, healthcare professions' educational needs, and healthcare workforce supplies. They must also provide adequate support to IMGs and INGs once they arrive to work and train in the United States.

Summary

This chapter discusses several aspects of a critical issue to U.S. healthcare managers: the globalization of the physician and nursing workforces. Given the essential role that foreign-trained physicians and nurses play in many U.S. healthcare organizations, an understanding of the history, current patterns, and factors that motivate physician and nurse migration is vital for managers. Physicians and nurses have sought work across international borders for several decades, and their movement is likely to continue long into the future, particularly in light of current healthcare workforce shortages in many receiving countries.

Many internationally trained physicians and nurses who work in the United States and other developed countries are trained in developing countries. Some of these sending countries—particularly those in sub-Saharan Africa and the Caribbean—face an uncontrolled "brain drain" of skilled health workers, while other countries such as India, Cuba, the Philippines, and possibly China purposely train physicians and nurses to work overseas. While these workers play a vital role in the health systems of many developed countries, their departure can have serious implications for the healthcare system in their home countries. Several international bodies and individual countries have adopted policies that attempt to manage the movement of physicians and nurses from developing to developed nations, but thus far no universal practices have been adopted.

In this context, U.S. healthcare organizations can recruit internationally trained physicians and nurses through a variety of mechanisms. Because the United States has not yet established a specific code of practice that governs international recruitment, employers themselves are responsible for providing a safe and transparent recruitment process for migrant workers. Additionally, managers must understand visa and credentialing regulations that apply to internationally trained healthcare workers as well as the challenges that these newly hired workers face as they adapt to working in the United States. Careful consideration of all these issues will help to ensure the fair hiring and successful incorporation of internationally trained physicians and nurses into the U.S. healthcare workforce.

Discussion Questions

1. Why is it important for healthcare managers to be aware of the trends in international migration of physicians and nurses?
2. What impact do these trends have on the U.S. healthcare system?
3. Sending countries experience two distinct situations as a result of international migration—brain drain and strategic deployment. What are the differences between the two? What are the advantages (if any) and disadvantages of each situation?
4. Suppose that U.S. policymakers are developing ethical international recruitment guidelines based on the National Health Service's Code of Practice on International Recruitment. What elements of the Code can be included in the guidelines, and what can be implemented in the context of the U.S. healthcare system?
5. What are the ethical issues that healthcare leaders and managers must consider when recruiting IMGs and INGs? What steps can be taken to deal with these issues?
6. Discuss the importance of orienting IMGs and INGs to their roles in the U.S. healthcare system. What obstacles (cultural, organizational, and professional) do they face, and what are the implications if these barriers are not addressed?

Experiential Exercise

Case   For the Philippines, exporting nurses has been a long-standing government strategy, part of a broad and concerted program of labor migration introduced in the 1970s during the administration of President Ferdinand Marcos (Tyner 2004). Although intended initially as a short-term solution to domestic unemployment and high foreign debt, this program has become a permanent strategy for generating income for the country through regular remittances from migrant workers.

The Philippines has a net surplus of nurses because of high production and relatively low demand, mainly because of underfunding of the country's health system. Because of nurse migration, the country has lost many of its most skilled nurses. For the last several years, the Philippines has been experiencing two trends that are causing concern among nursing leaders:

1. *An explosive growth in the number of nursing programs.* In the 1980s, only 40 nursing schools were in existence throughout the country; in 2007, the number was much higher: 460 programs in total. Some schools have sought rapid, drastic expansions to their enrollment, contributing to the vast and steady increase in the number of nursing students. The Philippines currently produces about 20,000 nurses per year (Lorenzo et al. 2007).

2. *A movement of physicians into "second course" nursing education.* Physicians are leaving their posts in public hospitals and rural areas to work abroad as nurses. Demand for medical education has declined, and some nursing schools have created special programs that allow physicians to pursue nursing education while continuing to practice as physicians.

Policymakers in the Philippines are concerned that the growth in the number of nursing programs has been accompanied by a decline in quality of education: In recent years, fewer than half of the nursing graduates passed the nursing licensure examination. This means that many nursing graduates cannot even work as nurses in the Philippines, much less in the United States and other overseas markets. Nonetheless, thousands of students enter nursing programs every year.

In this context, nursing leaders in the Philippines are struggling to maintain quality education and a sense of public service in a profession that is increasingly governed by business interests and influenced by individual aspirations for overseas employment. The country's Department of Health (DOH) has developed the Master Plan for Health Human Resources to address domestic healthcare human resources distribution, motivation (compensation—provision of living wages for government workers), and production. The DOH has attempted to be directly involved in improving the quality of nursing education and the process of nurse migration, but the department's efforts have been rebuffed by the president, who wants these issues to be handled by the Philippine Overseas Employment Administration, the division of the Department of Labor and Employment that manages overseas deployment of Filipino workers.

Case Exercise You are a consultant to a task force charged with overhauling nursing education and migration practices in the Philippines. You have been asked to recommend short-term and long-term strategies to achieve sustainable improvements in nursing education and to harmonize the nursing-deployment policy with domestic health system needs.

1. Who are your stakeholders, and from whom will you seek perspectives? What questions will you ask each of them?

2. Which issue—explosive growth of programs, declining quality, training of physicians to be nurses—will you address first? How will you engage the labor and health departments to implement your recommendations successfully?

3. What obstacles do you expect to face in this process? What strategies will you use to overcome them?

Note

1. IMGs who are U.S. citizens make up approximately 3 percent of the physician workforce in the United States (Mullan 2005). Many of these physicians are trained in "offshore" medical schools in the Caribbean or Central America. This phenomenon is not discussed in this chapter.

References

Aiken, L. H., J. Buchan, J. Sochalski, B. Nichols, and M. Powell. 2004. "Trends in International Nurse Migration." *Health Affairs* 23 (3): 69–77.

Andrews, D. R. 2004. "The Nurse Reinvestment Act: The Impact of Governmental and Nongovernmental Administrative Tools." *Journal of Professional Nursing* 20 (4): 260–69.

Arends-Kuenning, M. 2006. "The Balance of Care: Trends in the Wages and Employment of Immigrant Nurses in the U.S. Between 1990 and 2000." *Globalizations* 3 (3): 333–48.

Bagchi, A. D. 2001. "Migrant Networks and the Immigrant Professional: The Role of Weak Ties." *Population Research and Policy Review* 20 (1–2): 9–31.

Ball, R. E. 1996. "A Nation Building or Dissolution: The Globalization of Nursing—The Case of the Philippines." *Pilipinas* 27 (Fall): 67–91.

Bieski, T. 2007. "Foreign-Educated Nurses: An Overview of Migration and Credentialing Issues." *Nursing Economic$* 25 (1): 20–23, 34.

British Medical Journal (BMJ). 1968. "Emigration of British Doctors to United States of America and Canada. Report and Recommendations of a Ministry of Health Interview Board on Interviews and Discussions in North America with British Trained Doctors." *British Medical Journal* 1 (5583): 45–48.

Brush, B. L., J. Sochalski, and A. M. Berger. 2004. "Imported Care: Recruiting Foreign Nurses to US Health Care Facilities." *Health Affairs* 23 (3): 78–87.

Buchan, J. 2007. "International Recruitment of Nurses: Policy and Practice in the United Kingdom." *Health Services Research* 42 (3 Pt 2): 1321–35.

Buchan, J., T. Parkin, and J. Sochalski. 2003. *International Nurse Mobility: Trends and Policy Implications.* Geneva, Switzerland: World Health Organization.

Buchan, J., and G. Perfilieva. 2006. *Health Worker Migration in the European Region: Country Case Studies and Policy Implications.* Geneva, Switzerland: World Health Organization.

Buchan, J., and J. Sochalski. 2004. "The Migration of Nurses: Trends and Policies." *Bulletin of the World Health Organization* 82 (8): 587–94.

Cooper, R. A., and L. H. Aiken. 2006. "Health Services Delivery: Reframing Policies for Global Migration of Nurses and Physicians—A U.S. Perspective." *Policy, Politics, and Nursing Practice* 7 (3 Suppl): 66S–70S.

Dovlo, D. 2007. "Migration of Nurses from Sub-Saharan Africa: A Review of Issues and Challenges." *Health Services Research* 42 (3 Pt 2): 1373–88.

Educational Commission on Foreign Medical Graduates (ECFMG). 2007. "Certification Fact Sheet." [Online information; retrieved 9/21/07.] www.ecfmg.org/cert/certfact.pdf.

Fang, Z. Z. 2007. "Potential of China in Global Nurse Migration." *Health Services Research* 42 (3 Pt 2): 1419–28.

Feinsilver, J. M. 1989. "Cuba as a 'World Medical Power': The Politics of Symbolism." *Latin American Research Review* 24 (2): 1–34.

Forcier, M. B., S. Simoens, and A. Giuffrida. 2004. "Impact, Regulation, and Health Policy Implications of Physician Migration in OECD Countries." *Human Resources for Health* 2 (1): 12.

HSM Group, Ltd. 2002. "Acute Care Hospital Survey of RN Vacancy and Turnover Rates in 2000." *Journal of Nursing Administration* 32 (9): 437–39.

International Council of Nurses (ICN). 2007. "Ethical Nurse Recruitment: Position Statement." [Online information; retrieved 9/25/07.] www.icn.ch/psrecruit01.htm.

Janiszewski Goodin, H. 2003. "The Nursing Shortage in the United States of America: An Integrative Review of the Literature." *Journal of Advanced Nursing* 43 (3): 335–50.

Khadria, B. 2007. "International Nurse Recruitment in India." *Health Services Research* 42 (3 Pt 2): 1429–36.

Kingma, M. 2006. *Nurses on the Move: Migration and the Global Health Care Economy.* Ithaca, NY: Cornell University Press.

———. 2007. "Nurses on the Move: A Global Overview." *Health Services Research* 42 (3 Pt 2): 1281–98.

Kline, D. S. 2003. "Push and Pull Factors in International Nurse Migration." *Journal of Nursing Scholarship* 35 (2): 107–11.

Kuczkowski, K. M. 2004. "International Medical Graduates in American Medicine: Is There a 'Dark Side of the Moon'?" *Acta Obstetrica et Gynecologica Scandinavia* 83 (12): 1228–29.

Lee, N. 1996. "Cuban Doctors Take South Africa by Storm." *Lancet* 347 (9002): 681.

Lorenzo, F. E. M., J. Galvez-Tan, K. Icamina, and L. Javier. 2007. "Nurse Migration from a Source Country Perspective: Philippine Country Case Study." *Health Services Research* 42 (3 Pt 2): 1406–18.

Marchal, B., and G. Kegels. 2003. "Health Workforce Imbalances in Times of Globalization: Brain Drain or Professional Mobility?" *International Journal of Health Planning and Management* 18 (Suppl 1): S89–S101.

Martineau, T., K. Decker, and P. Bundred. 2004. " 'Brain Drain' of Health Professionals: From Rhetoric to Responsible Action." *Health Policy* 70 (1): 1–10.

Mautino, K. 2002. "Physicians and Immigration." *Journal of Immigrant Health* 4 (4): 167–69.

———. 2003. "Nurses and Immigration." *Journal of Immigrant Health* 5 (1): 1–3.

Mejía, A. 1978. "Migration of Physicians and Nurses: A Worldwide Picture." *International Journal of Epidemiology* 7 (3): 207–15.

Mullan, F. 2005. "The Metrics of Physician Brain Drain." *New England Journal of Medicine* 353 (17): 1810–18.

———. 2006. "Doctors for the World: Indian Physician Immigration." *Health Affairs* 25 (2): 380–93.

Muntaner, C., R. M. Guerra Salazar, J. Benach, and F. Armada. 2006. "Venezuela's Barrio Adentro: An Alternative to Neoliberalism in Health Care." *International Journal of Health Services* 36 (4): 803–11.

Padarath, A., C. Chamberlain, D. McCoy, A. Ntuli, M. Rowson, and R. Loewensen. 2004. "Health Personnel in Southern Africa: Confronting Maldistribution and the Brain Drain." EQUINET Discussion Paper #3. [Online information; retrieved 9/10/07.] www.equinetafrica.org/bibl/docs/DIS3hres.pdf.

Salmon, M. E., J. Yan, H. Hewitt, and V. Guisinger. 2007. "Managed Migration: The Caribbean Approach to Addressing Nursing Services Capacity." *Health Services Research* 42 (3 Pt 2): 1354–72.

Saravia, N. G., and J. F. Miranda. 2004. "Plumbing the Brain Drain." *Bulletin of the World Health Organization* 82 (8): 608–15.

Sherman, R. O. 2007. "Leadership Development Needs of Managers Who Supervise Foreign Nurses." *Leadership in Health Services* 20 (1): 7–15.

Tyner, J. A. 2004. *Made in the Philippines: Gendered Discourses and the Making of Migrants.* New York: RoutledgeCurzon.

Vujicic, M., P. Zurn, K. Diallo, O. Adams, and M. R. Dal Poz. 2004. "The Role of Wages in the Migration of Health Care Professionals from Developing Countries." *Human Resources for Health* 282 (1): 3.

Whelan, G. P. 2006. "Coming to America: The Integration of International Medical Graduates into the American Medical Culture." *Academic Medicine* 81 (2): 176–78.

Whelan, G. P., N. E. Gray, J. Kostis, J. R. Boulet, and J. A. Hallock. 2002. "The Changing Pool of International Medical Graduates Seeking Certification Training in US Graduate Medical Education Programs." *JAMA* 288 (9): 1079–84.

World Health Organization (WHO). 2007. *Taking Stock: Health Worker Shortages and the Response to AIDS.* Geneva, Switzerland: World Health Organization.

HEALTHCARE PROFESSIONALS

Kenneth R. White, PhD, FACHE; Dolores G. Clement,
DrPH, FACHE; and Kristie G. Stover, PhD

Learning Objectives

After completing this chapter, the reader should be able to

- understand the role of healthcare professionals in the human resources management function of healthcare organizations;
- define the elements of a profession, with an understanding of the theoretical underpinnings of the healthcare professions in particular;
- describe the healthcare professions, which include the majority of healthcare workers, and the required educational levels, scopes of practice, and licensure issues for each;
- relate knowledge of the healthcare professions to selected human resources management issues and systems development; and
- comprehend the changing nature of the existing and emerging healthcare professions in the healthcare workforce, particularly the impact of managed care.

Introduction

Healthcare professionals are central to the delivery of high-quality healthcare services. Extensive training, education, and skills are essential in meeting the needs and demands of the population for safe, competent healthcare. These specialized techniques and skills that healthcare professionals acquired through systematic programs of intellectual study are the basis for socialization into their profession. Additionally, the healthcare industry is labor intensive and is distinguished from other service industries by the number of licensed and registered personnel that it employs and the variety of healthcare fields that it produces. These healthcare fields have emerged as a result of the specialization of medicine, development of public health, increased emphasis on health promotion and prevention, and technological advances and growth.

Because of this division of labor within medical and health services delivery, many tasks that were once the responsibility of medical providers have been delegated to other healthcare personnel. Such delegation of duties raises important questions for the industry: Should healthcare providers other than those specifically trained to practice medicine be considered professionals in their own right? To what extent should their scope of practice be extended?

In this chapter, we respond to the aforementioned questions by defining key terms, describing the healthcare professions and labor force, explaining the role of human resources in healthcare, and discussing key human resources issues that affect the delivery of healthcare.

Professionalization

Although the terms "occupation" and "profession" often are used interchangeably, they can be differentiated.

An *occupation* enables workers to provide services, but it does not require skill specialization. An occupation is the principal activity that supports one's livelihood. However, it is different from a profession in several ways. An occupation typically does not require higher skill specialization. An individual in an occupation is usually supervised, adheres to a defined work schedule, and earns an hourly wage rate. An individual in an occupation may be trained for a specific job or function and, as a result, is less able to move from one organization to another.

A *profession* requires specialized knowledge and training that enable professionals to gain more authority and responsibility and to provide service that adheres to a code of ethics. A professional usually has more autonomy in determining the content of the service he or she provides and in monitoring the workload needed to do so. A professional generally earns a salary, requires higher education, and works with more independence and mobility than do nonprofessionals.

The distinction between an occupation and a profession is important because the evolving process of healthcare delivery requires professionals who are empowered to make decisions in the absence of direct supervision. The proliferation of knowledge and the skills needed in the prevention, diagnosis, and treatment of disease has required increasing levels of education. Undergraduate- and/or graduate-level degrees are now required for entry into virtually every professional field. Some professions, such as pharmacy and physical therapy, are moving toward professional doctorates (i.e., PharmD and DPT, respectively) for practice.

A countervailing force against the increasing educational requirements of the healthcare professions is ongoing change in the mechanisms for delivery and payment of services. With consolidation of the healthcare system and the rise of managed care, along with its demands for efficiency, fewer financial resources are available. As a result, healthcare organizations are pressured to replace highly trained—and, therefore, more expensive—healthcare professionals with unlicensed support personnel. Fewer professionals are being asked to do more, and those with advanced degrees are required to supervise more assistants who are functionally trained for specified organizational roles.

Functional training produces personnel who can perform tasks but who may not know the theory behind the practice; understanding theory is essential to becoming fully skilled and able to make complex management and patient care decisions. Conversely, knowing the theory without having the experience also makes competent practice difficult. When educating potential healthcare professionals, on-the-job training or a period of apprenticeship is needed, particularly in addition to basic coursework. Dreyfus and Dreyfus (1996) contend that both theoretical knowledge and practiced response are needed in the acquisition of skill in a profession. These authors lay out five stages of abilities that an individual passes as he or she develops a skill:

1. *Novice.* At this stage, the novice learns tasks and skills that enable him or her to determine actions based on recognized situations. Rules and guidelines direct the novice's energy and action at this stage.
2. *Advanced beginner.* At this stage, the advanced beginner has gained enough experience and knowledge that certain behaviors become automatic, and he or she can begin to learn when tasks should be addressed.
3. *Competent.* At this stage, the competent individual has mastered the practiced response of definable tasks and processes and has acquired the ability to deal with the unexpected events that may not conform to plans.
4. *Proficient.* At this stage, the proficient individual has developed the ability to discern a situation, intuitively assess it, plan what needs to be done, decide on an action, and perform the action more effortlessly than possible in the earlier stages.
5. *Expert.* At this stage, the expert can accomplish the goals without realizing that rules are being followed because the skill and knowledge required to reach the goal have become second nature.

Theoretical understanding is melded with practice in each progressive stage. Functional training can help an individual progress through the first three stages and can provide the individual with calculative rationality or inferential reasoning ability to be able to apply and improve theories and rules learned. For skill development at the proficient and expert levels, deliberative rationality or ability to challenge and improve theories and rules learned is required. Healthcare professionals need to become experts in fields where self-direction, autonomy, and decision making for patient care may be required (Dreyfus and Dreyfus 1996).

Healthcare Professionals

The healthcare industry is the largest and most powerful industry in the United States. It constitutes more than 6.5 percent of the country's total labor force and nearly 15 percent of the gross domestic product. Healthcare professionals include physicians, nurses, dentists, pharmacists, optometrists, psychologists, nonphysician practitioners such as physician assistants and nurse practitioners, healthcare administrators, and allied health professionals. The allied health professions are a huge group that consists of therapists, medical and radiologic technologists, social workers, health educators, and other ancillary personnel. Healthcare professionals are represented by professional associations. Table 4.1 provides a sample of professional associations in healthcare.

Healthcare professionals work in a variety of settings, including hospitals; ambulatory care centers; managed care organizations; long-term-care organizations; mental health organizations; pharmaceutical companies; community health centers; physician offices; laboratories; research institutions; and schools of medicine, nursing, and allied health professions. According to the Bureau of Labor Statistics (BLS 2007), healthcare professionals are employed by the following:

- hospitals (34.5 percent),
- nursing and personal and residential care facilities (23.0 percent),
- physician offices and clinics (17.1 percent),
- home health care services (6.9 percent),
- dentist offices and clinics (6.3 percent), and
- other health service sites (12.2 percent).

The U.S. Department of Labor recognizes about 400 different job titles in the healthcare sector; however, many of these job titles are not included in our definition of healthcare professionals. For example, almost one-third of those employed in the healthcare sector probably belong in the support staff category—that is, employees who are part of the patient care team or involved in delivering health services. These approximately 2.2 million nursing aides, home health aides, and personal attendants are critical to the delivery of healthcare services (BLS 2007).

The primary reasons for the increased supply and demand for healthcare professionals include the following interrelated forces:

- technological growth,
- specialization,
- changes in third-party coverage,
- the aging of the population, and
- the proliferation of new and diverse healthcare delivery settings.

Organization	Target Audience	Website
Health Professions		
Pew Health Professions Commission	Future health professions	http://futurehealth .ucsf.edu
American College of Healthcare Executives: Health Management Careers	Future healthcare managers and administrators	www.healthmanage mentcareers.org
Accrediting Organizations		
Accreditation Association for Ambulatory Health Care	Ambulatory healthcare facilities	www.aaahc .org
Accreditation Council for Graduate Medical Education	Graduate medical education programs	www.acgme .org
American Osteopathic Association	Osteopathic hospitals and health systems	www.osteopathic .org
Commission on Accreditation of Rehabilitation Facilities	Rehabilitation facilities	www.carf.org
The Joint Commission	Hospitals and health systems	www.joint commission.org
National Committee for Quality Assurance	Health plans	http://web .ncqa.org
American Association of Blood Banks	Blood banks	www.aabb.org
American College of Surgeons	Surgeons	www.facs.org
American College of Surgeons: Commission on Cancer	Cancer programs	www.facs.org/ cancer
College of American Pathologists	Clinical laboratories	www.cap.org
Professional Associations		
American College of Healthcare Executives	Healthcare executives	www.ache.org
National Association of Health Services Executives	African-American healthcare executives	www.nahse.org
Institute for Diversity in Health Management	Healthcare managers, students, organizations, diversity programs	www.diversity connection.org

TABLE 4.1
Resource Guide for the Healthcare Professional

(Continued)

TABLE 4.1
Continued

Organization	Target Audience	Website
Medical Group Management Association	Physician practice managers and executives	www.mgma.com
American Hospital Association: American Society for Healthcare Human Resources Administration	Healthcare human resources professionals	www.hrleader.org
American College of Physician Executives	Physician executives	www.acpe.org
American College of Health Care Administrators	Long-term-care administrators	www.achca.org
Association for Healthcare Documentation Integrity	Medical transcriptionists	www.ahdionline.org
American Association of Nurse Anesthetists	Nurse anesthetists	www.aana.com
American Association for Respiratory Care	Respiratory therapists	www.aarc.org
American Health Information Management Association	Medical records and information management professionals	www.ahima.org
American Medical Technologists	Medical technologists	www.amt1.com
American Nurses Association	Registered nurses	www.ana.org
American Association for Homecare	Homecare administrators	www.aahomecare.org
American Occupational Therapy Association, Inc.	Occupational therapists	www.aota.org
American Organization of Nurse Executives	Nurse executives	www.aone.org
National League for Nursing	Nurse faculty and educators	www.nln.org
American Physical Therapy Association	Physical therapists	www.apta.org
American Society for Clinical Pathology	Pathologists and laboratory professionals	www.ascp.org
American Society of Health-System Pharmacists	Health system pharmacists	www.ashp.org

Organization	Target Audience	Website	TABLE 4.1 Continued
American Society of Radiologic Technologists	Radiologic technologists	www.asrt.org	
American Speech-Language-Hearing Association	Speech-language pathologists; audiologists; and speech, language, and hearing scientists	www.asha.org	
Healthcare Financial Management Association	Controllers, chief financial officers, and accountants	www.hfma.org	
Healthcare Information and Management Systems Society	Health information and technology managers	www.himss.org	
National Cancer Registrars Association	Cancer registry professionals	www.ncra-usa.org	
Trade Associations			
American Hospital Association	Hospitals, health systems, and personal membership groups	www.aha.org	
Federation of American Hospitals	Investor-owned hospitals and health systems	www.fah.org	
Association of American Medical Colleges: Council of Teaching Hospitals and Health Systems	Teaching hospitals and health systems	www.aamc.org/members/coth	
Catholic Health Association of the United States	Catholic hospitals and health systems	www.chausa.org	
America's Health Insurance Plans	Health insurers	www.ahip.org	

This chapter focuses primarily on nurses, pharmacists, selected allied health professionals, and healthcare administrators.

Nurses

The art of caring, combined with the science of healthcare, is the essence of nursing. Nurses focus not only on a particular health problem but also on the whole patient and his or her response to treatment. Nurses work in many different areas, but the common thread of nursing is the nursing process, which has five steps (ANA 2008):

1. *Assessment.* This involves collecting and analyzing physical, psychological, and sociocultural data about a patient.
2. *Diagnosis.* This entails making a judgment on the cause, condition, and path of the illness.
3. *Planning.* This revolves around creating a care plan that sets specific treatment goals.
4. *Implementation.* This includes supervising or carrying out the actual treatment plan.
5. *Evaluation.* This focuses on continuous assessment of the plan.

Nurses also serve as patient advocates, multidisciplinary team members, managers, executives, researchers, and entrepreneurs.

Nurses make up the largest group of licensed healthcare professionals in the United States. According to the "National Sample Survey of Registered Nurses (NSSRN)," the United States has 2.9 million registered nurses (RNs), of whom more than 1.8 million (83.2 percent) are employed in healthcare organizations (HRSA 2006a). Approximately 56 percent of employed RNs, or 1.6 million, work in hospitals, while 15 percent, or 435,000, work in community or public health settings. Complementing this workforce are 749,000 licensed practical nurses, or licensed vocational nurses as they are known in some states (BLS 2006).

According to the demographic profiles from the NSSRN (HRSA 2006a), most nurses are women. In 2004, the average age of a nurse was 46.8 years old, nearly two years older than in 1997, when the average age was 44.5 years. The aging of the workforce is also reflected in the demographics of nurses: The RN population under 30 years old dropped, from 25 percent in 1980 to 8 percent in 2004. Meanwhile, the percentage of nurses older than 54 years increased to 25.2 percent in 2004, compared to 20.3 percent in 2000 and 16.9 percent in 1980. Only 5.8 percent of RNs are men, and only 11 percent of RNs come from racial/ethnic minority backgrounds.

Registered Nurses and Licensed Practical Nurses

All U.S. states require nurses to be licensed to practice. The licensure requirements include graduation from an approved nursing program and successful completion of a national examination. Educational preparation distinguishes the two levels of nurses.

RNs must complete an associate's degree in nursing (ADN), a diploma program, or a baccalaureate degree in nursing (BSN) to qualify for the licensure examination. ADN programs generally take two years to complete and are offered by community and junior colleges, and hospital-based diploma programs can be completed in about three years. The fastest growing avenue for nursing education is the baccalaureate preparation, which typically can be completed in four years and is offered by colleges and universities. Licensed practical nurses (LPNs), on the other hand, must complete a state-approved program in practical nursing and must achieve a passing score on a national examination. Each state maintains regulations and practice acts that delineate the scope of nursing practice for RNs and LPNs.

Among employed RNs, about 34 percent hold associate's degrees, 20 percent have hospital-based program diplomas, and 34 percent possess BSN degrees. In 2004, 13 percent of nurses reported having a master's degree or a doctoral degree (HRSA 2006a). In addition to licensure and educational achievements, some nurses obtain certification in specialty areas such as critical care, infection control, emergency nursing, surgical nursing, and obstetric nursing. The nursing field comprises many specialties and subspecialties; certification in these areas requires specialty education, practical experience, and successful completion of a national examination. Some nurses obtain certification in these specialty areas because certification helps them maintain their professional associations. To remain certified, continued employment, continuing education units, or reexamination may be required.

Advanced Practice Nurses

An advanced practice nurse (APN) is a nurse with particular skills and credentials, which typically include basic nursing education; basic licensure; a graduate degree in nursing; experience in a specialized area; professional certification from a national certifying body; and, if required in some states, APN licensure (National Council of State Boards of Nursing 2006). The APN specializes as a nurse practitioner, certified nurse midwife, certified registered nurse anesthetist, or clinical nurse specialist.

The APN role is defined by seven core competencies or skillful performance areas. The first core competency of direct clinical practice is central to and informs all of the other areas, as follows (Hamric 2005):

- Direct clinical practice (central)
- Expert guidance and coaching of patients, families, and other care providers
- Consultation
- Research skills, including use and implementation of evidence-based practice, evaluation, and conduct
- Clinical and professional leadership, which includes competence as a change agent
- Collaboration
- Ethical decision-making skills

Additional core competencies may be needed in each specialty area that an APN pursues. The largest number of APNs is made up of nurse practitioners (NPs), who may further specialize in acute care or community settings or for particular client groups such as adults, children, women, or psychiatric/mental health populations.

Each state maintains its own laws and regulations regarding recognition of an APN, but the general requirements in all states include licensure as an RN and successful completion of a national specialty examination. Some states permit certain categories of APNs to write prescriptions for certain classes of drugs. This prescriptive authority varies from one state to another and may be regulated by boards of medicine, nursing, pharmacy, or allied health. Some states require physician supervision of APN practices, although some managed care plans now include APNs on their lists of primary care providers.

APN
Specialization   Certified nurse midwives (CNMs) specialize in low-risk obstetric care, including all aspects of the prenatal, labor and delivery, and postnatal processes. Certified registered nurse anesthetists (CRNAs) complete additional education to specialize in the administration of various types of anesthesia and analgesia to patients and clients. Often, nurse anesthetists work collaboratively with surgeons and anesthesiologists as part of the perioperative care team. Clinical nurse specialists (CNSs) hold master's degrees, have successfully completed a specialty certification examination, and are generally employed by hospitals as nursing "experts" in particular specialties. The scope of the CNS is not as broad as that of the NP; CNSs work with a specialty population under a somewhat circumscribed set of conditions, and the management authority of patients still rests with physicians. In contrast, NPs have developed an autonomous role in which their collaboration is encouraged, and they generally have the legal authority to implement management actions.

Pharmacists

In the foreseeable future, the pharmacy profession will continue to undergo extensive change. Until the 1970s, pharmacists performed the traditional role of preparing drug products and filling prescriptions. In the 1980s, however, pharmacists expanded that role. Pharmacists now act as an expert for clients and patients on the effects of specific drugs, drug interactions, and generic drug substitutions for brand-name drugs.

To be eligible for licensure, pharmacists must graduate from an accredited bachelor-degree program in pharmacy, successfully complete a state board examination, and obtain practical experience or complete a supervised internship. After passing a national examination, a registered pharmacist (RPh) is permitted to carry out the scope of practice outlined by state regulations. The trend in pharmacy has been to broaden education to include the terminal degree Doctor of Pharmacy (PharmD). Many pharmacy schools offer this program for those interested in research careers, teaching, higher administrative responsibility, or being part of the patient care team. This educational preparation also requires successful completion of a state board examination and other practical clinical experience, as outlined by state laws.

Allied Health Professionals

The term "allied health professionals" is generally not well understood because of its ambiguous definition (O'Neil and Hare 1990) and a lack of consensus about what such a role constitutes. In general, allied health professionals complement the work of physicians and other healthcare providers, although one may also be a provider. The U.S. Public Health Service defines an allied health professional as follows (Health Professions Education Extension Amendments of 1992, Section 701 PHS Act):

> . . . a health professional (other than a registered nurse or a physician assistant) who has received a certificate, an associate's degree, a bachelor's degree, a master's degree, a doctoral degree, or post-baccalaureate training in a science related to health care; who shares in the responsibility for the delivery of health care services or related services, including (1) services relating to the identification, evaluation and prevention of disease and disorders, (2) dietary and nutrition services, (3) health promotion services, (4) rehabilitation services, or (5) health systems management services; and who has not received a degree of doctor of medicine, a degree of doctor of osteopathy, a degree of doctor of veterinary medicine or equivalent degree, a degree of doctor of optometry or equivalent degree, a degree of doctor of podiatric medicine or equivalent degree, a degree of bachelor science in pharmacy or equivalent degree, a graduate degree in public health or equivalent degree, a degree of doctor of chiropractic or equivalent degree, a graduate degree in health administration or equivalent degree, a degree of doctor of clinical psychology or equivalent degree, or a degree in social work or equivalent degree.

A debate on the exclusiveness and inclusiveness of this definition continues. Some healthcare observers consider nursing, public health, and social work to fall under the umbrella of allied health, but these professions are often categorized as separate groups. Figure 4.1 lists the major categories that compose the allied health profession and the job titles and positions that normally fall under each category.

According to the "2006 National Occupational and Wage Estimates for Healthcare Personnel," the allied health professions constitute 45.5 percent of the healthcare workforce in the United States (BLS 2007). This number excludes physicians, nurses, dentists, pharmacists, veterinarians, chiropractors, and podiatrists. The allied health profession is the most heterogeneous of the personnel groupings in healthcare.

The National Commission on Allied Health (1995) broadly divided allied health professionals into two categories of personnel: (1) therapists/technologists and (2) technicians/assistants. Some of the job titles presented in Figure 4.1 may not fit into these two categories. In general, the therapist/technologist category represents those with higher-level professional training

FIGURE 4.1
Major
Categories of
the Allied
Health
Profession and
Professional
Titles

Behavioral Health Services

- Substance abuse counselor
- Home health aide
- Mental health aide

- Community health worker
- Mental health assistant

Clinical Laboratory Sciences

- Laboratory associate
- Laboratory technician

- Laboratory microbiologist
- Chemist (biochemist)
- Microbiologist
- Associate laboratory microbiologist

Dental Services

- Dental assistant
- Dental laboratory technologist

- Dental hygienist

Dietetic Services

- Dietitian
- Dietary assistant

- Assistant director of food service
- Associate supervising dietitian

Emergency Medical Services

- Ambulance technician

- Emergency medical technician

Health Information Management Services

- Director of medical records
- Assistant director of medical records
- Medical record specialist

- Senior analyst of medical records
- Health information manager
- Data analyst
- Coder

Medical and Surgical Services

- Electroencephalograph technician
- Electroencephalograph technologist
- Operating room technician
- Biomedical equipment technician
- Biomedical engineer
- Cardiovascular technologist

- Medical equipment specialist
- Electrocardiograph technician
- Dialysis technologist
- Surgical assistant
- Ambulatory care technician

Occupational Therapy

- Occupational therapist
- Occupational therapy assistant

- Occupational therapy aide

Ophthalmology

- Ophthalmic technician
- Optometric aide

- Optician

FIGURE 4.1

Continued

Physical Therapy

- Physical therapist
- Physical therapy assistant

Radiological Services

- Nuclear medicine technician
- Radiation technician
- Ultrasound technician
- Medical radiation dosimetrist
- Nuclear medicine technologist
- Diagnostic medical sonographer
- Radiologic (medical) technologist

Rehabilitation Services

- Art therapist
- Exercise physiologist
- Recreational therapist
- Recreation therapy assistant
- Addiction counselor
- Addiction specialist
- Psychiatric social health technician
- Music therapist
- Dance therapist
- Rehabilitation counselor
- Rehabilitation technician
- Sign-language interpreter

Orthotics/Prosthetics

- Orthopedic assistant

Respiratory Therapy Services

- Respiratory therapist
- Respiratory therapy assistant
- Respiratory therapy technician

Speech-Language Pathology/Audiology Services

- Audiology clinician
- Staff speech pathologist
- Staff audiologist
- Speech clinician

Other Allied Health Services

- Central supply technician
- Podiatric assistant
- Health unit coordinator
- Home health aide
- Medical illustrator
- Veterinary assistant
- Chiropractic assistant

and who are often responsible for supervising those in the technician/assistant category. Therapists/technologists usually hold a bachelor's or a higher-level degree, and they are trained to evaluate patients, understand diagnoses, and develop treatment plans in their area of expertise. On the other hand, technicians/assistants are most likely to have two years or less postsecondary education, and they are functionally trained with procedural skills for specified tasks.

Educational and training programs for the allied health profession are sponsored by a variety of organizations in different academic and clinical settings. They range from degree offerings at colleges and universities to clinical programs in hospitals and other health facilities. Before 1990, one-third of allied health programs were housed in hospitals, although hospitals graduated only 15 percent of their students (O'Neil and Hare 1990). The Association of Schools of Allied Health Professions (ASAHP 2007) includes these among its membership: 112 academic institutions, 2 professional associations, and approximately 200 individual members. Junior or community colleges, vocational or technical schools, and academic health centers can all sponsor allied health programs. These programs can also be stand-alone when aligned with an academic health center, or they can be under the auspices of the school of medicine or nursing if a specific school of allied health professions does not exist. Dental and pharmacy technicians/assistants may or may not be trained in their respective schools or in a school of allied health professions.

A vast number of the undergraduate allied health programs are accredited by the Commission on Accreditation of Allied Health Education Programs (CAAHEP), a freestanding agency that in 1994 replaced the American Medical Association's Committee on Allied Health Education and Accreditation. The formation of CAAHEP was intended to simplify the accrediting process, to be more inclusive of allied health programs that provide entry-level education, and to serve as an initiator of more far-reaching change. Some key allied health graduate programs, such as physical therapy and occupational therapy, are accredited through specialty professional accreditation organizations.

Healthcare Administrators

Healthcare administrators organize, coordinate, and manage the delivery of health services; provide leadership; and guide the strategic direction of healthcare organizations. The variety and numbers of healthcare professionals they employ; the complexity of healthcare delivery; and environmental pressures to provide access, quality, and efficient services make healthcare institutions among the most complex organizations to manage.

Healthcare administration is taught at the undergraduate and graduate levels in a variety of settings, and these programs lead to a number of different degrees. The settings include schools of medicine, public health, healthcare business, and allied health professions. A bachelor's degree in health administration allows individuals to pursue positions such as nursing home administrator, supervisor, or middle manager in healthcare organizations. Most students who aspire to have a career in healthcare administration go on to receive a master's degree. (For a detailed description of various career paths and options, see Haddock, McLean, and Chapman 2002).

Graduate education programs in healthcare administration are accredited by the Commission on Accreditation of Healthcare Management

Education. Most common degrees include the master of health administration (MHA), master of business administration (MBA) with a healthcare emphasis), master of public health (MPH), or master of public administration (MPA). However, the MHA degree, or its equivalent, has been the accepted training model for entry-level managers in the various sectors of the healthcare industry. The MHA program, when compared to the MPH program, offers core courses that focus on building business management (theory and applied management), quantitative, and analytical skills and that emphasize experiential training. In addition, some MHA programs require students to complete three-month internships or 12-month residencies as part of their two- or three-year curricula. Some graduates elect to complete postgraduate fellowships that are available in selected hospitals, health systems, managed care organizations, consulting firms, and other health-related organizations.

A growing number of healthcare administrators are physicians and other clinicians. As evidence, membership in the American College of Physician Executives (ACPE 2007) has increased to more than 10,000 in 2007, up from 5,700 in 1990, although stable since 2000. Physicians, nurses, and other clinicians refocus their careers on the business side of the enterprise, getting involved in the strategy, decision making, resource allocation, and operations of healthcare organizations. A traditional management role for physician executives is the chief medical officer (or a similar position) in a hospital, overseeing the medical staff and serving as a liaison between clinical care and administration. Likewise, a typical management career path for nurses is to become the chief nursing officer, with responsibility for the clinical care provided by employed professional staff.

Typically, chief medical officers begin their careers practicing medicine, then they slowly transition into the operations side of healthcare. However, physician executives work at every level and in every setting in healthcare. Many physician executives earn a graduate degree such as an MHA or an MBA if interested in pursuing a formal educational program in healthcare administration and management. As of 2007, 49 medical schools offer a combined MD/MBA program, and two medical schools offer the MD/MHA dual degrees (AAMC 2007). Whether physician executives start as administrators or later shift to become executives after clinical practice, they represent for other doctors an alternative way to make an impact on healthcare delivery.

Nursing home administrator programs require students to pass a national examination administered by the National Association of Long Term Care Administrator Boards. Passing this examination is a standard requirement in all states, but the educational preparation needed to qualify for this exam varies from state to state. Although more than one-third of states still require less than a bachelor's degree as the minimum academic preparation, approximately 70 percent of the practicing nursing home administrators have, at a minimum, a bachelor's degree. As the population continues to live longer, the demand and educational requirements for long-term-care administrators are estimated to increase, along with the growth of educational programs targeted to this sector.

Considerations for Human Resources Management

The role of human resources management (HRM) in healthcare organizations is to develop and implement systems, in accordance with regulatory guidelines and licensure laws, that ensure selection, evaluation, and retention of healthcare professionals. In light of this role, human resources (HR) personnel should be aware that each of the healthcare professions, and often the subspecialties within those professions, has specific requirements that allow an individual to qualify for an entry-level job in his or her chosen profession. The requirements of national accrediting organizations (e.g., the Joint Commission), regulatory bodies (e.g., the Centers for Medicare & Medicaid Services), and licensure authorities (e.g., state licensure boards) should be considered in all aspects of HRM. In this section, we briefly discuss some of the issues that a healthcare organization's HR department must consider when dealing with healthcare professionals.

Qualifications

In developing a comprehensive employee-compensation program, HR personnel must include the specific skill and knowledge required for each job in the organization. Those qualifications must be determined and stated in writing for each job. The job description usually contains the level of education, experience, judgment ability, accountability, physical skills, responsibilities, communication skills, and any special certification or licensure requirements. HR personnel need to be aware of all specifications for all job titles within the organization. This knowledge of healthcare professionals is necessary to ensure that essential qualifications of individuals coincide with job specifications, and it is also necessary for determining wage and salary ranges (see Chapter 7).

Licensure and Certification

An HR department must have policies and procedures in place that describe the way in which licensure is verified on initial employment. Also, HR must have a system in place for tracking the expiration dates of licenses and for ensuring licensure renewal. Therefore, HR must be conscientious about whether the information it receives is a *primary verification* (in which the information directly comes from the licensing authority) or a *secondary verification* (in which a candidate submits a document copy that indicates licensure has been granted, including the expiration date). Certifications must be verified during the selection process, although certifications and licenses are generally not statutory requirements. Many healthcare organizations accept a copy of a certification document as verification. If the certification is a job requirement, systems must be in place to track expiration dates and to access new certification documents.

Career Ladders

In selecting healthcare professionals, HR personnel must consider past employment history, including the explanation of gaps in employment. To assess the amount of individual experience, evaluating the candidate's breadth and depth of responsibility in previous jobs is essential. Many healthcare organizations have career ladders, which are mechanisms that advance a healthcare professional within the organization. Career ladders are based on the Dreyfus and Dreyfus model of novice to expert (explained earlier in the chapter), and experience may be used as a criterion for assignment of an individual to a particular job category. In addition, healthcare organizations may conduct annual reviews of employees who have leadership and management potential. This review entails that HR works with senior management to assess the competency, ability, and career progression of employees on an ongoing basis.

Educational Services

Healthcare professionals require continuous, lifelong learning. Healthcare organizations must have in-house training and development plans to ensure that their healthcare professionals achieve competency in new technologies, programs, and equipment and are aware of policy and procedure changes. Certain competencies must be renewed annually in areas such as cardiopulmonary resuscitation, safety and infection control, and disaster planning.

In addition to developing specific training programs, healthcare organizations should provide orientation for all new employees. Such organization-specific training enables the leadership to share the values, mission, goals, and policies of the institution. Such clear communication often serves as a retention tool that enables employees to better understand how the organization works and how to be successful in that organization. Similarly, some professions and licensing jurisdictions may require continuing education that is profession specific.

A healthcare organization can provide training and development in a variety of ways. On one end of the spectrum, training and development can be outsourced to a firm that specializes in conducting educational programs. Conversely, another option is to consolidate all training and development in-house, which are managed typically by the HR department. Regardless of how each healthcare organization provides continuing education, training and development should be a priority. Strong programs can be viewed as recruitment and retention tools. As such, healthcare organizations must be cognizant of fiscal resources necessary to support these educational requirements.

Practitioner Impairment

Healthcare professionals are accountable to the public for maintaining high professional standards, and the governing body of a healthcare organization is, by statute, responsible for the quality of care rendered in the organization. This quality is easily jeopardized by an impaired practitioner. An *impaired practitioner* is a healthcare professional who is unable to carry out his or her professional duties with reasonable skill and safety because of a physical or mental illness, including deterioration through aging, loss of motor skill, or excessive use of drugs and alcohol.

The HR department must periodically evaluate the performance of all healthcare professionals in the organization to ensure their competence (i.e., the basic education and training necessary for the job) and proficiency (i.e., the demonstrated ability to perform job tasks). Mechanisms must be in place to identify the impaired practitioner, such as policies and procedures that describe how the organization will handle investigations, subsequent recommendations for treatment, monitoring, and employment restrictions or separation. Hospitals, for instance, usually have a process in place for the board of directors (which has the ultimate responsibility for the quality of care delivered in the organization) to review provider credentials and performance and to oversee any employment actions. Each national or state licensing authority maintains legal requirements for reporting impaired practitioners.

As a result of ever-increasing changes in the health professions, in the foreseeable future, new challenges and opportunities, such as the issues described in this section, will face the HR department of every healthcare organization.

Changing Nature of the Health Professions

In the 1990s, we entered a new era of uncertainty in healthcare, one faced with a quickening pace of change (Begun and White 2008). Within this framework, new ways of thinking are rewarded as the meaning of health is redefined, the boundaries of healthcare professionals are reshaped, and the outcomes of healthcare professional interventions are measured in terms of quality of life. Changes in the organization and financing of healthcare services have shifted delivery from the hospital to outpatient facilities, the home, long-term-care facilities, and the community. This is largely the result of three major forces: (1) a shift in managed care reimbursement to outpatient settings and a focus on cost containment; (2) technological advances, such as telemedicine and the electronic medical record; and (3) medical innovation—the science of medicine has progressed to the point that complicated procedures that once required several nights of stay can now be treated with a simple procedure or even solely with medication. These changes are intended to improve the delivery of healthcare while reducing cost and increasing access for patients.

As the setting for the delivery of care continued to change, so did arrangements between physicians and healthcare organizations. For instance, physicians can function as individual providers (either in solo or group practice) and refer patients to the hospital. Typically, these private-practice doctors have admitting privileges to the hospital but are not governed by the hospital, do not serve as attending physicians, and infrequently participate on hospital committees. Physicians considered "on staff" at any hospital are those who refer and treat patients at that hospital. They are credentialed by the hospital credentialing committee (usually managed by the chief of staff office) and are governed by the medical staff bylaws. This is a common type of hospital-provider arrangement.

However, a trend toward hospitals employing physicians has been growing. In this arrangement, physicians are on staff, referring to and treating at only the hospital that employs them. Because they are considered employees, physicians are not only held to the HR policies of the healthcare organization but are also governed by the medical staff bylaws. Physicians who are employed by a hospital can also maintain a private practice.

Finally, the field of hospitalists is also growing. Typically, these physicians do not run their own practice aside from their hospital employment. Hospitalists work full time for the hospital and are trained in delivering specialized inpatient care. Regardless of the type of arrangement, most hospitals have a chief medical officer, or a similar position, who oversees the roles and responsibilities of the hospitalist as a member of the medical staff; the hospitalist's employee issues and responsibilities are typically managed by the HR department. These hospital–physician arrangements get more complex in academic medical centers, which must integrate the roles and responsibilities of the physicians, the hospital, and the medical school.

As a result of the changing environment and decreased reimbursement, more primary care physicians are joining or forming group practices. Large physician-owned group practices offer several advantages to physicians, including competitive advantage with vendors and manufacturers, improved negotiating power with managed care organizations, shared risk and decision making, and improved flexibility and choice for patients. Physicians usually own or share ownership in the group practice and, therefore, are responsible for the business operations. Typically, group practices employ an office manager who works closely with the physicians to manage the day-to-day operations. Often, a full-time administrator is on staff not only to manage everyday issues but also to formulate strategies and oversee personnel, billing and collection, purchasing, patient flow, and other functions. Many group practices opt to outsource their business functions, including human resources, to specialized firms. For complete details on medical practice management, go to www.mgma.com.

These shifts in various healthcare settings and arrangements have changed the roles, functions, and expectations of the healthcare workforce and gave way to the emergence of the following issues.

Supply and Demand

Throughout the twentieth century, the nursing labor market cycled through periods of shortages and surpluses (Lynn and Redman 2005; Aiken et al. 2002; Kovner 2002; Coile 2001; Jones 2001; Buerhaus, Staiger, and Auerbach 2000). The beginning of the twenty-first century brought the nursing and allied health professions the challenge of keeping pace with the demand for their services. Indicators of demand include numbers of vacancies, turnover rates, and an increase in salaries. To fill positions, hospitals—the largest employers of nurses and allied health professionals—have raised salaries, provided scholarships, and given other incentives such as sign-on bonuses and tuition reimbursement.

The supply of nurses and allied health professionals is reflected in the number of students in educational programs and those available for the healthcare workforce. Future supply of such professionals continues to be threatened by the following factors:

- *The aging of the nursing workforce.* According to the results of the 2004 National Sample Survey of Registered Nurses (HRSA 2006a), the average age for all nursing faculty was 51.6, and for nursing faculty who have doctoral degrees, it was 55.4 (up from 53.5 in 2003).
- *The decline in available educational resources.* Almost two-thirds (68.5 percent) of the nursing schools that responded to the 2006 American Association of Colleges of Nursing (AACN 2007a) survey identified faculty shortages as a reason for not accepting all qualified applicants into entry-level baccalaureate programs. The survey also noted lack of classroom space and clinical facilities and budgetary restraints.
- *The decline in nursing school enrollees.* From 1995 through 2000, enrollment decreased by 21 percent. From 2001 through 2007, increases of 3.7 to 16.6 percent were observed, but more than 30,000 qualified applicants were turned away from baccalaureate nursing programs in 2007 (AACN 2007a).

As a result, recruitment of nursing and allied health professions students has become a major focus of practitioners, professional associations, and academic institutions. In response, healthcare organizations (in addition to increasing salaries) are developing innovative ways to recruit and retain nurses and allied health professionals. Such developments include opening or sponsoring new schools, offering shorter and more flexible shifts, and providing child care.

Alternative Therapies

Alternative therapies have gained more popularity, judging by the growing number of publications on this topic in the lay press and in academic literature. A turning point in this acceptance and increased respectability was the sentinel study of the prevalence of the use of alternative or unconventional therapies (Eisenberg et al. 1993). In the study, Eisenberg and colleagues concluded that one in three adults relied on treatments and interventions that are not widely taught at medical schools in the United States; examples of these alternative interventions included acupuncture and chiropractic and massage therapies. In a follow-up study, Eisenberg and colleagues (1998) determined that, from 1990 to 1997, visits to alternative medicine practitioners increased by 47.3 percent. Another study reported that 75 (60 percent) out of the 125 medical schools that participated in the survey offered a course in complementary or alternative medicine (Wetzel, Eisenberg, and Kaptchuk 1998). Additionally, consumers are demanding the use of alternative therapies, and hospitals have begun offering more of these services (Clement et al. 2006). As the use of alternative therapies continues to gain acceptance and to be integrated in medical school curriculum, this specialty area may be more and more considered as an emerging healthcare profession.

Nonphysician Practitioners

With the advent of managed care, greater reliance has been placed on nonphysician practitioners. Collaborative practice models with nurse practitioners, physician assistants, pharmacists, and other therapists are appropriate to both acute and long-term healthcare delivery. Strides have been made in the direct reimbursement for some nonphysician healthcare provider services, which is an impetus for further collaboration in practice. The consolidation and integration of the healthcare delivery system have not, however, eliminated slack and duplication of services. Although the changes attributed to managed care have led to the promotion and use of less-costly sites for care delivery, a larger impact on the division of labor among all healthcare professionals, and thus on health professions, may yet occur.

Licensure and Certification

The use of nonphysician practitioners at various sites may be viewed as an opportunity for the growth of nursing, pharmacy, allied health professions, and health administration. Alternatively, Hurley (1997) contends that it may lead to concerted efforts to repeal professional licensure and certification in healthcare. If policymakers jump on the bandwagon, this deregulation may lead to not only the demise of some healthcare professions but also the proliferation of functionally trained, unlicensed personnel. The use of personnel who have less education will have greater implications for the existence and growth of educational programs in academic medical centers. The use of unlicensed support personnel poses concerns about the intensity and quality of healthcare delivered. When fewer highly trained professionals are employed to oversee operations and care delivery, the potential for adverse outcomes increases. Aiken, Sochalski, and Anderson (1996) found that, although the percentage of RNs increased overall, fewer nurses per patient were available in the mid-1990s than in the 1980s to provide care for more acutely ill patients. The net effect was a relative increase in nonclinical personnel, which added stress for those who were expected to supervise unlicensed staff and to care for sicker patients. This is a trend that continues to affect the provision of healthcare (Aiken et al. 2002).

Recruitment and Retention

Recruitment and retention of healthcare professionals are important in the face of continuing shortages in key healthcare professions, including nursing and allied health professions. The American Hospital Association (2007) reported an average hospital nurse vacancy rate of 8.1 percent. The RN vacancy rate is projected to be 20 percent by 2020 (Buerhaus, Staiger, and Auerbach 2000; Heinrich 2001). This vacancy rate is related to an RN shortage, which is estimated to be in the range of 340,000 to 1 million nurses by 2020 (Auerbach, Buerhaus, and Staiger 2007; HRSA 2006b). Nearly 17 percent of RNs were not employed in nursing in 2004, which was a 26.2 percent increase over the 1992 rate (HRSA 2006a). Letvak (2002) predicted that one in five nurses planned to leave the profession and turnover costs could be up to two times a nurse's salary. Fifty-five percent of nurses reported their intention to retire between 2011 and 2020 in a survey released in 2006 (AACN 2007b), which would further contribute to the RN shortage. Similarly, the American Hospital Association (2007) reported vacancy rates among allied health professionals (e.g., occupational and physical therapists, laboratory technologists, imaging technicians) that range from 6 percent to 11 percent of needed positions. These shortages require current professionals to treat more patients and to work longer hours. Such conditions can contribute to emergency department diversions, increased patient wait times, and decreased patient safety.

In response, healthcare organizations need to develop and execute recruitment and retention programs. These programs require senior management support and dedicated financial and human resources. Such programs should focus on building a culture of retention. While salary is an important aspect of employee recruitment and retention, other aspects of work are also influential, such as leadership support, ability to contribute to the organization and provide quality care to patients, degree of autonomy, engaging in positive relationships with direct supervisors and peers, good working conditions, and ability to maintain a work–life balance. Additional tools for retaining employees include conducting employee-engagement surveys, providing mentoring, and making training programs available.

One innovative way to differentiate a hospital from its competitors, which helps in recruitment and retention, is to achieve Magnet status. In 1993, the American Nurses Credentialing Center's Magnet Recognition Program was developed as a way to specifically recognize excellence in nursing services at the institutional level and to benchmark best practices to be disseminated throughout the industry. Hospitals that apply for and achieve Magnet status have created and demonstrated a professional practice environment that ensures quality outcomes. These hospitals are recognized for their best practices in nursing care, improved patient outcomes, and increased workplace satisfaction. The actual evaluation process is based on nine Magnet standards, the completion of an intensive written application, and a two-day site visit by a team of nurse scholars. Hospitals that do not wish to engage in the application process can benefit greatly from using Magnet strategies to create a culture based on excellence in nursing and patient care (Pieper 2003). For more information on Magnet status, see www.nursecredentialing.org/magnet.

Entrepreneurship

Given the bureaucratic nature of organizations, the regulation of the healthcare industry, and additional constraints by payers and managed care, many healthcare professionals are choosing to pursue opportunities on their own. The service economy coupled with knowledge-based professions may encourage pursuit of new and different ventures for individuals who have the personality, skills, and tenacity to go into business for themselves. An entrepreneur must have a mix of management skills and the means to depart from a traditional career path to practice on one's own.

White and Begun (1998) characterize the entrepreneurial personality traits of a profession in terms of its willingness to take the risks associated with undertaking new ventures. Each profession may be categorized either as defending the status quo, which therefore entails little risk (defender professions), or as looking for new and different opportunities with greater risk (prospector professions). White and Begun view the more entrepreneurial professions as more diversified in terms of processes and services delivered. The accrediting bodies of such entrepreneurial professions encourage educational innovation that may extend to nontraditional careers. Each of the healthcare professions has, to greater or lesser extents, defender and prospector aspects.

Workforce Diversity

Each of the healthcare professions must continue to monitor and encourage diversity in its membership because the demographic shifts that the United States is going through will have an impact on the workforce composition in the coming decades. Although workforce diversity is a broad concept, it focuses on our differences in gender, age, and race; these aspects not only reflect the population that healthcare serves but also the people who provide the services. Some professions are dominated by one gender or the other, which is illustrated by the predominantly female field of nursing or the historically predominantly male field of health administration. The health administration profession, however, has made strides in recent years as more female administrators have entered the field. Labor shortages and employee turnover are common in the healthcare professions. Consequently, healthcare executives must balance the needs of new entrants into the profession and those already in the profession.

Changes in the ethnic and racial composition of the workforce are proportional to the changes in the size and age of the population (D'Aunno, Alexander, and Laughlin 1996). Because many healthcare professionals are racial/ethnic minorities, a concerted effort needs to be made to recruit and retain them because the diversity of the members of a profession should reflect the diversity of the members of the population.

Summary

Healthcare professionals are a large segment of the U.S. labor force. Historically, the development of healthcare professionals is related to the following trends:

- Supply and demand
- Increased use of technology
- Changes in disease and illness
- The impact of healthcare financing and delivery

The healthcare workforce is very diverse. The different levels of education, scopes of practice, and practice settings contribute to the complexity of managing this workforce. The coming decades will be characterized by some reforms within the healthcare professions because of increasing pressures to finance and deliver healthcare with higher-quality, lower-cost, and measurable outcomes.

Discussion Questions

1. Describe the process of professionalization. What is the difference between a profession and an occupation?

2. Describe the major types of healthcare professionals (excluding physicians and dentists) and their roles, training, licensure requirements, and practice settings.

3. Describe and apply the issues of human resources management and systems development to healthcare professionals.

4. How has managed care affected the healthcare professions?

5. Who are nonphysician practitioners who provide primary care? What is their role in the delivery of health services?

Experiential Exercise

The purpose of this exercise is to give you an opportunity to explore one healthcare profession in detail.

From all of the healthcare professions, select one for analysis. Table 4.1 provides a starting point for selection. Describe the following characteristics of the profession you selected:

- Knowledge base
- Collective goals
- Training
- Licensure (this varies by state)
- Number of professionals in practice by
  1. Vertical differentiation (position, experience, education level)
  2. Horizontal differentiation (geography, practice setting, specialty)
- History and evolution of the profession
- Professional associations and their roles
- Competitor professions
- Current strategic issues that face the profession and the profession's position on these issues

To get started on this exercise, you may wish to go to the websites of professional organizations and various state licensing boards. You may also interview members of the profession as well as leaders in the field.

References

Aiken, L. H., S. P. Clarke, D. M. Sloane, J. Sochalski, and J. H. Silber. 2002. "Hospital Nurse Staffing and Patient Mortality, Nurse Burnout, and Job Dissatisfaction." *JAMA* 288 (16): 1987–93.

Aiken, L. H., J. Sochalski, and G. F. Anderson. 1996. "Downsizing the Hospital Nursing Workforce." *Health Affairs* 15 (4): 88–92.

American Association of Colleges of Nursing (AACN). 2007a. "Enrollment Growth Slows at U.S. Nursing Colleges and Universities in 2007 Despite Calls for More Registered Nurses." [Online news release; retrieved 1/31/08.] www.aacn.nche.edu/Media/NewsReleases/2007/enrl.htm.

———. 2007b. "Nursing Shortage." [Online news release; retrieved 1/29/08.] www.aacn.nche.edu/Media/FactSheets/NursingShortage.htm.

American College of Physician Executives (ACPE). 2007. [Online information; retrieved 2/4/08.] www.acpe.org/Footer/AboutACPE.aspx.

American Hospital Association. 2007. "The 2007 State of America's Hospitals—Taking the Pulse: Findings from the 2007 AHA Survey of Hospital Leaders July 2007." [Online information; retrieved 1/31/08.] www.aha.org/aha/content/2007/PowerPoint/StateofHospitalsChartPack2007.ppt.

American Nurses Association (ANA). 2008. "The Nursing Process: A Common Thread Amongst All Nurses." [Online article; retrieved 2/6/08.] www.nursingworld.org/EspeciallyForYou/StudentNurses/Thenursingprocess.aspx.

Association of American Medical Colleges (AAMC). 2007. "Combined Degree Programs." [Online article; retrieved 7/16/07.] http:/services.aamc.org/currdir/section3/degree2.cfm.

Association of Schools of Allied Health Professions (ASAHP). 2007. [Online information; retrieved 2/4/08.] www.asahp.org/history.htm.

Auerbach, D. I., P. I. Buerhaus, and D. O. Staiger, 2007. "Better Late than Never: Workforce Supply Implications of Later Entry into Nursing." *Health Affairs* 26 (1): 178–85.

Begun, J. W., and K. R. White. 2008. "Positioning Nursing for Leadership in a Complex Healthcare System." In *On the Edge: Nursing in the Age of Complexity,* edited by C. Lindberg, S. Nash, and C. Lindberg. Allentown, NJ: Plexus Institute.

Buerhaus, P. I., D. O. Staiger, and D. I. Auerbach. 2000. "Implications of a Rapidly Aging Registered Nurse Workforce." *JAMA* 283 (22): 2948–54.

Bureau of Labor Statistics (BLS). 2006. "Licensed Practical and Licensed Vocational Nurses, 2006." [Online information; retrieved 2/5/08.] www.bls.gov/oco/ocos102.htm.

———. 2007. "Health Care." [Online information; retrieved 2/6/08.] www.bls.gov/oco/cg/cgs035.htm.

Clement, J. P., H. Chen, D. Burke, D. G. Clement, and J. L. Zazzali. 2006. "Are Consumers Reshaping Hospitals? Complementary and Alternative Medicine in US Hospitals 1999–2003." *Health Care Management Review* 31 (2): 109–18.

Coile, R. C. 2001. "Magnet Hospitals Use Culture, Not Wages, to Solve Nursing Shortage." *Journal of Healthcare Management* 46 (3): 224–28.

D'Aunno, T., J. A. Alexander, and C. Laughlin. 1996. "Business as Usual? Changes in Health Care's Workforce and Organization of Work." *Hospital & Health Services Administration* 41 (1): 3–18.

Dreyfus, H. L., and S. E. Dreyfus. 1996. "The Relationship of Theory and Practice in the Acquisition of Skill." In *Expertise in Nursing Practice: Caring, Clinical Judgment, and Ethics,* edited by P. Benner, C. A. Tanner, and C. A. Chesla. New York: Springer.

Eisenberg, D. M., R. B. Davis, S. L. Ettner, S. Appel, S. Wilkey, M. Van Rompay, and R. C. Kessler. 1998. "RC Trends in Alternative Medicine Use in the United States, 1990–1997: Results of a Follow-Up National Survey." *New England Journal of Medicine* 280 (18): 1569–75.

Eisenberg, D. M., R. D. Kessler, C. Foster, R. E. Norlock, D. R. Calkins, and T. L. Delbanco. 1993. "Unconventional Medicine in the United States." *New England Journal of Medicine* 328 (24): 246–52.

Haddock, C. C., R. A. McLean, and R. C. Chapman. 2002. *Careers in Healthcare Management.* Chicago: Health Administration Press.

Hamric, A. B. 2005. *Advanced Practice Nursing: An Integrative Approach,* Third Edition, edited by A. B. Hamric, J. A. Spross, and C. M. Hanson, 95–96. St. Louis, MO: Elsevier Saunders.

Health Professions Education Extension Amendments of 1992, Section 701 PHS Act. Washington, DC: Government Printing Office.

Health Resources and Services Administration (HRSA). 2006a. "The Registered Nurse Population: Findings from the 2004 National Sample Survey of Registered Nurses." [Online information; retrieved 1/29/08.] http://bhpr.hrsa.gov/health-workforce/rnsurvey04.

———. 2006b. "What Is Behind HRSA's Projected Supply, Demand, and Shortage of Registered Nurses?" [Online information; retrieved 1/29/08.] http://bhpr.hrsa.gov/healthworkforce/reports/behindrnprojections/index.htm.

Heinrich, J. 2001. *Nursing Workforce: Emerging Nurse Shortages Due to Multiple Factors.* GAO Report to Health Subcommittee on Health: GAO-01-944, pages i–15. Washington, DC: Government Accountability Office.

Hurley, R. E. 1997. "Moving Beyond Incremental Thinking." *Health Services Research* 32 (5): 679–90.

Jones, C. B. 2001. "The Future Registered Nurse Workforce in Healthcare Delivery." In *The Nursing Profession,* edited by N. L. Chaska, 123–38. Thousand Oaks, CA: Sage Publications.

Kovner, C. T. 2002. "CMS Study: Correlation Between Staffing and Quality." *American Journal of Nursing* 102 (9): 65–67.

Letvak, S. 2002. "Retaining the Older Nurse." *Journal of Nursing Administration* 32: 387–92.

Lynn, M. R., and R. W. Redman. 2005. "Faces of the Nursing Shortage: Influences on Staff Nurses' Intentions to Leave Their Positions or Nursing." *Journal of Nursing Administration* 35 (5): 264–70.

National Commission on Allied Health. 1995. *Report of the National Commission on Allied Health.* Rockville, MD: Health Resources and Services Administration.

National Council of State Boards of Nursing. 2006. [Online information; retrieved 7/16/07.] www.ncsbn.org.

O'Neil, E. H., and D. M. Hare (eds.). 1990. "Perspectives on the Health Professions." In *Pew Health Professions Programs.* Durham, NC: Duke University.

Pieper, S. K. 2003. "Retaining Staff the Magnet Way: Fostering a Culture of Professional Excellence." *Healthcare Executive* 18 (3): 12–17.

Wetzel, M. S., D. M. Eisenberg, and T. J. Kaptchuk. 1998. "Course Involving Complementary and Alternative Medicine at US Medical Schools." *JAMA* 280 (9): 784–87.

White, K. R., and J. W. Begun. 1998. "Nursing Entrepreneurship in an Era of Chaos and Complexity." *Nursing Administration Quarterly* 22 (2): 40–47.

THE LEGAL ENVIRONMENT OF HUMAN RESOURCES MANAGEMENT

Beverly L. Rubin, JD, and Bruce J. Fried, PhD

Learning Objectives

After completing this chapter, the reader should be able to

- understand the impact of legal considerations on key human resources management activities and functions;
- define employment-at-will and its public policy exceptions;
- enumerate the major pieces of federal equal employment opportunity legislation;
- explain the rationale for government intervention in the workplace to prevent discrimination;
- describe the strategies that organizations use to prevent and identify discrimination in the workplace;
- understand the concepts of disparate impact and disparate treatment and the types of evidence required to demonstrate each form of discrimination;
- discuss the key features of the Americans with Disabilities Act, including the concepts of undue hardship and reasonable accommodation;
- describe the complexities of the equal employment opportunity complaint process;
- discuss the requirements of the Uniformed Services Employment and Reemployment Rights Act;
- understand that sexual harassment is a form of employment discrimination, and describe the legal definitions of sexual harassment law;
- address employee rights and responsibilities, and distinguish among statutory, regulatory, and common-law rights;
- describe recent developments in the area of federal anti-retaliation law;
- list employee privacy issues, including the Health Insurance Portability and Accountability Act, and realize when to consult legal counsel when privacy issues arise;
- recognize the legal backdrop for a variety of healthcare-specific employee rights and responsibilities issues;

- discuss the contractual implications of employee handbooks, employment agreements, personnel manuals, separation agreements, and disciplinary documents;
- define the concepts of dismissal for cause and due process;
- explain the concept of progressive discipline, and know the steps required for employee termination; and
- enumerate the types and role of alternative dispute-resolution methods in the workplace.

Introduction

This chapter discusses the complex set of laws that affect human resources management (HRM). Understanding the basic premise of the legal environment is as critical in workforce management as it is in any other area of management and healthcare. Laws that address the workplace are rooted in the essential value system of the United States, which includes the right to privacy, freedom from discrimination, the right to self-determination, and the opportunity to live and work in a safe environment. We view the workplace as a part of our life and culture, and our laws aim to ensure that individual protections afforded to people in society at large are extended to the workplace. We also place a value on jobs as a form of property; that is, just as we have laws to prevent people from losing their homes and other property without due process, we protect people's jobs in a similar fashion.

The laws that govern the relationship between the employer and the employee reflect society's attempt to achieve a complex balance between keeping employees free from personal injury, prejudice, duress, and unwanted sexual advances and allowing management to pursue its business goals. Thus, while our legal system seeks to protect employee rights, the legal environment also protects management rights. However, given the relative power of employers in the employer–employee relationship, it is fair to say that our laws tend to "level the playing field" by emphasizing protection of the employee. Employee rights that are protected by legislation also extend to potential employees—that is, the job applicants. As discussed later in this chapter, our laws protect the rights of job applicants by outlawing employment discrimination based on race, gender, disability, and other characteristics.

Employment law is of course not the only area of law affecting life in healthcare organizations. Healthcare organizations are highly complex and operate within the constraints of numerous laws and regulations. It is not necessary for clinicians and managers to be lawyers, but it is essential that managers are aware of key legal issues that face the organization, including those involving the workforce. Managers have discretion in how they manage the workforce, but managers' adherence to legal requirements places significant constraints on their autonomy. It is particularly important that managers and supervisors in large healthcare organizations understand legal requirements and constraints. While senior managers in any organization need to understand the legal issues inherent in HRM, day-to-day application of these laws falls to line managers who may not have the same degree of awareness as members of the senior management do. This is an important consideration because senior managers and boards of directors may be the ones liable for violations that occur at any level of the organization.

Perhaps an even more compelling reason for managers to understand and comply with legal requirements is this: Compliance implies good management practice; this is most notably the case with regard to equal employment opportunity. While "equal opportunity" is often viewed as a regulatory challenge or at worst a quota-based scheme, adherence to mandated procedures is consistent with sound human resources practices. In fact, the literature provides evidence that many companies choose to continue affirmative action initiatives even when such programs are being dismantled through legislation and executive orders (Fisher 1994).

An important consideration concerning the legal and regulatory environment is the ambiguity of the actual laws and regulations. Virtually every employment-related law has been subject to extensive and far-reaching interpretation by the courts and quasi-judicial administrative agencies, such as the National Labor Relations Board and the Equal Employment Opportunity Commission (EEOC). For this reason, employment law cannot be understood by simply reading the text of existing laws. Furthermore, as with all legislation, application of employment law may have unintended consequences. For example, implementation, interpretation, or use of a particular law may be inconsistent with the original intent of the lawmakers. One example is the Americans with Disabilities Act (ADA). The ADA was intended to increase the employment potential of individuals with disabilities. However, the majority of complaints filed under the ADA deal with on-the-job injuries of employees. After the terrorist attacks in the United States on September 11, 2001, significant changes have been made to employment law that affect employee privacy. On the flip side, the privacy requirement of the Health Insurance Portability and Accountability Act of 1996 (HIPAA) offers greater privacy protection for personal health information.

Because of the constantly changing legal landscape, this chapter cannot present the most current court rulings and agency regulations. However, the chapter aims to sensitize the reader to the legal framework that currently governs the workplace, communicate the importance of keeping up with such laws and regulations, and emphasize that equal employment opportunity laws and good management practices should be compatible.

Employment Laws

The respective rights and responsibilities that govern the workplace are documented in federal and state statutes, administrative agency regulations, case law interpretations of various state and federal legislation and regulations, written and verbal employment agreements, and employee handbooks. Among the most important federal statutes that directly or indirectly affect the employment setting are the Civil Rights Act, the Age Discrimination in Employment Act, the Fair Labor Standards Act, HIPAA, and the ADA. Each of these is discussed later in the chapter.

Other key laws that deal directly or indirectly with employment include the following:

- *Consolidated Omnibus Budget Reconciliation Act (COBRA)* is an amendment to the Employee Retirement Income Security Act of 1974. COBRA gives employees and their families the right to choose to continue to receive health benefits provided by the employer's group health plan for a limited period of time in such circumstances as voluntary or involuntary job loss, reduction in hours worked, transition between jobs, death, divorce, and other life events.
- *Consumer Credit Protection Act (Title III)* prohibits an employer from discharging an employee because his or her earnings are subject to garnishment and limits the amount of wages that can be withheld for garnishment in a single week. Wage garnishment refers to a procedure whereby an employer withholds the earnings of an employee to pay a debt resulting from a court order or other procedure.
- *Drug-Free Workplace Act of 1988* requires that all organizations that receive federal grants in any amount or federal contracts of $25,000 or more must certify that they are providing a drug-free workplace. Drug-free workplace certification is a precondition of receiving a federal grant, and criteria for compliance include the organization establishing an explicit drug policy, implementing it, and publicizing it to all employees.
- *Employee Polygraph Protection Act of 1988* generally prohibits employers from using lie-detector tests either for pre-employment screening or during the course of employment. A number of people are exempt from this Act, including federal contractors engaged in national security intelligence or counterintelligence functions; employees suspected of involvement in an incident resulting in economic loss to the employer; employees of security firms; and prospective employees engaged in manufacturing, distributing, or dispensing controlled substances.
- *Employee Retirement Income Security Act of 1974 (ERISA)* regulates private pension plans and sets minimum standards for most voluntarily

established pension and health plans. ERISA requires plans to provide participants with information about plan features and funding, establishes fiduciary responsibilities for those who manage and control plan assets, orders plans to establish grievance and appeals procedures for participants, and gives participants the right to sue for benefits and breaches of fiduciary duty.

- *Equal Pay Act of 1963* (part of the Fair Labor Standards Act) requires employers to pay all employees equally for equal work, regardless of their gender. The intent of the Act was to correct wage disparities experienced by women workers because of sex discrimination. Jobs are considered equal if they involve equal levels of skill, effort, and responsibility and if performed under similar conditions.

- *Executive Order 11246 and Executive Order 11375* bar discrimination on the basis of race, color, religion, and national origin in federal employment and in employment by federal contractors and subcontractors. It also requires government contractors to develop a written affirmative action program to help identify and analyze problems in workforce participation by women and minorities.

- *Family and Medical Leave Act (FMLA) of 1993* requires employers to provide 12 weeks of unpaid leave for family and medical emergencies, childbirth, or serious health conditions. FMLA is discussed further in Chapter 12.

- *Genetic Information Nondiscrimination Act of 2007.* As of this writing, this Act has passed the U.S. House of Representatives but has yet to be voted on in the Senate, but it has garnered much support from policymakers and politicians alike. This Act prevents an employer from using a person's genetic information in its decision to hire, fire, or promote. Protection against genetic discrimination is already available for federal employees under Executive Order 13145.

- *Immigration Reform and Control Act of 1986,* amended in 1990, is intended to control unauthorized immigration to the United States and designates penalties for employers who hire people not authorized to work in the country. The Act also prohibits discrimination against individuals on the basis of national origin or citizenship. Given the current debate over immigration, the future of this area is somewhat uncertain. However, given the nurse shortage, any new legislation that restricts immigration will likely include an element that allows immigration of nurses (see Chapter 3). Such legislation will also likely continue to allow immigration of people who have scarce skill sets.

- *Occupational Safety and Health Administration (OSHA)* serves two regulatory functions: setting standards and conducting inspections to ensure that employers are providing safe and healthful workplaces. OSHA established the National Institute for Occupational Safety and Health as its research institution. OSHA addresses a broad range of health and safety issues, including exposure to toxic chemicals, excessive noise levels, mechanical dangers, heat or cold stress, and sanitation. OSHA is discussed further in Chapter 13.

- *Uniformed Services Employment and Reemployment Rights Act of 1994 (USERRA)* requires that, in most situations, employers are obligated to re-employ workers who are returning from military leave.
- *Worker Adjustment and Retraining Notification Act (WARN)* requires employers to provide notice to employees 60 days in advance of plant closings and mass layoffs. WARN's intent is to provide workers and their families transition time to adjust to the prospective loss of employment, to seek and obtain alternative jobs and, if necessary, to enter skill training or retraining.

A number of sources exist for further information about these and other federal laws. See, for example, the U.S. Department of Labor's website: www.dol.gov.

State law covers additional rights and responsibilities for employees. For example, in North Carolina, an employer may not withhold money from an employee's paycheck if that employee owes money to the employer unless the employee was given prior notice and has authorized the transaction (see NC Gen. Stat. § 95–25.8 to 95–25.10). Other states, such as California, have enacted statutes that are supplemental to federal statutes—for example, in the area of pregnancy leave (see CA Govt. § 12945). An employer familiar with well-publicized federal law inadvertently may ignore non-preempted state law and thereby deprive an employee of protected rights.

Employment Discrimination

The legal environment affects virtually all aspects of HRM; however, this was not always the case. Traditionally, the employee–employer relationship was guided by the *employment-at-will* principle, which assumes that both employee and employer have the right to sever the work relationship at any time without notice, for any reason, no reason, or even a bad or immoral reason (Bouvier 1996). Within this context, an employee may be terminated for trying to organize a union, for being a member of a particular race/ethnic group, or for refusing to participate in illegal activities. The employment-at-will principle was strengthened in 1908 in Adair v. United States (208 U.S.161) and continues to be the general standard for employee–employer relations in the private sector. Over the last decades, the employment-at-will principle has been eroded dramatically by a variety of laws and regulations. This principle will be discussed in more detail later in the chapter.

Before we begin our review of specific legislation, let us address two key concepts: discrimination and workplace regulation. *Illegal discrimination* means discrimination against a particular individual or group of individuals based on non-job-related characteristics such as race, ethnicity, age, gender, sexual orientation, or disability. A great deal of legislation is aimed at reducing non-job-related discrimination. The passage of laws that address illegal discrimination is, in effect, a form of workplace regulation. Whenever any type of regulatory legislation is considered, the question arises about whether such legislation is, in fact, required. Put another way, can market forces perform these regulatory functions? According to some economists, illegal discrimination is ineffective and inefficient over the long haul. The organization that hires highly qualified individuals regardless of, for example, race, gender, or age will win over the organization that hires individuals of its preferred race, gender, or age. According to this view, discriminating employers will lose and perhaps learn that discrimination does not serve the organization well. Presumably, such organizations will change their ways.

What leads organizations to engage in illegal discrimination practices? Some organizations and individuals have a "taste" for discrimination and may simply not want certain types of individuals in their workplaces. These organizations seem to be willing to pay for their preference with lower profits, diminished quality of service, and decreased market share that accompany the practice of hiring a preferred group (England 1994). Alternatively, employers may discriminate not because of their own preferences but those of their customers or employees (Becker 1957; Cooter 1994).

Others see a more deliberate application of discrimination—that is, *statistical discrimination,* in which a calculated decision is made about a particular individual based on one's perceptions about the larger group to which the individual belongs. For example, if an employer believes that newly married women in their early 20s are highly likely to leave work in the near future for family reasons, this view will be applied to all female job applicants who fit the category. This view puts all members of a particular group at a disadvantage. Employers may consciously or unconsciously use statistical generalizations about the group to which an individual belongs to make hiring and other employment decisions (England 1994). If an employer uses or administers selection tools (such as those listed in Figure 5.1) inconsistently or differently for certain groups, then the organization may be charged with systemic discrimination.

- Detailed application form

- Interview

- Honesty test

- Handwriting analysis

- Drug screening

- Criminal background check

- Credit report check

- Reference check

- Motor vehicle record check

- Educational records check

- Personality tests

Equal Employment Opportunity Legislation

In this section, the most important laws and regulations that deal with equal employment opportunity are outlined.

Equal employment opportunity (EEO) refers to governmental attempts to ensure that all individuals have an equal chance for employment, regardless of age, race, religion, disability, and other non-job-related characteristics. Employment is defined broadly and includes hiring, firing, fairness in promotions, compensation and benefits, training opportunities, and other employment activities. To accomplish EEO aims, the federal government has used constitutional amendments, legislation, executive orders, and courts and quasi-judicial bodies. Table 5.1 provides a summary of the major constitutional provisions, laws, and executive orders that support EEO. The table is not a comprehensive listing of relevant federal laws and does not include state and local ordinances.

The Fourteenth Amendment forbids the state from taking life, liberty, or property without due process of law and prevents states from denying equal protection of the laws. This amendment, passed immediately after the Civil War, was originally intended to protect blacks, but it has more recently been used in cases of alleged reverse discrimination. The most notable case was Bakke v. California Board of Regents of the University of California (438 U.S. 265) in 1978, in which a white applicant to a medical school alleged that he was not admitted because of a discriminatory quota system. The U.S. Supreme Court found in his favor, stating that the quota system had violated his right to equal protection under the law.

TABLE 5.1
Sources of EEO Law

Source	Purpose	Coverage	Administration
Fifth Amendment, U.S. Constitution	Protects against federal violation of due process	All individuals	Federal courts
Thirteenth Amendment, U.S. Constitution	Abolishes slavery	All individuals	Federal courts
Fourteenth Amendment, U.S. Constitution	Provides equal protection for all citizens, and requires due process in state action	State (actions, decisions) or governmental organizations	Federal courts
Civil Rights Acts of 1866 and 1871	Establishes the rights of all citizens to make and enforce contracts	All individuals	Federal courts
Equal Pay Act of 1963	Requires that men and women performing equal jobs receive equal pay	Employers engaged in interstate commerce	EEOC* and federal courts
Civil Rights Act of 1964, Title VII, as amended in 1991	Prohibits discrimination on the basis of race, color, religion, sex, or national origin	Employers with 15 or more employees working 20 or more weeks per year; labor unions; employment agencies	EEOC

(Continued)

TABLE 5.1
Continued

Source	Purpose	Coverage	Administration
Age Discrimination in Employment Act of 1967	Prohibits discrimination in employment against individuals 40 years of age and older	Employers with 15 or more employees working 20 or more weeks per year; labor unions; employment agencies	EEOC
Rehabilitation Act of 1973	Protects persons with disabilities against discrimination in the public sector, and requires affirmative action in the employment of individuals with disabilities	Government agencies; federal contractors and subcontractors with contracts of or greater than $2,500	OFCCP**
Americans with Disabilities Act of 1990	Prohibits discrimination against individuals with disabilities	Employers with more than 15 employees	EEOC
Executive Orders 11246 and 11375	Prohibits discrimination by contractors and subcontractors of federal agencies, and requires affirmative action in hiring women and minorities	Federal contractors and subcontractors with contracts of or greater than $10,000	OFCCP
Family and Medical Leave Act	Requires employers to provide 12 weeks of unpaid leave for family and medical emergencies, childbirth, and other serious personal events	Employers with more than 50 employees	Department of Labor

* Equal Employment Opportunity Commission
** Office of Federal Contract Compliance Program

The 1960s was a period of significant social activism in the United States. Federal legislation was passed to extend civil rights and equal opportunity in housing, voting, education, employment, and other areas. The basic premise of all of these laws is that employment decisions, including hiring, promotion, compensation and benefits, and training opportunities, should not be based on non-job-related characteristics such as age, gender, race, or disability. As a result of the complexity of these laws, the federal government has produced a useful document, entitled "Uniform Guidelines on Employee Selection Procedures," that summarizes and synthesizes the employment-related implications of these laws (EEOC 1978). This document provides basic guidance on compliance in virtually every human resources function and is a valuable tool for all management professionals (see www.uniformguidelines.com).

The Fair Labor Standards Act (FLSA) was originally passed in 1938 but has been amended many times since. The major provisions of the FLSA concern the minimum wage, overtime payments, child labor, and equal pay. With respect to EEO, the child labor and equal-pay provisions are most critical. The FLSA forbids the employment of children younger than 18 years in hazardous occupations such as mining, logging, woodworking, meatpacking, and certain types of manufacturing. Severe restrictions are placed on the employment of minors under age 16 years in most other industries. Minors aged 14 to 15 years may work outside school hours under the following restrictions (29 CFR 570.119):

- No more than 3 hours on a school day, 18 hours in a school week, 8 hours on a non-school day, or 40 hours in a non-school week
- Work may not begin before 7 a.m. nor end after 7 p.m., except between June 1 and Labor Day, when 9 p.m. is the ending time

The Equal Pay Act of 1963, an amendment to the FLSA, requires that men and women in the same organization who perform equal jobs receive equal pay. This act outlaws the once-prevalent practice of paying women less because of their gender, not the work they perform. This practice was commonly defended on the theory that a married man needed a higher salary to support his family. Sometimes, determining what constitutes "equal work" may be difficult. The Equal Pay Act specifies that jobs are the same if they are equal in terms of skill, effort, responsibility, and working conditions. If pay differences are the result of differences in seniority, merit, quantity or quality of work, or any other factor other than gender, then differences in compensation are allowable (Greenlaw and Kohl 1995). Although the Equal Pay Act has been law for more than 40 years, substantial gaps in earnings between men and women still exist. In 2006, women earned about 76.9 cents on the dollar of what men made, compared with 73.8 cents in 1996 (National Committee on Pay Equity 2008).

Because of the difficulty in eradicating wage differences between men and women, some jurisdictions have adopted comparable worth legislation (Ledvinka and Scarpello 1991). *Comparable worth* is a concept that calls for equal or comparable pay for jobs that require similar skills, effort, and responsibility and that are performed in comparable working conditions. In the healthcare environment, this concept is particularly salient because of the large concentration of female employees in certain occupations. If the work of hospital nurses, for example, is only compared to that of other nurses, it would be difficult to remedy gender-based wage discrepancies. If, however, the wages of nurses are compared to the wages of employees whose contribution or worth is comparable to that of nurses, wage disparities may be discovered and addressed.

Title VII of the Civil Rights Act of 1964 is clearly the most far-reaching and significant of all antidiscrimination statutes. The Act prohibits discrimination in a variety of areas, including voting, public accommodations, use of public facilities, public education, and employment. In terms of employment, the Act bars discrimination in hiring, promotion, compensation, training, benefits, and other aspects. Discrimination is specifically prohibited on the basis of race, color, religion, gender, and national origin.

As amended by the Equal Employment Opportunity Act of 1972 and the Civil Rights Act of 1991, the jurisdiction of Title VII includes the following:

- All private employers involved in interstate commerce that employ 15 or more employees for 20 or more weeks per year
- State and local governments
- Private and public employment agencies
- Joint labor-management committees that govern apprenticeship or training programs
- Labor unions that have 15 or more members or employees
- Public and private educational institutions
- Foreign subsidiaries of U.S. organizations that employ U.S. citizens
- Federal government employees covered by section 717 of the Civil Rights Act and Civil Service Reform Act

A large majority of employers in the United States are covered by the Civil Rights Act, except for government-owned corporations, tax-exempt private clubs, religious organizations that employ persons of a specific religion, and companies that hire Native Americans on or near a reservation. Title VII is quite specific in its definition of discrimination. Section 703a states the following:

(a) It shall be an unlawful employment practice for an employer—

    (1) to fail or refuse to hire or to discharge any individual, or otherwise to discriminate against any individual with respect to his compensation,

terms, conditions, or privileges of employment, because of such individual's race, color, religion, sex, or national origin; or

(2) to limit, segregate, or classify his employees or applicants for employment in any way which would deprive or tend to deprive any
individual of employment opportunities or otherwise adversely affect his status as an employee, because of such individual's race,
color, religion, sex, or national origin.

While gender discrimination is illegal under Title VII, discrimination
based on sexual orientation is not prohibited under U.S. federal law. However, 17 states and the District of Columbia have passed laws that prohibit sexual-orientation discrimination in private employment. In addition, six states
have laws that prohibit sexual-orientation discrimination in public workplaces
only. On the local level, more than 180 cities and counties have passed laws
prohibiting sexual-orientation discrimination in some workplaces. State laws
on this issue vary, however. For example, while Michigan does not have a law
that prohibits discrimination based on sexual orientation, it has statutes that
apply only to employment in healthcare facilities. Minnesota is among the
most progressive of states in this area, with laws that prohibit discrimination
in public employment, public accommodations, private employment, education, housing, credit, and union practices. Minnesota state law also provides
protection for transgendered people (Lambda Legal 2007).

The Civil Rights Act is a far-reaching law with strong enforcement provisions, particularly after the 1991 amendments. Before 1991, Title VII limited damage claims to equitable relief, such as back pay, lost benefits, front pay
in some cases, and attorney's fees and costs. The 1991 amendments allow
compensatory and punitive damages when intentional or reckless discrimination is proven. Compensatory damages may include future pecuniary loss,
emotional pain, suffering, and loss of enjoyment of life. Punitive damages are
intended to discourage discrimination by providing for payments to the plaintiff beyond actual damages suffered. Maximum damages are limited by the
number of employees in the organization and range from $50,000 to
$300,000 (Kobata 1992).

The Age Discrimination in Employment Act (ADEA) of 1967 forbids
discrimination against men and women aged 40 years and older by employers, unions, employment agencies, state and local governments, and the federal government. As with Title VII, enforcement of the ADEA is the responsibility of the EEOC. The U.S. Supreme Court has ruled that employees may
sue on the basis of a *disparate impact theory* of intentional discrimination because of age. However, the Supreme Court also ruled that employers are not
liable if the disparate impact was a result of non-age factors, such as seniority
(see Smith v. City of Jackson Mississippi). In another case, the Supreme
Court ruled that providing preferential treatment for older workers is not a

violation of the ADEA. Thus, an employer may not show preferential treatment for younger workers, but it may do so for older workers (see General Dynamics Land Systems v. Cline). As with all EEO laws, an employer is not liable if an age requirement (or other job requirement) is a bona fide occupational qualification.

The Older Workers Benefit Protection Act (OWBPA), passed in 1990, is an amendment to the ADEA. OWBPA protects employees when they sign liability waivers for age discrimination as part of a severance package. Specifically, the legislation establishes minimum standards for a waiver to be considered valid. Among other requirements, a valid ADEA waiver must be in writing and be understandable, must specifically refer to ADEA rights or claims, may not waive rights or claims that may arise in the future, must offer the employee value beyond that which the employee would have received without the package, must advise the individual in writing to consult an attorney before signing the waiver, and must provide the individual at least 21 days to consider the agreement and at least 7 days to revoke the agreement after signing it (EEOC 1997).

Discrimination against individuals with disabilities was first prohibited in federally funded activities by the Vocational Rehabilitation Act of 1973. Because individuals with disabilities were not covered by Title VII, they were not protected from employment discrimination. The ADA, which covers various segments of life, offers substantial protections for individuals with disabilities who are either employed or potentially employable. The Act applies to private-sector organizations and departments or agencies of state or local governments that employ 15 or more employees. Of the many federal EEO laws, the ADA is unique in that its establishment received unanimous support from both Republicans and Democrats. The ADA prohibits discrimination against individuals with disabilities in all aspects of the employee–employer transaction, including job application procedures, hiring, termination, promotions, compensation, and training. After the ADA's passage, most large organizations were motivated to examine their procedures and, in many cases, to modify them to ensure compliance.

The language of the ADA, like other legislation, is somewhat vague and thus is open to interpretation. Section 3(2)(a) of the Act defines a disability as "(a) a physical or mental impairment that substantially limits one or more of the major life activities of such individual; (b) a record of such impairment; or (c) being regarded as having such impairment." Each of these clauses is obviously open to considerable debate and interpretation. Part (a) of this definition includes individuals who have serious disabilities, such as epilepsy, blindness, deafness, or paralysis, that affect their ability to carry out major life activities. Part (b) includes individuals with a history of a disability, such as history of cancer, heart disease, or mental disorder. Part (c) deals with people who are regarded as having an impairment, such as burn victims and individuals with disfiguring conditions. For example, Part (c) protects individuals who may be denied employment because an employer feels that coworkers will have negative reactions to that individual's physical appearance (*Employment Law Update* 1991). While these categories are rather broad, the ADA specifically excludes the following from the definition of a disability:

- Homosexuality and bisexuality (State and local legislation may provide protection against discrimination based on sexual orientation.)
- Gender-identity disorders that do not result from physical impairment or other sexual-behavior disorders (e.g., transvestitism, transsexualism)
- Compulsive gambling, kleptomania, or pyromania
- Psychoactive substance abuse disorders
- Current illegal use of drugs

One of the biggest areas of review by the EEOC has been the definition of a disability. In the area of obesity, for example, the EEOC has determined that only severely obese (i.e., weight in excess of 100 percent of the norm for a particular height) persons or those whose weight can be linked to a medical disorder can be covered by the ADA. In addition, because almost 13 percent of all complaints filed with the EEOC between 1993 and 1997 were related to emotional and mental disorders, the EEOC released guidelines in 1997 that deal specifically with this type of issue.

The ADA does not require an organization to hire someone who has a disability but is otherwise not qualified for a job. For an employee or a prospective employee to be protected under the ADA, the person must be qualified. In the language of the ADA (42 U.S.C. § 12111[8]), "the term 'qualified individual with a disability' means an individual with a disability who, with or without reasonable accommodation, can perform the essential functions of the employment position that such individual holds or desires." This definition, first of all, requires the organization to have a good and defensible understanding of the essential functions of the job, with accurate and current job descriptions. The "qualified individual" definition simply implies that an employer cannot discriminate against an individual with a disability if that person can do the job with or without reasonable accommodation.

This leads us to the next dilemma in the ADA: the concept of *reasonable accommodation*. The ADA specifically states that it is the employer's responsibility to make reasonable accommodation to the physical or mental limitations of an employee with a disability, unless doing so will impose an undue hardship on the organization. Reasonable accommodation may be defined as an attempt by employers to adjust, without undue hardship, the working conditions or schedules of employees with disabilities. (Note that the reasonable accommodation concept may also be applied to Civil Rights Act issues concerning individuals with religious preferences.) This rule, again, is ambiguous in that reasonable accommodation may be interpreted in many ways. Reasonableness is determined on a case-by-case basis and typically includes relatively noncontroversial accommodations, such as making existing facilities accessible to individuals with disabilities. However, it may also be reasonable to restructure jobs, alter work schedules, reassign individuals to different tasks, adjust training materials, and provide readers or interpreters.

Defining reasonable accommodation depends on determining the level of undue hardship to the organization. No strict guidelines exist for determining the threshold of undue hardship, but the law suggests this: Compare the cost of the accommodation with the employer's operating budget. The law also stipulates that the overall size of the organization may be considered as well as the type of operation and the nature and cost of the accommodation. The cost of most accommodations is not great. In fact, a study of Sears Roebuck & Company revealed that 69 percent of all accommodations cost nothing, 28 percent cost less than $1,000, and only 3 percent cost more than $1,000 (Reno and Thornburgh 1995). The EEOC published "A Technical Assistance Manual," which suggests the following process for assessing reasonable accommodation:

1. Examine the particular job involved, and determine its purpose and essential job function.
2. Consult the individual with the disability to identify potential accommodations that may be needed. If several accommodations are available and possible, deference should be given to the individual's preferred accommodation.

Rulings by the U.S. Supreme Court have sought to curtail what many consider abuses of the ADA. Policymakers and managers should understand this Act so that they can anticipate and deal with both its intended and unintended consequences. Legislation that protects employee leaves, such as FMLA or USERRA, also requires input from human resources and legal personnel.

Over the years, the types of discrimination cases brought before the EEOC have been relatively consistent. Between 1997 and 2006, the total number of claims ranged from 75,428 in 2005 to 84,442 in 2002. About 35 percent of charges were brought on the basis of race, and this proportion has been stable in the last ten years. Similarly, charges based on sex discrimination have accounted for 30 percent to 31 percent of all complaints. Of all the bases for charges, discrimination based on national origin has seen the most consistent increase: 6,712 charges (8.3 percent of all charges) were filed in 1997, and this number grew to 8,327 (11 percent of all charges) in 2006 (EEOC 2007a).

Implementing EEO Principles

In this section, the implications of EEO laws on HRM practices, including hiring, training, and discipline, are examined.

Implementation of these laws is affected by two interacting aspects: (1) the legal requirements associated with compliance and (2) the mechanisms that ensure legal compliance. The first aspect involves tasks such as completing affirmative action plans and filling out the annual AA-1 government reporting form. The second aspect deals with ensuring that the organization's human resources systems, including job design, employee selection, and performance appraisal, comply with requirements.

An *affirmative action plan* is required under Executive Order 11246: Federal contractors and subcontractors must "take affirmative action to ensure that all individuals have an equal opportunity for employment, without regard to race, color, religion, sex, national origin, disability or status as a Vietnam era or special disabled veteran" (DOL 2002). Specifically, an affirmative action plan must be developed and implemented by all federal contractors and subcontractors. This plan must then be integrated into the organization's written personnel policies. The goal of such a plan is to demonstrate the positive steps an organization will take to recruit and advance qualified minorities, women, persons with disabilities, and covered veterans. The plan may include such activities and initiatives as training programs and outreach efforts. In addition, the law requires these plans to be implemented and updated on an annual basis.

The U.S. Department of Labor specifically indicates that affirmative action plans are not quota systems. Rather, they allow organizations to work toward greater inclusion by setting goals and timetables related to their good-faith efforts. A complete affirmative action plan will contain a number of components, including the following:

- Workforce analysis, by department, job title, salary level, and promotion
- External availability analysis
- Internal utilization analysis, including calculation of disparate impact
- Goals and timetables
- Procedures for internal auditing and reporting

Affirmative action is frequently misunderstood as a quota-driven system that requires companies to hire and promote individuals based on demographic characteristics rather than on job qualifications. However, affirmative action simply asks employers to analyze their workforce and relevant labor markets and then determine the steps needed to improve the representation of their workforce. For detailed information about affirmative action plans and their components, see "Facts on Executive Order 11246—Affirmative Action" on the U.S. Department of Labor's website (DOL 2002).

Interview Questions

Exhibiting cultural sensitivity is important when framing interview questions and posing them to potential employees. If the appropriateness of an interview question is inconclusive, then avoiding the question altogether is prudent.

Furthermore, the same questions should be asked of all interviewees. If a question can only be posed to certain job candidates, then the appropriateness of the question is dubious. For example, a question regarding plans for becoming pregnant or for retirement is not appropriate for two reasons: (1) It can only be asked of female and older candidates, and (2) it delves too deeply into personal issues that have no bearing on the candidate's ability to perform the job.

Screening

Effective screening of potential employees is a necessary step in minimizing employer liability and in preventing employee discipline in the future. The amount of screening to be performed must be balanced against the level of risk associated with the open position. Employers are expected to perform more thorough screening on candidates for positions that carry greater risk, including those that give the employee access to master keys, narcotics, finances, children, the elderly, and disabled individuals.

Many pre-employment screening tests (see Figure 5.1) pose risks or may be objectionable to applicants; thus, the employer must consider such screenings as well and apply them consistently and with consideration for any adverse impact on protected classes (see, for example, the case of Georgia-Pacific, OFCCP audit [Aug. 8, 2007] regarding a test of adult basic education and also the case of EEOC v. Dial Corp., 8th Cir. [Nov. 17, 2006] regarding physical strength tests). Alternatively, to avoid claims of negligent hiring, employers (especially in healthcare) have an obligation to prescreen employees, at a minimum, for references, education, and professional license status.

Selection

As noted earlier, the federal government created "Uniform Guidelines on Employee Selection Procedures" to assist employers in the areas of hiring, retention, promotion, transfer, demotion, dismissal, and referral. The document, published in the *Federal Register* and posted on www.uniformguide-lines.com, is the most readily accessible and useful interpretation of the rules, helping employers comply with federal antidiscrimination statutes. The guidelines define the circumstances under which an employee selection procedure may be discriminatory (EEOC 1978):

> The use of any selection procedure which has an adverse impact on the hiring, promotion, or other employment or membership opportunities or members of any race, sex, or ethnic group will be considered to be discriminatory and inconsistent with these guidelines, unless the procedure has been validated in accordance with these guidelines (or, certain other provisions are satisfied).

This definition implies that all the elements in the selection process (e.g., job qualifications, tests, interviews) must be job related and positively associated with job success. The guidelines also describe different methods of validating a test (these methods are discussed further in Chapter 8). A selection procedure may be found discriminatory if it measures factors unrelated to job success, which adversely affects an individual or group.

The landmark discrimination case in this area was Griggs v. Duke Power Company in 1971 (401 U.S. 424), in which an employee's request for a promotion was denied because he was not a high school graduate. Griggs, an African American, claimed that this job standard was discriminatory because it did not relate to job success and because the standard had an adverse impact on a protected class. *Protected class* refers to a group of individuals (e.g., women, minorities, people with disabilities) protected under a particular law. The U.S. Supreme Court decided in favor of Griggs and established two important principles. First, employer discrimination need not be overt or intentional to be present and illegal. Second, employment selection practices must be job related, and employers have the burden of demonstrating that employment requirements are job related or constitute a business necessity. In this case, the employment practices had the effect of excluding protected classes and were thus found illegal, even if they appeared racially neutral (Dobbin 2004). This is called *disparate impact.*

More common than discrimination based on disparate impact is disparate treatment. *Disparate treatment* exists when individuals in similar employment situations are treated differently because of race, color, religion, sex, national origin, age, or disability. The most obvious case of disparate treatment is when an employer decides whom to hire on the basis of one of these criteria. Disparate treatment may also be more subtle, such as asking female job applicants to demonstrate a particular skill when male applicants are not asked to do the same. The defining case in this area was McDonnell Douglas Corp. v. Green in 1973 (411 U.S. 792), in which a member of a protected class applied for a job and was rejected, but the company continued to advertise for this position. This case established the four-part guideline for determining disparate treatment:

1. The person is a member of a protected class.
2. The person applied for a job and is qualified.
3. The person was rejected for the job.
4. The position remained open to applicants with equal or fewer qualifications.

The most important difference between disparate impact and disparate treatment is that motive is irrelevant in disparate impact cases. In disparate treatment cases, however, proof must exist that an intent to discriminate is present. In a disparate impact case, the plaintiff must prove that a particular employment practice disproportionately affects a particular group; whether the employer intends to discriminate is not necessary to demonstrate disparate impact. In fact, disparate impact can be proven where employment practices appear quite innocuous. A minimum height requirement, for example, may appear quite neutral; however, height is not distributed equally among sexes and ethnic groups, and if this requirement is not linked to job performance, a disparate impact case can be made. With disparate treatment, it must be proven that a discriminatory intent is behind the employment procedure.

A number of legitimate defenses can be made against charges of disparate treatment. One defense is that while a candidate may have had the qualifications for a particular job, the employer hired someone else with superior qualifications. Another defense is that a protected class characteristic (e.g., gender) is in fact a *bona fide occupational qualification* (BFOQ). A clear example of a BFOQ is requiring a woman to work as an attendant in a women's restroom. However, a great debate brews over what constitutes a BFOQ, and court rulings are inconsistent in this area. The courts have rejected the argument that because most women cannot lift 50 pounds, all women should be eliminated from consideration for jobs that require heavy lifting. On the other hand, citing safety concerns, the U.S. Federal Court of Appeals upheld the Federal Aviation Administration policy of forced retirement of pilots at age 60 years (Castaneda 1977).

Generally, liability for the employee's conduct rests with the employer and, therefore, with the manager. The legal concept of this relationship is that of *agency*. The employer empowers the employee under his or her supervision to perform duties, services, or work in the name of the organization. The employee's conduct while in this charge is a direct reflection of the employer or organization. Legally, the employee's actions are of potential equal liability to the employer. Specifically, the legal doctrine of *respondeat superior* (Furrow et al. 1997) holds the employer liable for the conduct of its employees because the employer enables the employee and is thus responsible for managing and supervising that employee. In this age of technology, employers may be liable even for the employee's use of a company computer for sex-related crimes and violation of securities laws (Davis 2002; see Haybeck v. Prodigy Services, 944 F. Supp. 326 S.D.N.Y. 1996).

Therefore, it is of utmost importance that managers not only provide training in appropriate workplace conduct but also supervise the subsequent behaviors. An employer should not assume that employees are knowledgeable about equal opportunity, discrimination, and sexual harassment legalities. However, an employer should assume the burden of employee education to promote organizational compatibility and to prevent future litigation.

Defenses Against Discrimination

A healthcare organization's best defense against lawsuits is creating and following a set of policies that are nondiscriminatory in nature. Disseminating organizational policies serves multiple purposes. First, it is an initial step in educating employees of what behavior is expected and accepted by the organization. Specifying unacceptable behavior and its consequences at the onset of employment is likely to decrease future inappropriate conduct. Second, standard policies will promote consistent employee conduct that lends itself to fair and nondiscriminatory employee treatment. In other words, employees trained with uniform methods are likely to conduct themselves in a relatively similar manner. Third, publicizing desired employee conduct is a preemptive step against litigation. A set of policies allows an organization, to a certain extent, to separate a specific employee action from the standard rules of employee conduct established by the organization. Legally, it is important to distinguish between what the employee does through autonomous choices and what the employee does through organizational support or inattention. Policies permit the organization to delineate the behaviors it endorses. However, simply having in place a set of policies is not a substantial defense. For them to be effective, policies must be monitored and enforced, and this is a fact recognized by the courts. Tacit, unpoliced policies are ineffective defenses against discrimination.

Sexual Harassment

Increased awareness about sexual harassment came about as a result of feminism and the women's movement, greater societal attention to diversity and equal accommodation in the workplace, and the growth in the number of women in the workplace. Certainly, well-publicized cases, such as those involving President Bill Clinton and Supreme Court Justice Clarence Thomas, have also amplified the public's familiarity with sexual harassment. Although sexual harassment in the workplace has been occurring for a long time, surprisingly, the prevalence and impact of this issue have only been recognized within the last 30 years by employers and courts. To put it simply, sexual harassment was not acknowledged as an important workplace concern.

The major statute governing sexual harassment is Title VII of the Civil Rights Act. Under this statute, sexual harassment is considered a violation of an individual's civil rights, and several cases that reached the Supreme Court provide a richer understanding of sexual harassment issues. Many ambiguities surround sexual harassment charges. To clarify ambiguities, the EEOC has established a definition of sexual harassment to help courts, employers, and employees understand the scope of this issue (see Figure 5.2).

Consistent with the EEOC's definition are two recognized types of sexual harassment: (1) quid pro quo and (2) hostile environment. *Quid pro quo sexual harassment* occurs when a job-related benefit is made contingent on an employee's submission to sexual advances. A typical case is that of an employee at the University of Massachusetts Medical Center who was awarded $1 million in 1994 after she testified that her supervisor had forced her to engage in sex once or twice a week over a 20-month period as a condition of keeping her

FIGURE 5.2

EEOC's
Definition
of Sexual
Harassment

Unwelcome sexual advances, requests for sexual favors, and other verbal or physical contact of a sexual nature constitute sexual harassment when

1. Submission to such contact is made, either explicitly or implicitly, a term of condition of an individual's employment

2. Submission to or rejection of such conduct by an individual is used as the basis for employment decisions affecting such individual

3. Such conduct has the purpose or effect of unreasonably interfering with an individual's work performance or creating an intimidating, hostile, or offensive work environment

job (BNA 1994). Of greater magnitude was a class-action lawsuit on behalf of a group of female employees at Lutheran Medical Center in Brooklyn, New York (EEOC v. Lutheran Medical Center, No. 01-5494, E.D.N.Y., April 24, 2003). In this case, a physician engaged in inappropriate practices with female employees during the employment-related exams. The EEOC ordered the hospital to pay more than $5.425 million and significant remedial relief on behalf of these employees. Like other sexual harassment cases, "the EEOC alleged that Lutheran knew or should have known of the sexual harassment and failed to take adequate measures to prevent such harassment" (EEOC 2003). In a recent case, the top official of Caritas Christi Health Care Systems—the second largest healthcare provider in New England—was forced to resign after the board voted to fire him as a result of sexual harassment accusations by at least six women (Zezima 2006). For a recent example of a mixed sexual/racial harassment case and retaliation settlement, see EEOC v. R.T.G. Furniture Corp., No. 8:04-CV-2155-T24-TBM (M.D. Fla. May 16, 2006).

The second type of sexual harassment is more subtle. *Hostile environment sexual harassment* occurs when the behavior of anyone in the work setting is perceived by another person as offensive and undesirable. While the law is not explicit about what constitutes this type of harassment, some examples may include posting sexually explicit pictures, using sexually laden jokes, and using sexually explicit language. While some cases of sexual harassment are relatively clear cut, the clarity of other cases is contingent on the particular workplace and the individuals involved.

In a 2003 case, the Supreme Court stated that the distinction between quid pro quo and hostile environment is not the controlling factor for determining liability (Gabel and Mansfield 2003). The determining factor in such cases is whether a "tangible employment action" (i.e., an action that changes the employment status) was taken against the employee. If no tangible employment action exists, the employer may use the following affirmative defense: "(a) that the employer exercised reasonable care to prevent and correct promptly any sexually harassing behavior, and (b) that the plaintiff employee unreasonably failed to take advantage of any preventive or corrective opportunities provided by the employer or to avoid harm otherwise" (see Burlington Indus., Inc. v. Ellerth, 524 U.S. 742, 746 [1998]). This defense is not available to the employer if tangible employment action was taken.

For employers, an important concern is liability. In sexual harassment cases, courts typically address three issues in determining whether harassment occurred and whether the employer is liable. First, the plaintiff cannot have invited the sexual advances; sexual advances must be unwelcome. Courts typically have looked for repetitiveness in the harassment. A plaintiff is more likely to be successful if it can be demonstrated that the harassment was not a one-time event but was in fact persistent and pernicious. Second, the harassment needs to have been severe enough to have altered the terms, conditions, and privileges of employment. Basically, significant consequences for the employee must have occurred. Particularly in hostile environment cases, it is often difficult to objectively assess whether an environment is actually "hostile." The Supreme Court has established several questions to help courts decide on hostile environment sexual harassment cases:

- How frequent is the discriminatory conduct?
- How severe is the discriminatory conduct?
- Is the conduct physically threatening or humiliating?
- Does the conduct interfere with the employee's work performance?

Third, courts need to examine the extent of employer liability for the harassment. Two questions are typically considered here: (1) Did the employer know about the harassment, or should it have known? and (2) Did the employer take steps to stop the behavior? In most instances, if the employer knew about the harassment and the behavior did not stop, courts will decide that the employer did not act appropriately to curtail the behavior. Table 5.2 provides a summary of the most important precedent-setting sexual harassment court cases within the last 27 years.

Sexual harassment charges continue to be filed with the EEOC. In 2007, the EEOC received 12,510 sexual harassment complaints. More than 16 percent of those charges were filed by males. In that same year, the EEOC resolved 11,592 sexual harassment allegations and recovered $49.9 million in monetary benefits for charging parties and other aggrieved individuals; this dollar amount does not include monetary benefits obtained through litigation (EEOC 2007b). The magnitude of this problem in the workplace has been documented:

- A report by the National Council for Research on Women concludes that 42 percent to 67 percent of working women can expect to be sexually harassed during their careers (Lee and Greenlaw 1995).

TABLE 5.2
Key Court
Decisions
on Sexual
Harassment in
the Workplace

Case	Key Finding and Precedent
Bundy v. Jackson, 641 F.2d934, 24 FEP 1155, D.C. Cir. (1981)	A quid pro quo harassment case, it extended the idea of discrimination to sexual harassment.
Meritor Savings Bank v. Vinson, Supreme Court of the United States, 40 FEP 1822 (1986)	The U.S. Supreme Court ruled that sexual harassment can constitute unlawful sex discrimination under Title VII if the harassment is so severe as to alter the conditions of the victim's employment and create an abusive working environment.
Ellison v. Brady, United States Court of Appeals, Ninth Circuit, 924 F.2d 872 (1991)	The Supreme Court ruled that sexual harassment must be viewed from the perspective of a "reasonable woman" and not people in general; employers must take positive action to eliminate sexual harassment from the workplace.
Harris v. Forklift Systems, Inc., 114 S. Ct. 367 (1993)	An abusive work environment can be demonstrated even when the victim does not suffer serious psychological harm; the case adopted the idea that harassment occurs if a "reasonable person" would find that the behavior leads to a hostile or abusive working environment.
Oncale v. Sundowner Offshore Services, Inc., 523 US 75 (1998)	Same-sex harassment is actionable under Title VII.
Burlington Industries v. Ellerth, 524 U.S. 742 (1998)	Employers are vicariously liable for supervisors who create hostile working conditions for subordinates even if threats are not carried out and the harassed employee suffers no adverse, tangible effects. Employers may defend themselves by demonstrating that they acted quickly to prevent and correct harassment and that the harassed employee failed to utilize their protection.
Faragher v. Boca Raton, 524 U.S. 775 (1998)	Employers are vicariously liable under Title VII of the Civil Rights Act of 1964 for discrimination caused by a supervisor.
Lockard v. Pizza Hut, Inc., 1998 10CIR 1472, 162 F.3d 1062 (1998)	Employers can be liable when a nonemployee harasses one of their employees.

- Nearly two-thirds of college students experience sexual harassment at some point during college; nearly one-third of first-year students have been the subject of harassment (Hill and Silva 2005).
- Sexual harassment in healthcare is coming to light globally; see, for example, data on sexual harassment among nurses in Turkey and Japan (Yusuf and Yusuf 2007; Hibino, Ogino, and Inagaki 2006).
- Sexual harassment is as prevalent, or more so, in healthcare as in other industries. A study indicates that nearly three-fourths of women in healthcare have been sexually harassed (Walsh and Borowski 1995).
- A study conducted by the American Medical Association reveals that 81 percent of female medical students in the study endured sexual slurs and 50 percent were direct targets of sexual advances, with the worst harassment occurring in academic medical centers (Decker 1997).
- *Fortune* 500 companies spend an average of $1.6 million each year to manage sexual harassment claims (Sherer 1995).

Furthermore, courts have recently awarded damages to plaintiffs and allowed other cases to proceed based on same-sex harassment (see Beach v. Yellow Freight System, Inc., 312 F.3d 391 [8th Cir. 2002]; Rene v. MGM Grand Hotel, Inc., 305 F.3d 1061 [9th Cir. 2002] [en banc], cert. denied, 123 S. Ct. 1573 [2003]).

Although sexual harassment is unfortunately common in virtually all organizations, it is particularly problematic in healthcare organizations. The American Nurses Association's House of Delegates declared a resolution denouncing sexual harassment in the workplace and called on the industry to adopt and enforce sexual harassment policies (Mikulenak 1992). Several factors may explain why sexual harassment is so prevalent in healthcare organizations. First, sexual harassment almost always includes an important element of power and control. Because of the hierarchical nature of many healthcare organizations and the traditional gender dynamics of the doctor–nurse relationship, the professional and organizational authority is imbalanced between male and female healthcare professionals. From a gender perspective, hospitals are unique: The majority of hospital employees are women, but those in positions of authority (i.e., physicians and administrators) are predominantly men. This differential in authority is frequently the precursor to sexual harassment. Controlling sexual harassment in hospitals is also difficult because of the ambiguous lines of authority in hospitals. While every nurse certainly has a formal supervisor in the organization, many people are unclear about who supervises physicians.

Second, the nature of healthcare work entails a certain amount of intimacy among care providers. Strong, collegial relationships often form in the high-stress environment of healthcare, engendering sexual jokes and off-color humor. Indeed, discussion of the human body and sexuality is central to much of healthcare, and it is not difficult to envision how such discussion can evolve in an abusive, condescending, or suggestive manner. The first line of defense against sexual harassment is putting in place a sexual harassment policy that is fully supported by management. Typically, this policy includes the following elements (Segal 1992):

- A statement against sexual harassment, including a definition of sexual harassment and a strong statement indicating that it will not be tolerated
- Extensive training of all employees on the policy, with particular focus on employees with management and supervisory authority
- Instructions on how to report complaints, including procedures to bypass a supervisor if he or she is involved
- Assurances of confidentiality and protection against retaliation
- A guarantee of prompt investigation
- A statement that disciplinary action will be taken against harassers up to and including termination

Such a policy needs to be reinforced with strong communications and training. Supervisors must understand clearly the requirements of Title VII as well as their duty to provide an environment free of sexual harassment. Supervisors also need to know the investigative procedures to be used when charges occur. If a complaint arises, management needs to respond immediately; launch an investigation; and, after an investigation proves the allegations true, discipline the offender according to policy. As done with violations of any other human resources policy, sexual harassment discipline has to be carried out consistently across similar cases and among managers and hourly employees alike.

Retaliatory Discharge

When an employer takes any materially adverse action that is likely to deter an employee from asserting a claim, such action could give rise to an employee's charge of retaliatory discharge. In 2006, the Supreme Court finally clarified the standards for retaliation; the standards appear in the Sarbanes-Oxley Act, FLSA, ADEA, OSHA, ERISA, FMLA, USERRA, Title VII, ADA, and numerous other federal statutes. The case before the Supreme Court was Burlington Northern & Santa Fe Railway Co. v. White, 126 S. Ct. 2405 (2006). In the Burlington case, Sheila White was hired to work as a forklift driver in an all-male rail yard. After several months of employment, she lodged a claim for sexual harassment and discrimination with management at Burlington Northern. In response, the company transferred White to the more difficult job of general track laborer. White then filed a complaint with the EEOC, alleging that the change in her position was unlawful gender discrimination and retaliation. Burlington Northern then suspended White for 37 days without pay. After exhausting her EEOC administrative remedies, White filed suit under Title VII, alleging retaliation because of her transfer and later suspension. A jury and en banc (with all the judges of the appellate court) Sixth Circuit found in favor of White. The Supreme Court unanimously determined that White's reassignment and suspension constituted retaliatory discrimination. Previously, the standard for retaliation usually required termination to be successful.

The Burlington case decision requires substantial change in the actions of employers in implementing and enforcing guidelines that prohibit retaliation. If an employee does file a claim under one of the many federal statutes that prohibit retaliation, the employer must be cautious about a change in schedule, reassignment, transfers, or exclusion from group activities. Employees must be trained in this area, because it is human nature to react negatively toward a coworker who has filed a claim against the person or organization.

Workplace Searches

Employers have an interest in monitoring employees for theft and attendance because they may be held accountable for the misconduct of their employees (Davis 2002). An employee of a private company has limited privacy rights against the search of a desk, office, or work area. In Schowengerdt v. General Dynamics Corp. (823 F.2d 1328 [9th Cir.], cert. denied 117 L.Ed.2d 650), the court ruled that a private employee who has no property interest in an area searched continues to have privacy rights. Workplace searches conducted without employee consent or a search warrant may still be valid if the search meets a "standard of reasonableness under all of the circumstances" (see O'Connor v. Ortega, 480 U.S. 709, 720, 94 L.Ed2d714, 725, 107 S.Ct 1492 [1987]). In O'Connor v. Ortega, the desk and file cabinet of a state-employed physician (a public employee) were searched. Most of the Supreme Court justices agreed that the physician had a reasonable expectation of privacy in his office and that there was a reasonable expectation of privacy in the physician's desk and file cabinet.

Electronic Monitoring

Employers use monitoring in the workplace to investigate organizational problems, particularly loss of productivity as a result of wasted time e-mailing coworkers, friends, and family. Use of company computer systems to send discriminatory or harassing materials can also lead to litigation if the employer fails to take proper precautionary or corrective measures. Figure 5.3 lists some reasons that employers may choose to undertake an employee surveillance program. Monitoring techniques that employers use can be as simple and obvious as a desk search or can involve sophisticated hidden cameras and microphones. Some employers will install such devices, for example, when an employee is suspected of a particular inappropriate act or when inventory is

FIGURE 5.3

Why Do
Employers
Monitor
Employees?

- Ensure and promote safety
- Protect trade secrets
- Enhance productivity
- Prevent theft or other unlawful activity
- Assess the quality and regularity of customer service
- Search for drug use
- Limit employer liability by detecting and recording discriminatory or illegal behavior

missing. Figure 5.4 lists some common monitoring techniques most often used by employers.

The Employee Polygraph Protection Act (EPPA) is a legislative attempt to provide direction in this area and to monitor potential for abuse. The EPPA prohibits an employer from doing the following:

- Requiring employees to take a lie-detector test
- Using the results of a lie-detector test
- Taking action against an employee for refusing to take a lie-detector test or for the results of such a test
- Retaliating against the employee for complaining about any of the above

Significant exemptions to the EPPA are applicable to the healthcare industry and to the handling of controlled substances (see 29 U.S.C. §§ 2001–2009).

Surveillance of employees is widespread and is increasing, as evidenced by research conducted by the American Management Association (AMA 2005). Following are some of the findings of its 2005 survey of 526 companies:

- Twenty-six percent have fired workers for misusing the Internet, 25 percent have terminated employees for e-mail misuse, and 6 percent have let go of employees for misusing office telephones.
- Seventy-six percent monitor workers' website connections, and 65 percent use software to block connections to inappropriate websites.
- Thirty-six percent track computer use, including document content, keystrokes, and time spent at the keyboard; 50 percent store and review employees' computer files; and 55 percent retain and review e-mail messages.
- Among companies that engage in such monitoring, about 85 percent inform employees of their monitoring practices.

FIGURE 5.4

Common Surveillance and Monitoring Techniques

- Placing hidden cameras and microphones
- Monitoring e-mail, voicemail, and fax use
- Recording telephone conversations
- Monitoring incoming and outgoing mail
- Searching desk or drawers
- Examining computer use
- Searching company property such as lockers or personal property such as briefcases

SOURCE: Ramsey (1999)

As is the case with technology, the point at which the employer's security concerns run up against the employee's civil liberties and right to privacy is unclear. Certainly, the use of various monitoring techniques suggests that this line has already been crossed. While the idea may seem improbable, some companies are experimenting with implanting RFID (radio frequency identification) chips in employees who are in highly sensitive positions as a way to monitor their movement and to positively identify them when necessary. RFID chips are routinely used to track pets, payment of highway tolls, and packages. One Australian casino attaches RFID chips in employee uniforms to prevent theft. A private video-surveillance company recently embedded silicon chips in four of its employees to assess the effectiveness of the technology when used in accessing a room filled with security video for government agencies and police (McGraw 2006). How widespread the use of this and other technologies will be in coming years is uncertain. However, given the modern world's propensity to adopt new technologies, along with its ongoing concerns about security and safety, the use of existing and emerging devices is constrained only by those who want to protect the civil liberties of society.

Drug Testing

Healthcare employees have access to many controlled substances, a fact that may account for significant problems with substance abuse among employees in this field. Healthcare organizations may initiate a pre-employment policy for cause and a random drug-testing program. A number of states have established laws that regulate the circumstances under which an employer may test for drugs. Thus, if an employer (e.g., a multisystem organization) has employees in multiple states, it must check for the specific requirements of each state. Testing must be done on a confidential basis, and employers must determine its next steps if the employee's results reveal drug use. An employer's options include disciplining the employee, referring the employee to an employee assistance program, or ordering the employee to attend a treatment or rehabilitation program.

Before initiating an employee drug-testing program, employers should consult with human resources personnel or a legal counsel who has experience in such matters. In addition, employers should use an independent, certified laboratory and medical review officer to conduct and interpret the testing. Using an outside laboratory will reduce the likelihood of employee claims for invasion of privacy.

HIPAA Compliance

To protect the health and medical information of an individual, the U.S. Department of Health and Human Services promulgated new regulations under HIPAA. HIPAA went into effect on April 14, 2003 (April 14, 2004 for smaller health plans) to ensure that employees have health insurance coverage after leaving a job and to provide a standard for electronic healthcare transactions. The HIPAA Privacy Rules regulate the use of protected health information that is electronically transmitted or maintained by health plans, healthcare clearinghouses, and healthcare providers.

The goal of the Privacy Rules is to protect the use and disclosure of protected health information in this age of technology. Employers who provide self-insured health coverage for employees may be unaware that the complex HIPAA regulations apply to them. These organizations should seek legal assistance when releasing such information to Worker's Compensation carriers or other third parties. Figure 5.5 offers tips on this and other violations.

Employment-at-Will Principle and Its Exceptions

In the United States, employment is generally at-will. This means that either party to the employment relationship may terminate the relationship for any

---

FIGURE 5.5
Measures to
Minimize
Litigation Over
Privacy
Violations

- Develop a policy statement that clarifies to employees that privacy in the workplace should not be assumed

- Use private information for justifiable reasons only

- Restrict the distribution of employees' personal information to company officials on a need-to-know basis

- Maintain employee medical records separately from the employee file

- Obtain a signed consent or waiver when using the employee's name or picture in an advertisement, a promotional material, or a training film

reason, without cause, and without notice. A substantial caveat to this rule, however, is that an employer cannot terminate an employee for a reason the law has deemed illegal. Examples of illegal grounds for termination include pregnancy, race and age, disability status, and the violation of federal and state restrictions.

Whistle-Blowing

An at-will employee may challenge termination based on violation of public policy. An employee, for instance, can claim wrongful discharge when terminated solely for refusing to commit perjury or for reporting the employer's violation of OSHA standards. Such challenges become difficult to handle if the employee's performance is also poor, as the employer may need to provide evidence that the termination is based solely on performance and not on the employee's whistle-blowing activities.

Many wrongful discharge cases also arise from an employer asking an employee to violate federal or state law on its behalf. Courts have allowed employees to pursue such claims because there is a public interest in protecting individuals who speak up about an employer's illegal acts. Such employers are viewed as harmful to the public in general (as in the case of unsafe practices at nuclear reactors that can pose dangers to communities) or to employees within the company (as in the case of locked fire and emergency exits that can result in injuries and deaths to workers). This public policy exception creates a cause of action for wrongful discharge when an employer fires a worker for reasons that violate or offend public policy (Yamada 1998).

A *whistle-blower* is an employee who discloses or otherwise exposes to law enforcement or a government agency any illegal activity in the workplace. Such illegal acts may involve, among other things, discrimination, fraud, or embezzlement. Employees who "blow the whistle" on their employers are protected by the law. It is illegal for an employer to retaliate against or mistreat an employee for whistle-blowing (see a case example in Figure 5.6). The False Claims Act (31 U.S.C. §§ 3729–33 [1991]), the only one of myriad laws in this area, governs actions in cases in which a company or an individual has financially defrauded the federal government. In 2005, the U.S. government recovered about $1.1 billion in healthcare fraud. In that same year, whistle-blowers were awarded $166 million (Stephenson 2005). Among the largest whistle-blower settlements in healthcare were the $900 million paid by Tenet Healthcare and the $1.7 billion that HCA paid between 2000 and 2003 (Walsh 2007). Various state whistle-blower laws only provide protection to the whistle-blower if the individual has reported the problem to his or her supervisor, allowing for a reasonable amount of time to correct the problem or if the individual has reason to believe the problem will not be corrected if reported (see Title 26 Maine Revised Statutes Annotated, § 833[2]).

Consider the scenario of a company that is hiring individuals who are not author-ized to work in the United States. An at-will employee reports this illegal practice to the Immigration and Naturalization Service (now known as the U.S. Citizenship and Immigration Services). The employer subsequently terminates the complain-ing employee. In this situation, the complaining employee may be successful in pursuing a claim for wrongful or bad-faith discharge based on the public policy exception.

Whistle-blowers often face an ethical and a moral dilemma when decid-ing whether to disclose the untoward information. They must consider the consequences of being deemed "disloyal" to their company and whether the disclosure benefits the public. The decision by an employee to blow the whis-tle clearly is difficult, as it presents a potential career detriment and the per-sonal stakes are high. The laws in this area seek to alleviate such concerns.

Personnel Policies

An employer's personnel policies, contained in handbooks or other corporate documents, that imply promises of continued employment may restrict the employer's ability to discharge employees at-will. Disciplinary documents prepared by inexperienced managers or human resources personnel may con-tain language that implies a promise of continued employment as well. For in-stance, consider an employee who has been absent from work for several con-secutive days without excuse. Her manager prepares a disciplinary document stating that the employee must maintain a better attendance record over the subsequent 12-month period to keep her job. This document may be inter-preted as the employee can stay on the job for 12 months providing she main-tains a good attendance record. One way to avoid such an implied promise is for a manager, with assistance from human resources or with legal advice, to use language such as the following: "Nothing contained herein alters the at-will nature of your employment or constitutes a promise of future employ-ment." Employee handbooks and personnel policies must contain similar lan-guage in an acknowledgment page signed by the employee and placed in the employee's personnel file.

Employment Agreements

Another notable exception to at-will employment is the employment agree-ment, with a specified term of employment. The terms of these agreements are either oral or written, or a combination of both. An employer may tell an employee upon hire, transfer, or promotion that the employee has a guaran-teed position for one year. However, this type of agreement is not recommended for either party. Typically, an employment agreement is in writing and is signed by both parties. Depending on the employee's position, an employment

1. Start date

2. Job title

3. Salary

4. Reporting relationships

5. Job duties or description

6. Term of employment

7. Notice and renewal periods

8. Termination-for-cause provisions

9. Severance payments

10. Bonus information

11. Fringe benefits

12. Confidentiality and work-product provisions

13. Noncompetition and nonsolicitation provisions

14. Assignment clauses

15. Choice of law

FIGURE 5.7

Standard Items in Employment Agreements

agreement can range from 1 page to as many as 25 or 50 pages in length. Some standard items in employment agreements appear in Figure 5.7.

Early termination of a fixed-term employment agreement usually entitles the employee to collect severance payments or liquidated damages specified under the agreement or to pursue a breach-of-contract claim in court. An employer has few rights when an employee terminates an employment agreement before the end of the term, because the courts will not force an employee to continue working against his or her will. Damages caused by the employee's departure also may be difficult to calculate.

Noncompetition and *nonsolicitation clauses* may be the only way to protect the employer against an employee whose departure may pose a competitive risk, confidentiality breach, or product-imitation issue to the employer. An employee presented with an agreement that contains these clauses should consult an attorney before signing the documents, given that these clauses often significantly limit an employee's ability to work after termination of employment. Likewise, employers should seek legal counsel in preparing contracts with such clauses, given that these clauses may be unenforceable under state law. (See the language provided in the California Business and Professional Code § 16600, "Except as provided in this chapter, every contract by which anyone is restrained from engaging in a lawful profession, trade or business of any kind is to that extent void" or because they are unreasonable.)

FIGURE 5.8
Case Example:
Covenant Not
to Compete
and Public
Policy

To be enforceable, most courts require that noncompetition clauses protect a legitimate business interest of the employer and are reasonable in terms of geography, time, and scope. For example, a hospital that prohibits a payroll clerk from working for any hospital in the United States for three years following termination probably is not protecting its legitimate business interest, and the court will find the clause unreasonable in terms of geography, time, and scope.

In Medical Specialist, Inc. v Sleweon (652 N.E.2d 517 [Ind. App. June 1995]), the plaintiff was an infectious disease specialist employed by a physician group practice. His employment agreement with the practice included a covenant not to compete. After resigning from his position, the defendant group practice sought to enforce the covenant not to compete. The plaintiff brought suit against his former employer, alleging the covenant was unenforceable based on public policy grounds. The court ruled against the doctor because there was no evidence of a shortage of such specialists in the restricted area.

Furthermore, in the healthcare context, noncompete clauses may be against public policy for physicians in specialty practice areas, where the availability of the service provided by the specialty physician is limited in the geographic region. See Figure 5.8 for an example of legal interpretation of a covenant not to compete.

Termination Procedures

Termination is rarely a happy event in an organization. Documentation of the circumstances surrounding the termination is as important as the reason for the termination itself. An employee, barring extreme circumstances in which the well-being of the organization is jeopardized, has the right to receive ample notice and an explanation of the employer's dissatisfaction with the employee's attempts to remedy the problematic issues. Documentation of all incidents, requests for changes in conduct, employee evaluations, and employee responses to evaluations is the responsibility of the employer. Sufficient documentation of the choice to sever an employer–employee relationship is one of the best strategies to demonstrate the fair handling of a termination.

Although not required by law or otherwise, some employers will provide at-will employees an opportunity to correct a performance problem before termination. Under the concept of progressive discipline, an employee is made aware of the problems and the steps required to correct them. The employee sometimes has a reasonable amount of time to correct the problem and is made aware of the consequences of inaction. Many organizations implement a termination-at-will policy that, in theory, permits the employer or the employee to sever employment relations at any time and for any reason. While these types of policies allow a heightened degree of employer discretion in termination matters, state and federal equal opportunity and discrimination standards supercede any private policies. A termination-at-will policy does not permit an employer to terminate an employee–employer relationship on non-work-performance grounds. An employee has the right to contest a termination, even if a termination-at-will policy exists, if he believes that he was fired for discriminatory reasons.

Furthermore, a prudent employer may regard termination-at-will policies lightly for any termination circumstance. Organizational termination-at-will policies have been likened to contract termination-without-cause clauses. Courts have pierced the veil of termination-without-cause policies even in cases when the termination was not of a discriminatory nature. In Harper v. Healthsource New Hampshire, Inc. (140 N.H. 770, 674 A.2d 962 [1996]), the termination of an employee without a specified reasonable cause was found to be against public policy. In this particular case, a physician was terminated without a cause or stated reason. Although this case stands alone in its findings, the ruling was intended to discourage bad-faith decisions that may endanger public welfare. Additionally, terminating without stating a cause was said to hamper the employee from properly responding to the termination. With these findings in mind, an employer may not retain much protection in termination at-will policies.

If termination is the proper course of action, several principles must be considered, including the following:

- *Analyze risk before termination.* Review carefully the personnel file and examine all facts and circumstances surrounding the termination. Ensure that human resources or management has investigated all valid complaints raised by the employee. Also, examine the employee's personal situation or status (e.g., pregnancy, disability, age).
- *Avoid procrastination.* Do not delay an employee's termination after satisfying the risk analysis.
- *Strategically choose the termination date.* Employees who are fired on Friday have the weekend to think about the termination and about possible recourse against the employer. Therefore, termination should be avoided on Fridays. Significant dates to the employee, such as a birthday, an anniversary, or a holiday, should also be avoided.
- *Consult human resources personnel.* Human resources requires advance notification to consider the possibility of a severance agreement or the necessity of communicating the termination to other affected employees

to avoid service disruption. The department can also process final paychecks and answer benefits questions.

- *Take action.* The individual who informs the employee of termination should be direct and to the point.

Separation Agreements

At the termination of employment, the employee and employer occasionally will enter into a separation or severance agreement. Such agreements often are required as a condition of receiving certain post-termination benefits, such as severance, health benefit payments, or outplacement services. The separation or severance agreement will be enforceable in court only if supported by valid consideration. This means that each party to the agreement must receive some benefit to which he or she otherwise was not entitled under a law, a regulation, a personnel policy, or an employment agreement.

The benefits to an employer in obtaining a severance agreement are that (1) it is a release of legal claims and (2) it is a covenant with the terminated employee not to sue. Because of the highly technical requirements of such a release, the employer should consult experienced human resources personnel or legal counsel. For example, in certain states, the severance agreement must specify state statutes to serve as a valid release of particular claims. Furthermore, to obtain a valid release for an age-discrimination claim, an employer must follow the ADEA (29 U.S.C. §§ 621–34) requirements: The employer must provide (1) a written agreement, (2) consideration, (3) advice in writing to seek counsel prior to signing, (4) 21 days to consider before signing, and (5) seven days to revoke after signing (29 U.S.C. § 626(f)[1]). Severance agreements also can require the employee to reaffirm or the employer to waive employment obligations, such as noncompetition and nonsolicitation provisions.

Dismissal for Cause

In the absence of an agreement or representation to the contrary, employers are not required to show cause to dismiss an employee. In many employment agreements, circumstances constituting a basis for "for-cause" termination are defined (see Figure 5.9).

FIGURE 5.9
Basis for For-Cause Termination

- Misconduct, including fraud, embezzlement, and commission of a criminal act
- Violation of corporate policy or practice
- Material failure to perform employment obligations
- For professionals, loss of license

Grievance Procedures

EEO Complaint Process

Under the EEO guidelines, no employee can be discriminated against based on the person's protected class status or as a result of reprisal. An employee or a class of employees, under such circumstances, must first file an administrative complaint with the EEOC. The first three phases—counseling, formal complaint, and appeal—are all part of the EEO process. The process exacts deadlines for complainants that are similar to statutes of limitations. If the EEOC finds no cause for the complaint, then the complainant has leave to file a judicial proceeding. The EEOC website is very helpful on all aspects of the process; see www.eeoc.gov.

Public Employees' Right to Due Process

Despite the many exceptions described earlier, at-will employment prevails for private employees. The same is not true, however, for public-sector employees, even in at-will states. Public employees enjoy certain due process rights and cannot be fired without a good reason or without notice and a hearing.

When considering the discharge of a public employee, an employer must remember that all public employees are protected by specific federal and state statutes and the federal and state constitutions. Both federal and most state governmental employees must be provided with written notice of the basis for any proposed disciplinary action. These employees also may be entitled to a hearing to allow them to defend against termination for cause. Because of these additional rights, management must seek professional assistance when terminating a public employee.

Alternative Dispute Resolution

Given the volume of employment litigation, some employers are attempting to control the escalating costs and media attention associated with litigation by including mandatory arbitration or *alternative dispute resolution* (ADR) clauses in employment contracts. These types of clauses mandate that any disagreement or claim that arises under the terms of employment will be subject to ADR. ADR agreements, however, do not preempt any rights of the EEOC or various state employment-rights commissions to investigate claims of discrimination. ADR agreements also do not apply to unemployment or Worker's Compensation claims, nor do they relieve an employer of its obligation to conduct investigation of claims such as racial discrimination or sexual harassment.

ADR has two main types: mediation and arbitration. *Mediation* is generally a nonbinding process in which opposing parties conduct semiformal settlement negotiations assisted by a neutral third-party mediator. *Arbitration,* much like a trial, is a more formal process in which both sides can present evidence and call witnesses; this form of ADR is typically binding on the parties and is enforceable by the courts. Employers usually exempt from ADR clauses their right to seek injunctive relief for violation of noncompetition and nonsolicitation provisions.

Other Employment Issues

Employers, especially in the healthcare industry, cannot allow their employees to perform job duties while impaired or suffering from extreme stress. Public health and liability problems arise for employers that do not take proactive measures in this regard. Employers should have confidential employee assistance programs available free of charge to all employees. Managers, with assistance from human resources or the legal department, also should discipline or terminate employees who work while impaired.

Job-Related Stress

Healthcare professionals and support staff experience great levels of stress because of the nature of their work (Rowe 1998). Such stressful conditions can be exacerbated if employees suffer from depression or anxiety, as those who suffer from these disorders are less likely to have a person to confide in and have greater incidences of prior psychiatric disorders. Other work-related stress inducers include job insecurity, managers who are not supportive, and limited potential for job promotion.

Workplace Substance Abuse

Substance abuse is characterized as the unlawful, unauthorized, or improper use of alcohol, over-the-counter drugs, or products with mind-altering properties. Changes in the impaired individual's performance, appearance, and behavior are likely to be obvious. The impact that these changes have on the employee's ability to carry out work-related duties without endangering his or her own safety or that of patients and coworkers is substantial (McAndrew and McAndrew 2000).

Impaired Professionals

A unique and challenging set of circumstances faces healthcare professionals who have substance abuse and dependence problems. Some of these issues are as follows:

- Fear of self-reporting because of the potential loss of licensure
- Positions of accountability and high visibility (Consequences of addiction problems are both personal and isolating, which conflict with public personas. Such problems also eventually affect people's work and the care of their patients.)
- Access to prescription medications that are highly addictive (Even when these professionals enter a treatment program and are highly motivated to change, their ongoing exposure and access to these medications put them at considerable risk for relapse.)
- Tendency to self-treat and self-prescribe (Professionals view their illness as a weakness and failure, preventing them from accepting and complying with medical advice from other professionals.)

Summary

Many of the laws and regulations discussed in this chapter are complex, interdependent, and often conflicting. The legal environment surrounding HRM is under constant federal scrutiny and reform. Additionally, the legal requirements imposed on an organization often shift according to industry- and state-specific regulations. Blanket policies and regulations are imposed on all employers, but there are regulations that apply specifically to segments of employers.

To accommodate the complexity of the workplace, managers must learn as much as possible about work environment regulations and should not rely on instinct alone when faced with dilemmas in areas such as whistleblowing, discrimination, or other types of highly sensitive situations. Because of the intricacy and specificity of workplace regulations, no single resource exists that managers can rely on. Instead, managers must acquire knowledge in specific and general areas of workplace laws; Table 5.3 lists resources available on the Internet.

Mishandling any situation can harm the employer's ability to attract and retain good employees and can lead to costly litigation and negative publicity. In general, a wise manager realizes the convoluted nature of his or her job and concedes to the necessity of ongoing education. An insightful manager executes thoughtful, deliberate choices. To make prudent law-abiding decisions, an employer must know the rights of both employer and employees. When dealing with employment issues, management should seek advice from experienced human resources personnel, in-house legal counsel, or external legal advisors.

TABLE 5.3
Internet
Resources for
Employment
Law

Web Site	Content
www.dol.gov	General site for the U.S. Department of Labor; contains labor statistics, DOL online library, current news, listing of programs and services, and contacts
www.eeoc.gov	General site for the U.S. Equal Employment Opportunity Commission; contains information regarding filing of charges, enforcement and litigation, enforcement statistics, small business information, and the Freedom of Information Act
www.access.gpo.gov	General site for the Government Printing Office; allows access to any public document printed by the federal government
www.nlrb.gov	General site for the National Labor Relations Board, the organization charged with administering the National Labor Relations Act. Its main duties include (1) the facilitation of fair relations between unions and employers and (2) the prevention and remedies of unfair labor practices by both parties
www.business.gov	General site of the U.S. Small Business Administration, the organization that provides guidance in all general business practices overseen by the government in some capacity
www.fmcs.gov	General site for the Federal Mediation and Conciliation Service, an independent agency created by Congress to facilitate strong and stable labor–management relations; contains information regarding dispute mediation, preventive mediation, alternative dispute resolution (litigation alternatives), arbitration services, and labor management grants

Discussion Questions

1. Is affirmative action still necessary to ensure equal employment opportunity? Given the diversity in the United States, should we begin to think about class-based rather than race-based affirmative action?

2. Has concern about sexual harassment gotten out of hand, and has political correctness replaced common sense?

3. Why is mental disability so difficult to define in the context of the Americans with Disabilities Act?

4. Should there be a uniform definition of reasonable accommodation in the Americans with Disabilities Act?

5. Why is sexual harassment so prevalent in the healthcare environment? What can be done to break this historical pattern?

6. Have federal antidiscrimination laws gone too far? Should public policy in the United States seek a return to employment-at-will?

7. What does public policy exception to employment-at-will mean?

8. Because employee handbooks may be used to contest a disciplinary procedure, what advice would you give to a work group that is assembling an employee handbook?

9. Under what circumstances would you use a progressive discipline process? When would you choose not to use such a procedure?

10. Given the great risks to the public that can result from the work of an impaired healthcare worker, should random drug testing be used in all healthcare organizations?

11. Consider the case of a physician who has been practicing for 15 years and is one of the few well-established physicians in a small community. How would you deal with information about this physician's abuse of alcohol or drugs?

12. Has the law against retaliation gone too far? How can an employer prevent the "shunning" of an employee who remains in the workplace and has filed a claim against the employer?

Experiential Exercises

Case 1   Dr. Mind, a prominent psychiatrist at the Mensa Medical Center, a Department of Veterans Affairs (VA) Hospital, treated Ms. Puppet for anxiety and panic disorder. Dr. Mind used recognized techniques for treating Ms. Puppet, including medication, psychotherapy, and hypnosis. During the many hypnosis sessions, Dr. Mind began a sexual relationship with Ms. Puppet. She did not remember having relations with Dr. Mind, as Dr. Mind, during hypnosis, had instructed her to have no memory of her thoughts.

On one occasion, however, Ms. Puppet noticed that, after she left Dr. Mind's of-fice, her undergarments were on backwards and her skirt was not buttoned properly. She became suspicious of Dr. Mind, so she forced herself to not fall into a hypnotic state at her next session with Dr. Mind. At this session, when Dr. Mind believed Ms. Puppet was in a hypnotic state, he began undressing her. She then broke her silence, confronted him, and left his office.

Following the confrontation, Dr. Mind was placed on paid administrative leave pending an investigation, which resulted in his admission of guilt and termination. Ms. Puppet then sued the United States, because the actions occurred at a VA hospital, under the Federal Torts Claim Act (28 U.S.C. Section 2675[a]). Ms. Puppet's attorney argued that Dr. Mind's acts took place during regularly scheduled therapy sessions, during working hours, and in an office provided to Dr. Mind by the VA hospital. Accordingly, under the doctrine of respondeat superior, the United States was liable for Dr. Mind's acts. The United States contended that it was not liable because Dr. Mind's motives were not intended to benefit the employee and that criminal and/or tortuous acts clearly fall outside the scope of employment.

Case Questions

1. Is the United States liable based on a theory that the wrongful acts of Dr. Mind took place within the scope of his employment?
2. What other theories may apply, such as the foreseeability of transference?
3. What can employers do to prevent such wrongful acts?

For helpful information on this situation, see the basis for the hypothetical case: Doe v. United States of America (912 F. Supp. 193 [E.D. Va. 1995]). Also, for study of transference, see Allen (2003).

Case 2   Dr. Zhivago grew up in a small town in North Carolina. He was extremely intelligent and did well in college and medical school. After a fellowship in thoracic surgery, he was offered positions, with extremely good employment terms and conditions, in various reputable medical practices throughout the United States.

Feeling some duty to his hometown, however, Dr. Zhivago decided to return to his local community to practice medicine. He was offered and accepted employment with a multispecialty group practice. The practice paid his expenses to relocate back to his hometown and required him to sign an employment agreement that contained a noncompetition provision. Being a trusting person, Dr. Zhivago did not seek an attorney's advice before signing the agreement. After several years of working at this practice, Dr. Zhivago fell in love with a patient who resided in another small town about 30 miles away. After this patient's recovery, Dr. Zhivago proposed marriage and agreed to move and to work in his fiancé's hometown. He opened a private practice in this town.

After giving notice to his employer, however, Dr. Zhivago received a stern letter from the employer's counsel, reminding him of his employment agreement. The agreement's noncompetition provision prevented him from working as a thoracic surgeon within a 60-mile radius of his current employer for one year after leaving employment. Given the rural nature of the community, Dr. Zhivago was the only thoracic surgeon within a 90-mile radius of either practice. He would have to move to the big city to practice medicine, leaving all the residents of his hometown (as well as those of his new wife's hometown) without a practicing thoracic surgeon.

Case Questions

1. Given that such agreements restrict competition, under what circumstances should a court enforce a covenant not to compete?
2. In general, courts will enforce a covenant not to compete if it is (1) in writing, (2) entered into at the time of employment as part of the employment contract, (3) based on reasonable consideration, (4) reasonable with respect to time and territory, and (5) not against public policy. Using this as a guide, how should the court decide in this case?

For additional information, see Iredell Digestive Disease Clinic, P.A., v. Petrozza, 92 N.C.App. 21, 373 S.E.2d 449 (1988), aff'd per curiam, 324 N.C.327, 377 S.E.2d 750 (1989).

Case 3   Among those who took the Civil Service Exam, Mr. Imelda received the highest score on the written portion. Feeling confident, he applied for a position with the city of Cary. The position required the preparation of written reports and the handling of complaints from the public, either by telephone or face to face. Mr. Imelda is a native of the Philippines, and English is his second language. When he was interviewed for the position, the two interviewers had difficulty understanding him because of his thick Filipino accent. The city of Cary decided not to hire Mr. Imelda because it believed that his heavy accent would impede his verbal capability to respond to complaints, which was an integral part of the position.

Upon learning that he did not receive the job, Mr. Imelda exhausted his administrative remedies and then filed an action under Title VII of the Civil Rights Act. He claimed he was discriminated against because of his accent and, thus, his national origin.

Case Questions
1. Is the city of Cary liable under the disparate treatment theory?
2. What could the city of Cary have done to mitigate the risk of this claim?
3. What defenses are available to the city of Cary?

For helpful information on this situation, see the basis for the hypothetical case—Fragrante v. City and County of Honolulu, 888 F.2d 591 (9th Cir. 1989).

Case 4   Mr. Jones and Ms. Meyers were employed by Lester & Meyer, PLLC, the only law firm in a small town in Oregon. After working on an employment class-action suit under FLSA for several years, Mr. Jones and Ms. Meyers grew closer and fell in love. They decided to marry, and both excitedly announced their intentions to the partners of Lester & Meyer, PLLC. Instead of being congratulated, the firm asked which of the two would resign following the wedding. Ms. Meyers was a partner and Mr. Jones was an associate, and, under the firm's antinepotism policy, Mr. Jones could no longer work for the firm. Additionally, the firm also had a nonfraternization policy, which both Mr. Jones and Ms. Meyers violated by dating. Mr. Jones is considering suing Lester & Meyer, PLLC.

Case Questions
1. Does the antinepotism policy serve a valid purpose in avoiding favoritism or conflict of interest?
2. Does the nonfraternization policy serve an important purpose in protecting the firm from claims of sexual harassment?
3. Do policies that require one person to quit upon marriage have a disparate impact on a protected group?
4. Would the situation be easier to address if the couple lived in a town where many other law firms existed?

For additional information, see Love at Work, 13 Duke J. Gender L. & Pol'y 237 (2006); Yuhas v. Libbey-Owens-Ford Co., 562 F.2d 496 (7th Cir. 1977).

References

Allen, T. 2003. "Notes and Comments: The Foreseeability of Transference: Extending Employer Liability Under Washington Law for Therapist Sexual Exploitation of Patients." *Washington Law Review* 78: 525.

American Management Association (AMA). 2005. "2005 Electronic Monitoring and Surveillance Survey: Many Companies Monitoring, Recording, Videotaping—and Firing—Employees." [Online information; retrieved 1/22/08.] www.amanet.org/ press/amanews/ems05.htm.

Becker, G. 1957. *The Economics of Discrimination.* Chicago: University of Chicago Press.

BNA. 1994. "Medical Center Employee Awarded $1 Million in Massachusetts Suit." *Employee Relations Weekly* 12 (January 31): 111–12.

Bouvier, C. 1996. "Why At-Will Employment Is Dying." *Personnel Journal* 75 (5): 123–28.

Castaneda, C. 1977. "Panel Backs FAA on Retire-at-60 Rule." *USA Today* (July 16): 11.

Cooter, R. 1994. "Market Affirmative Action." *San Diego Law Review* 31: 133–68.

Davis, E. 2002. "Comment: The Doctrine of Respondeat Superior: An Application to Employers' Liability for the Computer or Internet Crimes Committed by Their Employees." *Albany Law Journal of Science & Technology* 12: 683–713.

Decker, P. J. 1997. "Sexual Harassment in Health Care: A Major Productivity Problem." *The Health Care Supervisor* 16 (1): 1–14.

Dobbin, F. 2004. "The Social Sciences: Do the Social Sciences Shape Corporate Anti-Discrimination Practice: The United States and France." *Comparative Labor Law and Policy Journal* 23 (3): 829–63.

EEOC v. Lutheran Medical Center, No. 01-5494, E.D.N.Y. (2003).

Employment Law Update. 1991. "ADA: The Final Regulations (Title I): A Lawyer's Dream/An Employer's Nightmare." *Employment Law Update* 16 (9): 1.

England, P. 1994. "Neoclassical Economists' Theories of Discrimination." In *Equal Employment Opportunity: Labor Market Discrimination and Public Policy,* edited by P. Burstein. New York: Aldine de Gruyter.

Equal Employment Opportunity Commission, Civil Service Commission, Department of Labor, and Department of Justice. 1978. "Uniform Guidelines on Employee Selection Procedures." *Federal Register* 43 (166): 38290–315.

Equal Employment Opportunity Commission (EEOC). 1997. "Facts About Age Discrimination." [Online information; retrieved 1/22/08.] www.eeoc.gov/facts/age.html.

———. 2003. "Hospital in New York to Pay Over $5 Million to Settle Sexual Harassment by Doctor." [Online information; retrieved 1/22/08.] www.eeoc.gov/press/4-9-03.html.

———. 2007a. "Charge Statistics FY 1997 Through FY 2006. [Online information; retrieved 1/22/08.] www.eeoc.gov/stats/charges.html.

———. 2007b. "Sexual Harassment." [Online information; retrieved 3/21/08.] www.eeoc.gov/types/sexual_harassment.html.

Fisher, A. B. 1994. "Businessmen Like to Hire by the Numbers." In *Equal Employment Opportunity: Labor Market Discrimination and Public Policy,* 269–73, edited by P. Burstein. New York: Aldine de Gruyter.

Furrow, B. R., T. L. Greaney, S. H. Johnson, T. Jost, and R. L. Schwartz. 1997. *Health Law: Cases, Materials and Problems,* 3rd Edition, 237–307. St. Paul, MN: West Publishing Co.

Gabel, J., and N. Mansfield. 2003. "The Information Revolution and Its Impact on the Employment Relationship: An Analysis of the Cyberspace Workplace." *American Business Law Journal* 40 (2): 301–53.

General Dynamics Land Systems v. Cline 540 U.S. 581 (2004).

Greenlaw, P. S., and J. P. Kohl. 1995. "The Equal Pay Act: Responsibilities and Rights." *Employee Rights and Responsibilities Journal* 8 (4): 295–307.

Hibino, Y., K. Ogino, and M. Inagaki. 2006. "Sexual Harassment of Female Nurses by Patients in Japan." *Journal of Nursing Scholarship* 38 (4): 400–05.

Hill, C., and E. Silva. 2005. *Drawing the Line: Sexual Harassment on Campus*. Washington, DC: American Association of University Women Educational Foundation.

Kobata, M. 1992. "The Civil Rights Act of 1991." *Personnel Journal*, p. 48.

Lambda Legal. 2007. [Online information; retrieved 11/07.] www.lambdalegal.org.

Ledvinka, J., and V. G. Scarpello. 1991. *Federal Regulation of Personnel and Human Resource Management*, 2nd Edition. Boston: PWS-Kent.

Lee, R. D., and P. S. Greenlaw. 1995. "The Legal Evolution of Sexual Harassment." *Public Administration Review* 55 (4): 357–64.

McAndrew, K. G., and S. J. McAndrew. 2000. "Workplace Substance Abuse Impairment: The Occupational Health Care Provider's Role." *Journal of the American Association of Occupational Health Nurses* (January): 32–45.

McGraw, M. 2006. "Positive ID?" [Online article on *Human Resource Executive Online*; retrieved 1/22/08.] http://hre.lrp.com/HRE/story.jsp?storyId=5669707&query=hurts.

Mikulenak, M. 1992. "House Takes Stand Against Harassment, Discrimination." *The American Nurse* 1 (July–August): 13.

National Committee on Pay Equity. 2008. "The Wage Gap Over Time: In Real Dollars, Women See a Continuing Gap." [Online information; retrieved 3/30/08.] www.pay-equity.org/info-time.html.

Ramsey, R. 1999. "The 'Snoopervision' Debate: Employer Interest vs. Employee Privacy." *Supervision* 60 (8): 40–45.

Reno, J., and D. Thornburgh. 1995. "ADA—Not a Disabling Mandate." *Wall Street Journal* (July 26): A12.

Rowe, M. M. 1998. "Hardiness as a Stress Mediating Factor of Burnout Among Healthcare Providers." *American Journal of Healthcare Studies* 14 (1): 16–20.

Segal, J. A. 1992. "Seven Ways to Reduce Harassment Claims." *HR Magazine* (January): 84–85.

Sherer, J. L. 1995. "Sexually Harassed." *Hospitals & Health Networks* 69 (2): 54–57.

Smith v. City of Jackson Mississippi, 125 U.S. 1536 (2005).

Stephenson, C. E. 2005. "Health Care Whistleblower Suits Under False Claims Act on the Rise." *Daily Record* and the *Kansas City Daily News-Press*, November 23.

U.S. Department of Labor (DOL). 2002. "Facts on Executive Order 11246—Affirmative Action." [Online information; retrieved 1/22/08.] www.dol.gov/esa/regs/compliance/ ofccp/aa.htm.

Walsh, A., and S. C. Borowski. 1995. "Gender Differences in Factors Affecting Healthcare Administration Career Development." *Hospital & Health Services Administration* 40 (2): 263–77.

Walsh, M. W. 2007. "Blowing the Whistle, Many Times." *New York Times,* November 18.

Yamada, D. C. 1998. "Voices from the Cubicle: Protecting and Encouraging Private Employee Speech in the Post Industrial Workplace." *Berkeley Journal of Employment and Labor Law* 19 (1): 1–51.

Yusuf, Ç., and S. S. Yusuf. 2007. "Sexual Harassment Against Nurses in Turkey." *Journal of Nursing Scholarship* 39 (2): 200–06.

Zezima, K. 2006. "Archdiocese Hospital Chief Quits After Harassment Accusations." *New York Times,* May 26.

WORKFORCE DIVERSITY

Rupert M. Evans, Sr., DHA, FACHE

Learning Objectives

After completing this chapter, the reader should be able to

- understand how proactive use of diversity principles can transform the organization's culture;
- understand the business case for diversity and inclusion in healthcare organizations;
- work toward creating an inclusive organizational culture;
- define the roles that healthcare providers, management, and governance play in building a business imperative for diversity within the organization; and
- discuss how healthcare leaders can develop a diversity program in their organizations.

Introduction

When you hear the term "diversity," what comes to mind? To some, the word means the differences between human beings related to race or ethnicity. To others, it means the uniqueness of each individual. A few people still may jump up to argue that diversity is just a code word for affirmative action.

Healthcare organizations across the United States are beginning to move toward embracing and fostering workforce diversity. This cultural change means adopting new values that are inclusive and appropriately managing a diverse workforce. In the future, diversity will drive the business practices of hospitals and other healthcare organizations, and this dynamic will require strong leadership. This change will take time, but in the words of Reverend Jesse Jackson, "Time is neutral and does not change things. With courage and initiative, leaders change things."

In this chapter, we provide a definition of diversity and a framework for understanding the different ways people view the term. In addition, we highlight several studies and legal issues pertaining to this topic and enumerate methods for building a case for and establishing a diversity program.

A Definition of Diversity

People define diversity in many ways, depending on the way they live in and view society. In his book, *The 10 Lenses: Your Guide to Living and Working in a Multicultural World*, author Mark Williams (2001) discusses the framework that explains the way people see the world:

1. The *assimilationist* wants to conform and fit in with the group to which he or she belongs.
2. The *colorblind* ignores race, color, ethnicity, and other cultural factors.
3. The *cultural centrist* seeks to improve the welfare of his or her cultural group by accentuating its history and identity.
4. The *elitist* believes in the superiority of the upper class and embraces the importance of family roots, wealth, and social status.
5. The *integrationist* supports breaking down all barriers between racial groups by merging people of different cultures together in communities and in the workplace.
6. The *meritocratist* lives by the adage, "cream rises to the top"—the belief that hard work, personal merit, and winning a competition determine one's success.
7. The *multiculturist* celebrates the diversity of cultures, seeking to retain the native customs, languages, and ideas of people from other countries.
8. The *seclusionist* protects himself or herself from racial, cultural, and/or ethnic groups in fear that they may diminish the character and quality of his or her group's experiences within society.
9. The *transcendent* focuses on the human spirit and people's universal connection and shared humanity.
10. The *victim/caretaker* views liberation from societal barriers as a crucial goal and sees oppression as not only historical but also contemporary.

With this framework in mind, it is easier to understand why so many interpretations of the same idea exist. For our purposes, we describe diversity in the context of three key dimensions: (1) human diversity, (2) cultural diversity, and (3) systems diversity. Each dimension needs to be understood and managed in the healthcare workplace.

Human diversity includes the attributes that make a human being who he or she is, such as race, ethnicity, age, gender, family status (single, married, divorced, widowed, with or without children), sexual orientation, physical abilities, and so on. These traits are what frequently come to mind first when individuals consider the differences in people. Human diversity is a core dimension because it defines who we are as individuals. This dimension is with us throughout every stage of our lives, guiding how we define ourselves and how we are perceived by others. A workplace definition of diversity includes human diversity as a minimum.

Cultural diversity encompasses a person's beliefs, values, family structure practice (nuclear or extended family, independent living), and mind-set as a result of his or her cultural, community, and environmental experiences. This dimension includes language, social class, learning style, ethics or moral compass, religion, lifestyle, work style, global perspectives, and military views. Cultural diversity is a secondary dimension, but it can have a powerful impact on how a person behaves in the workplace. The cultural norms vary from one culture to another and influence how individuals interact with their work environments. For example, some religious groups are forbidden from working on the Sabbath, and this exemption has an impact on work scheduling and even hiring decisions.

Systems diversity relates to the differences among organizations in work structure and pursuits. This dimension includes teamwork reengineering, strategic alliances, employee empowerment, quality focus, educational development, corporate acquisitions, and innovation. Systems diversity deals with systems thinking and the ability to recognize how functions in the work environment are connected with diversity. In a multicultural, diverse, and inclusive workplace, organizational systems are integrated to enhance innovation, encourage teamwork, and improve productivity.

All of these dimensions are important and are present in the healthcare workplace, and all leaders should recognize them. The challenge is in seeing not only our differences but also our similarities as individuals, as professionals, and as members of a group. Leaders must develop effective strategies to manage the differences (and highlight similarities), and this will lead to building effective teams and a higher-performing organization (Guillory 2003).

Managing diversity is not an easy task, as a number of barriers often get in the way of achieving a harmonious working environment. Some of these barriers, which revolve around the diversity dimensions mentioned earlier, can be a great source of tension and conflict. For instance, a person's culture can be a barrier to a work team when other members of the group are not respectful of or misunderstand the person's values, beliefs, or even clothing, which that person gained through his or her cultural background. Examples of a cultural difference may be the person's hairstyle or affinity to wear religious artifacts. The education, race/ethnicity, work style, empowerment, and relationship/task orientation of an individual can also become barriers if they are not properly understood and managed.

Prejudice in the Workplace

Prejudice is a set of views held by individuals about members of other groups. Prejudice is pre-judgment; hence, it is not based on facts and/or experience.

It affects the way people react toward and think of other people, and it can be as innocent as children choosing to not play with children they deem different from themselves or as harmful as adults not associating with certain people because English is not their native language.

Formally, prejudice can be defined as a set of institutionalized assumptions, attitudes, and practices that has an invisible-hand effect in systematically advantaging members of more powerful groups over members of less dominant groups. This type of prejudice occurs in many healthcare institutions. Some examples include culturally biased assessment and selection criteria, cultural norms that condone or permit racial or sexual harassment, lower performance expectations for certain groups, and a collective misconception about a specific group that relegates the group's members to unfair positions. An example of the latter is stereotyping.

Stereotypes are generalizations about individuals based on their identity, group membership, or affiliations (Dreachslin 1996). A common stereotype in the healthcare management field is the assumption that black executives are not as qualified as their white counterparts. Thus, African-American executives are tested more often to prove their competence, while their white contemporaries are assumed to be capable from the start. (This fact is substantiated in the race/ethnic surveys discussed later in the chapter.)

The concept of "comfort and risk" relates to a human being's natural need to feel comfortable and to avoid risk. People tend to prefer to work with others from similar racial or ethnic backgrounds because doing so provides them with a certain amount of comfort and shields them from a certain amount of risk. Although subordinate–superior relationships that involve people from different backgrounds work sufficiently to allow people to get the job done, they often fail to lead to the close bonds that form between a mentor and a protégé.

Given the systemic existence of prejudice and the way it influences people's mind-set and behavior in the workplace, the fair and accurate assessment of minority employees (caregivers, support staff, and managers alike) remains an organizational dilemma rather than an established practice. For instance, existing literature provides evidence that managers systematically give higher performance ratings to subordinates who belong to the same racial group as they do, while high performers from minority groups remain comparatively invisible in the managerial/leadership selection process (Thomas and Gabarro 1999).

The Business Case for Diversity

In 1900, one in eight Americans was non-white; today, this ratio is one in four. By 2050, the ratio will be one in three (IOM 2004). The healthcare industry needs physicians, nurses, and other providers, but it also needs caregivers who reflect the diversity of the population, who, at one point or another, become patients. The same is true for healthcare managers and executives. Therefore, healthcare organizations must ensure that their caregivers and leaders represent the backgrounds of the communities they serve. In addition, healthcare executives must look for new insights, examples, and best practices to help navigate their organizations through a diversity journey. A key challenge in this journey is establishing a business case for having a diverse workforce.

The business case for diversity is unique for each organization. The circumstances, environment, and community demographics of one organization cannot be generalized to another institution. However, some elements are common in all organizations, which can be the basis of a diversity program: the healthcare marketplace, employee skills and talent, and organizational effectiveness. These elements will drive the institution's investment in and commitment to diversity. An organization can achieve and sustain growth and profitability by doing the following:

- Expand market share by adding or enhancing services that target diverse populations.
- Link the marketplace with the workplace through recruiting, developing, and retaining employees with diverse racial/ethnic backgrounds.
- Create and implement workplace policies and management practices that maximize the talent and productivity of employees with diverse backgrounds.

The facts are that all minority groups buy and consume healthcare services, many of them are educated and trained to either provide healthcare services or manage operations, and many of them currently work within the field and understand its complexities. Hospitals and other healthcare organizations cannot afford to miss such opportunities. They can seek, cultivate, and retain minority talent to help them compete in today's diverse healthcare environment. Failure to take advantage of these opportunities will mean the difference between being a provider and employer of choice and losing ground to competitors.

Governance Impact

The organization's board of governance can help in this regard. Members of the board or trustees are the ultimate links to the communities served by a healthcare organization. They know the makeup of the population the organization serves and seeks to target, and they have insights into their communities' healthcare needs. Because board members are part of the community, they have an interest in making sure that the organization that they represent is not only providing inclusive services but is also being a fair and equitable employer and neighbor. With this perspective in mind, governance should support a business strategy that promotes community goodwill, encourages growth, considers present social and demographic transformations and hence future needs, and emphasizes culturally competent and sensitive healthcare. Most importantly, members of the board should also reflect the multicultural mix of the surrounding communities.

Considering all of the challenges faced by any healthcare board, why should it be concerned with diversity? One of the many reasons is to protect the organization's bottom line. The financial impact of problems stemming from racial discrimination and discriminatory practices can be substantial. Well-publicized cases of large organizations committing or turning their backs on such practices provide evidence of the extent of cost consequences. For example, in 2007, two Equal Employment Opportunity Commission lawsuits were filed alleging racial and sexual discrimination. The first was filed in South Florida claiming that a manager at two Nordstrom stores in Palm Beach County harassed a Hispanic woman and other "similarly situated individuals" based on these individuals' national origin and race and that the company failed to take prompt action (*Puget Sound Business Journal* 2007). The second was a lawsuit against United HealthCare of Florida that accused a male executive of subjecting another male executive to repeated verbal sexual harassment (EEOC. 2007). This latter case resulted in a $1.8 million settlement and an order for United HealthCare to distribute a new antiharassment policy to all of its employees (EEOC 2007). Another reason that the board should support diversity initiatives is to encourage and strengthen employee commitment to the organization. Simply, a diverse workforce is an asset. It differentiates an organization in the marketplace, giving it an edge against its competitors in terms of inclusiveness, cultural sensitivity and competency, and even progressive practice.

Board commitment to the principles of diversity may lead to shifts in the corporate culture as well, allowing all stakeholders to contribute to the overall success of the organization and its mission. Trustees should hold organizational leaders and managers accountable for setting and following high diversity standards. This practice will lead to an improved organization and to healthy communities.

Legal Issues

The debate continues over whether having a diversity program is the right thing to do or whether it enhances shareholder/stakeholder value. The answer is both—not only is it the right thing to do, but it also adds value to the organization. Educated, skilled, and experienced professionals and workers who are considered in the minority (including but are not limited to women, racial and ethnic minorities, and people with physical challenges) bring strategic and unique perspectives into their roles, generate productive dialogue, and challenge the status quo. All of these are essential to the practices, products and services, and operations of a healthcare organization. If these are not reasons enough to maintain a diverse workforce, various laws also prohibit employment discrimination.

The Civil Rights Act of 1964 was signed into law on July 2, 1964. This legislation was intended to ensure that the financial resources of the federal government would no longer subsidize racial discrimination (Smith 1999). This law bans discrimination in any activities, such as training, employment, or construction, that are funded by federal monies. Discrimination is also prohibited in entities that contract with organizations that receive federal funds. Every recipient of federal funds is required to provide written assurances that nondiscrimination is practiced throughout the institution. Among the first major tests of the Civil Rights Act was the decision of the U.S. Court of Appeals for the Fourth Circuit on the case of Simkins v. Moses Cone Memorial Hospital. The decision struck down the separate-but-equal provisions of the Hill-Burton Act and gave the federal government the necessary power to enforce the Civil Rights Act (Smith 1999).

The Civil Rights Act also protects individuals whose native language is not English. The U.S. Department of Justice has issued the "National Origin Discrimination Against Persons with Limited English Proficiency (LEP) Guidance." This guidance, intended for recipients of federal funds, prohibits discrimination of people who have limited English-language proficiency. It requires federally funded entities to ensure that people whose primary language is not English can access and understand services, programs, and activities provided by these organizations. This mandate has made a serious impact in the way healthcare organizations, especially those in areas with large numbers of individuals who speak English as a second language (ESL), frame their service offerings. The National Council on Interpreting in Health Care has put together "The Terminology of Health Care Interpreting," a glossary of terms intended to help healthcare leaders in developing programs for ESL patients; visit www.ncihc.org for more information on this glossary.

See Chapter 5 for a comprehensive discussion of the Civil Rights Act and other laws that protect groups who are considered in the minority.

Diversity in Healthcare Leadership: Two Major Studies

Despite the demographic changes in the U.S. population, and hence in the healthcare field, few minorities are present in the executive suite. Within the last decades, two major studies were undertaken to understand the factors behind minorities' difficult climb on the healthcare management ladder. As the findings of these studies indicate, although improvements are continually being made in terms of how workforce and leadership diversity is viewed and valued in healthcare organizations, a lot of work is left to be done.

Study 1: A Race/Ethnic Comparison of Career Attainments in Healthcare Management

In 1992, the American College of Healthcare Executives (ACHE) and the National Association of Health Services Executives (NAHSE) conducted a study that compared the career attainment of Caucasian and African-American healthcare executives. The study found that among executives with similar training and experience, African Americans were in lower-level positions, made less money, and had lower levels of job satisfaction (ACHE 2002). The results of this study made way for the creation of the Institute for Diversity in Health Management (IFD), the only organization committed exclusively to promoting managerial diversity within the healthcare field.

In 1996, ACHE, with assistance and support from NAHSE, IFD, the Association of Hispanic Healthcare Executives (AHHE), and the Executive Leadership Development Program of the Indian Health Services (IHS), conducted a follow-up survey using many of the items included in the first survey. This second survey, completed and published in 1997, revealed that 23 percent of the U.S. hospital workforce was made up of African Americans and Hispanics. Unfortunately, less than 2 percent of these minority groups held the positions of president, chief executive officer, and chief operating officer.

The third cross-sectional study, released in 2002, was conducted to determine if the race/ethnic disparities in healthcare management careers had narrowed since the 1997 release of the second survey and was based on the observations and experiences of a similar pool of respondents. In planning this study, leaders of ACHE, AHHE, IFD, and NAHSE invited the collaboration of the Executive Leadership Development Program of the IHS so that the career attainments of Native-American executives could also be assessed.

Following is a summary of the most important findings of the third study (ACHE 2003):

- More white administrators than minority administrators worked in hospital settings.
- White female administrators earned more than female minority administrators. When controlling for education and experience, compensation earned by white women remained higher than the compensation for male and female members of minority groups.
- White male administrators earned more than male minority administrators. When controlling for experience and education, the total compensation of male African-American and Hispanic administrators was approximately equal to that of their white counterparts.
- Minority administrators expressed lower levels of job satisfaction than did white administrators. The items with which low satisfaction was reported included the following:
  1. Pay and fringe benefits were not proportionate to the minority administrators' contribution to their organization.

2. The degree of respect and fair treatment that minority administrators received from their leaders was inadequate.

3. The sanctions and treatment that minority administrators faced when they made a mistake were more severe than their action called for.

- Fewer minority administrators than white administrators expressed that their organizations had great personal meaning to them.

- More minority administrators than white administrators stated that they experienced racial/ethnic discriminatory acts in the past five years, such as not being hired or being evaluated with inappropriate standards.

- Only about 15 percent of female minority administrators aspired to be chief executive officers. More white male administrators had such aspirations than male minority administrators.

- The majority of minority administrators endorsed efforts to increase the percentage of racial/ethnic minorities in senior healthcare management positions. Nearly half of their white counterparts were neutral or opposed to such efforts.

Recommendations to address the disparities found between the white and minority groups are being developed. A fourth race/ethnic survey is expected to be conducted in 2008.

Study 2: Advancing Diversity Leadership in Healthcare

In 1998, Witt/Kieffer, an executive search firm, conducted a national survey of healthcare leaders (e.g., chief executive officers, presidents, human resources executives) to determine the advances in and barriers to recruiting and retaining women and minority leaders in the industry. The survey revealed divergences in opinions between nonminority and minority respondents. Nonminority respondents reported that minority leaders were hard to find, while minority respondents claimed that these leaders were not looking either hard enough or in the right places. Another significant difference in perspective was on the issue of whether organizational or even individual resistance to minority leadership was part of the problem (Witt/Kieffer 2006).

In 2006, Witt/Kieffer conducted a follow-up survey that involved human resources executives and minority leaders in hospitals and health systems nationwide. Seventy-one percent of respondents were nonminorities, and 29 percent were from minority groups. The project also included phone interviews with respondents who were willing to share additional thoughts regarding diversity leadership (Witt/Kieffer 2006).

The following are the main findings of the 2006 study:

- Eighty-two percent of the nonminority respondents and 81 percent of the minority group agreed or strongly agreed with the statement, "Internal diversity programs support the organization's overall mission/vision."

- Seventy-nine percent of minority and 68 percent of nonminority respondents agreed that "Internal diversity programs are strategic to organizational success."
- Virtually all respondents agreed that "Internal diversity programs demonstrate the value of cultural differences in an organization." By and large, both groups also shared the belief that organizations commit to diversity recruiting because they want to achieve "cultural competence" organization-wide.
- Seventy-two percent of minority and 63 percent of nonminority respondents agreed that "Internal diversity programs provide diversity staffing that mirrors the diversity of the patient population."
- Only 28 percent of nonminority respondents and 12 percent of the minority group agreed that "Healthcare organizations have been effective in closing the diversity leadership gap over the past five years."
- Nearly 73 percent of nonminority respondents personally believed that opportunities for diversity in leadership have improved over the past five years. Only 34 percent of minorities shared that personal belief. Also, 67 percent of nonminorities agreed that "The availability of diversity leadership positions in healthcare organizations has improved over the past five years," but only 30 percent of minority respondents agreed.
- Minority respondents remained unconvinced that they are "well represented today in healthcare organization management teams."
- Both respondent groups agreed that internal diversity programs drive organizational success and cultural competence. However, respondents, particularly minorities, expressed skepticism about whether hospitals and healthcare systems commit to diversity recruiting because those organizations believe diversity is good for business.
- Seventy-two percent of nonminorities and 53 percent of minorities agreed that healthcare organizations are effective in diversity recruiting because they have a genuine interest in it. Seventy-three percent of nonminorities and about 50 percent of minorities believed healthcare organizations are effective at diversity recruiting because they take their responsibility to do so seriously.
- Respondents held widely divergent views on the most important barriers to diversity recruitment, retention, and leadership development. The only barrier for which general agreement was reached was the "lack of commitment by top management."

Diversity Management

According to the Institute for Diversity in Health Management (2007), managing a diverse workforce involves the following elements:

- *Employee perspective.* Diversity management creates an environment where every hospital or health system employee feels valued, appreciated and respected and who, in turn, talks about the organization within the community with pride. Diversity management allows 100 percent of employees, whatever their capabilities, to achieve 100 percent of their potential 100 percent of the time.

- *Patient focus.* Diversity management creates an environment where because all patients feel valued, they are highly satisfied and loyal. Diversity management means understanding the cultural and ethnic values within a community. As a result, community members choose the organization, which increases market share.
- *Inclusion.* Diversity management means sending a message to minorities that there are leaders within the organization to champion their medical needs. If a minority patient knows the COO [chief operating officer] shares his or her ethnicity, for example, then that patient likely assumes his or her best interests will be served.
- *Community perspective.* Diversity management means bringing the community into the organization, specifically at the governance level. Putting prominent minority leaders on the hospital or health system board forges a bond with the community, which in turn creates patient comfort with and loyalty to the organization.

The Impact of Diversity on Care Delivery

According to the National Institutes of Health, "the diversity of the American population is one of the nation's greatest assets; one of its greatest challenges is reducing the profound disparity in health status of America's racial and ethnic minorities" (Smedley and Stith 2002). The Institute of Medicine's landmark report in 2002, entitled *Unequal Treatment*, reveals the presence of significant disparities in the way white and minority patients receive healthcare services, especially in treatment for heart disease, cancer, and HIV (Smedley and Stith 2002). Addressing such disparities in care, including the disproportionate recruitment and selection of a minority workforce, and ensuring cultural competence of caregivers are interconnected. To minimize care disparities, institutions and providers have to develop cultural competence. To develop cultural competence, a diverse group of providers, support staff, and managers needs to be in place and diversity training and policies for all employees and caregivers have to be established. Simply, the lack of a culturally competent healthcare workforce is a possible contributor to the disparities in care.

Having examined how a diverse physician community also benefits healthcare, researchers Cohen, Gabriel, and Terrell (2002) posited at least four practical reasons for attaining greater diversity: (1) it advances cultural competency, (2) it increases access to high-quality care, (3) it strengthens the medical research agenda, and (4) it ensures optimal management. These findings are relevant and applicable to healthcare management and leadership as well. As stated by Cohen, Gabriel, and Terrell, "the first and perhaps most compelling reason for increasing the proportion of medical students and other prospective health care professionals who are drawn from underrepresented minority groups: preparing a culturally competent health care workforce."

Cultural competence may be defined as a set of complementary behaviors, practices, attitudes, and policies that enables a system, an agency, or individuals to effectively work and serve pluralistic, multiethnic, and linguistically diverse communities. The demographic makeup of this country will continue to change in the years ahead, and culturally competent and sensitive care is and will be expected from current and future healthcare professionals. To effectively provide such care, leaders, clinical staff, and all the employees in between must have a firm understanding of how and why belief systems, personal biases, ethnic origins, family structures, and other culturally determined factors influence the manner in which patients experience illness, adhere to medical advice, and respond to treatment. Such factors ultimately affect the outcomes of care. Physicians and other healthcare professionals who are not mindful of the potential impact of language barriers, religious taboos, unconventional views of illness and disease, or alternative remedies are not only unlikely to satisfy their patients but, more important, are also unlikely to provide their patients with optimally effective care (Cohen, Gabriel, and Terrell 2002).

A study finds that although African-American physicians make up only 4 percent of the total physician workforce in the United States, they care for more than 20 percent of African-American patients in the United States (Saha et al. 2000). The study suggests that African Americans prefer to get care from black physicians, and a contributing factor to this may be that many African-American physicians locate their practices in predominantly black communities and are, therefore, more geographically accessible to African-American healthcare consumers. If the hypothesis is true that minority consumers prefer care from physicians of their own race simply because of geographic accessibility, then organizational policies aimed at better serving the needs of minority communities need not consider physician race and ethnicity in the equation. If, however, minority patients have this preference because of a shared language or culture, for example, then increasing the supply of underrepresented minority physicians is justifiable and necessary.

An understanding of the factors that influence the disparities in healthcare is essential in developing effective strategies to minimize the problem. Figure 6.1 presents two sets of factors: patient-related factors and health-system-related factors. Patient-related factors are cultural characteristics of patients that prevent them from getting fair and adequate treatment in an organization that is not culturally competent or sensitive. Health-system-related factors are organizational dynamics (e.g., employee attributes and biases) that influence the methods used to treat patients.

Patient-Related Factors	*Health-System-Related Factors*	**FIGURE 6.1**
Socioeconomic Low income and education	**Cultural competence** Insufficient knowledge of and sensitivity to cultural differences	Factors that Influence Disparities in Healthcare
Health education Lack of knowledge of health symptoms, conditions, and possible treatments	**Language** Inability to communicate sufficiently with patients and families whose native language is not English	
Health behavior Patient willingness and ability to seek care, adhere to treatment protocols, and trust and work with healthcare providers	**Discrimination** Healthcare system and provider bias and stereotyping	
	Workforce diversity Poor racial and ethnic match between healthcare professionals and the patients they serve	
	Payment Insufficient reimbursement for treating Medicare, Medicaid, and uninsured patients	

SOURCE: Smedley and Stith (2002)

Components of an Effective Diversity Program

Healthcare leaders can establish a diversity program that will lead to a more diverse and inclusive organization (see Figure 6.2). Some actions that leaders can take toward this goal include, but are not limited to, the following:

- Ensure that senior management and the governing board are committed to the development and implementation of a diversity program.
- Broaden the definition of diversity to include factors beyond race and ethnicity.
- Recognize the business case for bringing in diversity at the leadership level.
- Tie diversity goals to business objectives.
- Hold recruiting events that target racial and ethnic groups, women, people with disabilities, older but capable workers, and others who are considered minorities.
- Encourage senior executives to mentor minorities.
- Develop employee programs that emphasize and celebrate diversity and inclusivity.

FIGURE 6.2
How to
Create an
Inclusive
Culture

1. Study the culture, climate (i.e., what employees are thinking, feeling, or hearing about diversity issues), and demographics of the organization.

2. Select the diversity issues that allow the greatest breakthrough.

3. Create a diversity strategic plan.

4. Secure leadership's financial support for the plan.

5. Establish leadership and management accountabilities for the plan.

6. Implement the plan.

7. Provide continual training related to the new skills and competencies necessary to successfully achieve the plan goals.

8. Conduct a follow-up survey one or one-and-one-half years after implementing the plan.

The business imperatives and organizational necessities for aggressively creating a diversity program include, but are not limited to, the following:

1. *Reflection of the service population.* The healthcare organization's caregivers and support staff should mirror the diversity of the population that the institution serves. Toward this end, the organization should attract and take advantage of the talents, skills, and growth potential of minority professionals within the community.

2. *Workforce utilization.* Minority employees have a lot to contribute to the organization. Leaders should recognize this fact and should be open to, sensitive to, knowledgeable about, and understanding of the cultures, mind-set, and practices of the organization's diverse workforce. Doing so will not only enhance staff productivity and overall performance but will also boost staff morale.

3. *Work–life quality and balance.* Leaders should recognize that work and personal activities are interrelated, not separate preoccupations. Both are performed on the basis of necessity, practicality, efficiency, and spontaneity.

4. *Recruitment and retention.* Attracting and retaining a diverse workforce have a lot to do with the state of the workplace. Leaders should create an environment in which minorities feel included, professionally developed, and safe.

5. *Bridging generations.* Generational differences in expectations, education, and values exist between younger and older staff. Such gaps should be acknowledged, and attention should be paid to the physical, mental, and emotional well-being of all caregivers and staff at all ages regardless of backgrounds.

6. *Cultural competence.* This competence is an in-depth understanding of and sensitivity to the values and viewpoints of minority staff, patients,

and other customers. Leaders should master the skills necessary to work with and serve these groups and should provide training in this matter to all employees to ensure provision of culturally competent care.

7. *Organization-wide respect.* Leaders should create an environment in which the differences in title, role, position, and department are valued and respected but not held too lofty above everything else. Each employee, regardless of his or her level within the organization, should be viewed as integral to the overall success of the team.

Summary

Healthcare organizations in the United States are beginning to make a commitment to embracing and fostering workforce diversity. This cultural change means adopting new values in terms of being inclusive and attracting a diverse workforce. The business case for diversity is unique for each organization, as circumstances, the environment, and community demographics of one organization vary from those of another. However, elements (such as the marketplace and organizational effectiveness) that are common in all organizations can be the basis of a diversity program.

One of the many reasons that senior management and the governing board should pay attention to diversity issues is to protect the organization's bottom line. The financial costs of problems that stem from racial discrimination and discriminatory practices can be substantial. Studies have found disparities in two areas: (1) minority healthcare administrators ascend in rank more slowly within their organizations than do their white counterparts, and (2) patients who belong to minority groups receive different medical treatments than patients who are white. Such disparities may be bridged with the development of a diversity program.

Discussion Questions

1. While this chapter discussed the many benefits of diversity, an alternative view suggests that no empirical evidence exists that a diverse workforce has a positive effect on organizational performance, employee commitment, and employee satisfaction. In fact, anecdotal evidence indicates that diversity can negatively affect business performance because of the possibility for internal conflict, dissension, and turnover. What is your reaction to this perspective in light of the content of this chapter? Do these arguments have merit? Why or why not?

2. Respond to this statement: Diverse leadership is a competitive advantage. What is the most compelling business

argument for or against diverse leadership teams?

3. What are the legal, moral, and ethical consequences that prohibit hospitals from turning away patients based on race?

4. Why are there are no such consequences to patients who demand doctors, nurses, or workers of a specific race to administer their healthcare?

5. Can hospitals that adhere to gender- or race-based patient demands face discrimination lawsuits from their employees?

6. When an employer denies an employee (or a group of employees) his or her full employment opportunity based on the racial bias of customers, is the employer violating the employee's civil rights?

7. Does workforce diversity enhance organizational performance? Explain your answer.

8. Can an internal diversity program support an organization's overall mission and vision? How?

Experiential Exercise

Note: This case was adapted from Davis, R. A. 2003. "No African Americans Allowed: White Patient's Racism Rules at Pennsylvania Hospital." DiversityInc.com, October 9.

Case Abington Memorial Hospital is a 508-bed hospital located in Abington, Pennsylvania. It services patients from Philadelphia and the surrounding suburbs of Bucks and Montgomery counties. The hospital's mission "is to provide patients with the highest quality care possible, regardless of the health-care professionals' race. . . ."

Supervisors at the hospital told African-American healthcare professionals, as well as food-service and housekeeping staff, not to enter a certain white patient's room or interact with the family. This caused an outrage among the African-American staff. Abington administrators said they broke hospital policy to avoid a potentially "volatile situation" by adhering to the request of the pa-

tient's husband: Only white employees could enter his wife's room on the maternity ward. "We were wrong," said Meg McGoldrick, a vice president at Abington Memorial Hospital. "We should have followed our policy. The whole incident has greatly upset many of our employees who perceived that we were acquiescing to the family's wishes." Despite the hospital's policy that states, "care will be provided on a nondiscriminatory basis," the administrators' actions seemed as though patients were allowed to discriminate. Catholic Health Care West's medical ethicist, Carol Bayley, said that Abington failed in its responsibility to its employees and the community to accommodate a patient's racial preference: "This was a fundamental disrespect of these professionals' skills and their fundamental dignities . . . a hospital needs to stand against this undercurrent of racism in our society."

The Philadelphia office of the Anti-Defamation League (ADL) said that prohibiting African-American employees from carrying out the full scope of their duties is reprehensible. "I don't see why and how a hospital could justify accommodating a request that the professionals attending to a patient be of a particular background," said Barry Morrison, director of the Philadelphia chapter of the ADL; he added, "Certainly, it's demoralizing for the people who work there." The American Hospital Association (AHA), the largest hospital association in the United States, acknowledged that no hard-and-fast industry guidelines exist for hospitals to follow when a patient or a family member makes a racially biased request. AHA does not offer hospitals a suggestion on how to address this situation. "It's subjective," said Rick Wade, senior vice president at the AHA. "I'm sure the person who made the decision at Abington thought they were doing the right thing." McGoldrick said supervisors at Abington were acting with good intentions and sought to deflect any confrontation between its African-American staff and the Caucasian family. No incident was reported during the patient's stay.

Since then, Abington's president, Richard L. Jones, sent a letter to all its employees and volunteers apologizing for the situation, which he termed "morally reprehensible." In addition to creating a diversity task force at the 508-bed hospital, Abington has hired consultants and revised its antidiscrimination policy. The AHA bestowed on Abington the Quest for Quality Award for raising awareness of the need for an organizational commitment to patient safety and quality. Wade said hospitals are constantly evaluating how to provide the best treatment for their patients, while protecting and maintaining the dignity of their employees. He said that a hospital's constant patient turnover sometimes subjected workers to society's underbelly. "Perhaps Abington could have been more protective of their employees," Wade said. "Patients come and go, [but] the most important thing at a hospital is the work-force," he said.

References

American College of Healthcare Executives (ACHE). 2002. *A Race/Ethnic Comparison of Career Attainments in Healthcare Management*. Chicago: ACHE.

———. 2003. "Increasing and Sustaining Racial/Ethnic Diversity in Healthcare Management." *Healthcare Executive* 18 (6): 60–61.

Cohen, J., B. Gabriel, and C. Terrell. 2002. "The Case for Diversity in the Healthcare Workforce." *Health Affairs* 21 (5): 90–102.

Dreachslin, J. L. 1996. *Diversity Leadership*. Chicago: Health Administration Press.

Equal Employment Opportunity Commission (EEOC). 2007. "United Healthcare of Florida to Pay $1.8 Million for Same-Sex Harassment and Retaliation." [Online information; retrieved 2/4/08.] www.eeoc.gov/press/10-1-07.html.

Guillory, W. 2003. "The Business of Diversity: The Case for Action." *Health & Social Work* 28 (1): 3–7.

Institute for Diversity in Health Management (IFD). 2007. [Online information; retrieved 11/12/07.] http://www.diversityconnection.org/diversityconnection_app/homepage/index.jsp?SSO_COOKIE_ID=0a2f011430daf6dc821f57c54388ae60bb29ec14700b.

Institute of Medicine (IOM). 2004. *In the Nation's Compelling Interest: Ensuring Diversity in the Health Care Workforce.* Washington, DC: National Academies Press.

Puget Sound Business Journal. 2007. "EEOC Sues Nordstrom in South Florida Over Harassment." [Online information; retrieved 6/1/07.] http://seattle.bizjournals.com/seattle/stories/2007/10/01/daily6.html.

Saha, S., S. Taggart, M. Komaromy, and A. Bindman. 2000. "Do Patients Choose Their Own Race?" *Health Affairs* 19: 76–83.

Smedley, B. D., and A. Y. Stith. 2002. *Unequal Treatment, Confronting Racial and Ethnic Disparities in Health Care.* Washington, DC: Institute of Medicine, National Academies Press.

Smith, D. B. 1999. *Health Care Divided: Race and Healing a Nation.* Ann Arbor, MI: University of Michigan Press.

Thomas, D., and J. J. Gabarro. 1999. *Breaking Through: The Making of Minority Executives in Corporate America.* Boston: Harvard Business School Press.

Williams, M. 2001. *The 10 Lenses: Your Guide to Living and Working in a Multicultural World.* Sterling, VA: Capital Books.

Witt/Kieffer. 2006. *Advancing Diversity Leadership in Health Care: A National Survey of Healthcare Executives.* Oak Brook, IL: Witt/Kieffer.

JOB ANALYSIS AND JOB DESIGN

Myron D. Fottler, PhD

Learning Objectives

After completing this chapter, the reader should be able to

- distinguish between job analyses, job descriptions, and job specifications;
- describe the methods by which job analyses are typically accomplished;
- discuss the relationship of job requirements (as developed through job analyses, job descriptions, and job specifications) to other human resources management functions;
- enumerate the steps involved in a typical job analysis as well as the methods of job analysis;
- address the relationship between job analyses and strategic human resources management; and
- understand the changing nature of jobs and how jobs are being redesigned to enhance productivity.

Introduction

The interaction between an organization and its environment has important implications for the organization's internal organization and structure. For example, the environment affects how the institution organizes its human resources to achieve specific objectives and to perform different functions necessary in carrying out the organization's mission and goals. The organization formally groups the activities to be performed by its human resources (HR) into basic units referred to as jobs.

A *job* consists of a group of activities and duties that entail natural units of work that are similar and related. Jobs should be clear and distinct from other jobs to minimize misunderstandings and conflict among employees and to enable employees to recognize what is expected of them. Some jobs are required to be performed by several employees, each of whom occupies a separate position. A *position* consists of different duties and responsibilities that are performed by only one employee. For example, in a hospital, 40 registered nurses fill 40 positions, but all of them perform only one job—that of a registered nurse. Different jobs that have similar duties and responsibilities may be grouped into a job family for purposes of recruitment, training, compensation, or advancement opportunities. For example, the nursing job family may be performed by registered nurses, the nursing supervisor, and the director of nursing services.

Healthcare organizations are continually restructuring and reengineering in an attempt to become more cost effective and customer focused. They have put emphasis on smaller scale, less hierarchy, fewer layers, and more decentralized work units. As these changes occur, more managers want their employees to operate more independently and flexibly to meet customer demands. To do this, decisions must be made by employees who are closest to the information and who are directly involved in the service delivery. The objective is to develop jobs and basic work units that are adaptable and can thrive in a world of high-velocity change.

In this chapter, we define the terms job analysis, job description, and job specification; indicate the processes that may be used to conduct job analyses; and identify the relevance of and relationship between the results of job analysis (i.e., job descriptions and job specifications) and other human resources management functions. In addition, we emphasize that these job processes provide the organization with a foundation for making objective and legally defensible decisions in managing human resources. We discuss how healthcare jobs have been redesigned to contribute to organizational objectives while simultaneously satisfying the needs of the employees, and we review several innovative job design and employee-contribution techniques to enhance job satisfaction and organizational performance.

Definitions

Job analyses are sometimes called the cornerstone of strategic human resources management because the information they collect serves so many HR functions. *Job analysis* is the process of obtaining information about jobs by determining the job's duties, tasks, and/or activities. The procedure involves undertaking a systematic investigation of jobs by following a number of predetermined steps specified in advance of the analysis (Ash 1988). When the analysis is completed, a written report is created that summarizes the information obtained from studying 20 or 30 individual job tasks or activities. HR managers use these data to develop job descriptions and job specifications.

A *job description* is a written explanation of a job and the types of duties the job involves. Because no standard format for job descriptions exists, these documents tend to vary in appearance and content from one organization to another. However, most job descriptions contain the job title, a job identification section, and a job duties section. They may also include a job specification section; sometimes a job specification is prepared as separate documents, but sometimes it is a part of the job description. A specific job description is a detailed summary of a job's tasks, duties, and responsibilities, emphasizing efficiency, control, and detailed work planning. This type of description fits best with a bureaucratic organizational structure, where well-defined boundaries separate functions and different levels of management.

A general job description, which is fairly new on the HR scene, emphasizes innovation, flexibility, and loose work planning. This type of job description fits best with an organization with a flat structure, where few boundaries exist between functions and levels of management (Leonard 2000). Only the most generic duties, responsibilities, and skills for a position are documented in a general job description (Johnson 2001).

A *job specification* describes the personal qualifications an individual must possess to perform the duties and responsibilities contained in a job description. Typically, the job specification describes the skills required to perform the job and the physical demands the job places on the employee performing it. Skills relevant to a job include education and experience, specialized knowledge or training, licenses, personal abilities and traits, and manual dexterity. The physical demands of a job refer to the condition of the physical work environment; workplace hazards; and the amount of walking, standing, reaching, and lifting required by the job. Appendix A (at the end of this chapter) provides an example of a combined job description/job specification document for the position of staff nurse in a hospital's labor and delivery department.

The Job Analysis Process

Figure 7.1 indicates how a job analysis is performed, including the functions for which it is used. Analysis involves a systematic, step-by-step investigation of jobs. The end product of the analysis is a document that summarizes information about the various job tasks or activities examined. This information is then used by HR managers in developing job descriptions and job specifications, which in turn are used to guide performance and to enhance different HR functions, such as developing performance appraisal criteria or the content of training classes (Clifford 1994). The ultimate purpose of a job analysis is to improve organizational performance and productivity.

Steps
The process of conducting a job analysis involves a number of steps. Although healthcare organizations may perform their job analysis differently,

FIGURE 7.1

The Process of
Job Analysis

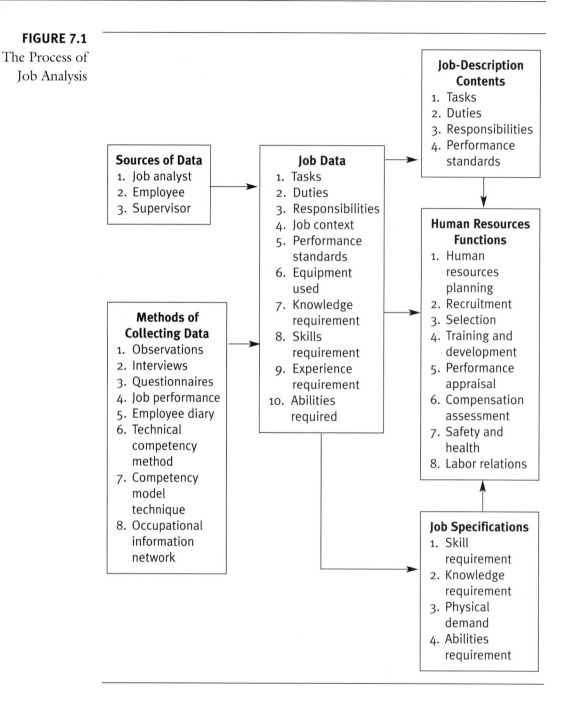

they follow a general guide such as that listed below (Anthony, Perrewe, and Kacmar 1993):

1. *Determine the purpose of the job analysis.* As a result of rapid growth or downsizing, jobs may have changed in their content. Such changes may cause employee salaries to be inequitable. The purpose of conducting the analysis should be explicit and tied to the organization's overall

business strategy to increase the probability of a successful job analysis program.

2. *Identify the jobs to be analyzed.* All jobs are analyzed if no previous formal job analysis has been performed. If the organization has undergone changes that have affected only certain jobs or if new jobs have been added, then only those jobs are analyzed.

3. *Explain the process to employees, and determine their levels of involvement.* Employees should be informed of who will conduct the analysis, why the analysis is needed, whom to contact to answer questions and concerns, when the analysis will take place, and what roles they are expected to play in the process. In addition to receiving good communication, employees may elect a committee to serve as a verification check and to reduce anxiety. Such a committee can also help answer employee questions and concerns.

4. *Collect the job analysis information.* Managers must decide which method or combination of methods will be used and how the information will be collected. Various alternatives are discussed in the next section of this chapter.

5. *Organize the job analysis information into a form that will be useful to managers and employees.* This form consists of job descriptions and job specifications. The job descriptions can vary from very broad to very specific and precise; the level of detail depends on the needs of the organization. The job specifications must be linked directly to the job description—that is, they must be relevant to the job.

6. *Review and update the job analysis information frequently.* Particularly in a dynamic environment such as healthcare, jobs seldom go unchanged for long periods of time. Even if no major changes have occurred within the organization, a complete review of all jobs should be performed every three years (Mathis and Jackson 1985). More frequent reviews are necessary when major organizational changes occur.

Data Sources and Data-Collection Methods

Conducting job analyses is usually the primary responsibility of the HR department or the individuals charged with this function. Although job analysts are typically responsible for the job analyses program, they usually enlist the cooperation of the employees and supervisors in the departments in which jobs are being analyzed. These supervisors and employees are the sources of much of the job information generated through the process.

Job information is collected in several ways, depending on the purpose identified by the organization. Typically, the organizational chart is reviewed to identify the jobs to be included in the analysis. Often, restructuring, downsizing, merger, or rapid growth initiates the job analysis. A job may be selected because its content has undergone undocumented changes. As new job demands arise and the nature of the work changes, compensation for the job also may have to change. The employee or the manager may request a job analysis to determine the appropriate compensation. The manager may also be interested in documenting change for recruitment selection, training, and performance appraisal purposes.

Managers should consider a number of different methods to collect information because it is unlikely that any one method will provide all of the necessary data needed for a job analysis. Among the most popular methods of data collection are observing tasks and behaviors of jobholders, interviewing individuals or groups, using structured questionnaires and checklists, performing the job, reviewing employee work diaries, asking job experts through the technical conference method, using a competency model, and referring to the Occupational Information Network. Each method is described as follows:

- *Observations* require job analysts to observe jobholders performing their work. The observations may be continuous or intermittent based on work sampling—that is, observing only a sampling of tasks performed. For many jobs, observation may be of limited usefulness because the job does not consist of physically active tasks. For example, observing an accountant review an income statement may not provide valuable information. Even with more active jobs, observation does not always reveal vital information such as the importance or difficulty of the task. Given the limitations of observation, it is helpful to incorporate additional methods for obtaining job analysis information.

- Employees who are knowledgeable about a particular job (i.e., the employee holding the job, supervisors, or former jobholders) may be *interviewed* concerning the specific work activities of the job. Usually a structured interview form is used to record information. The questions correspond to the data needed to prepare a job description and job specification. Employees may be suspicious of the interviewer and his or her motives, especially if the interviewer asks ambiguous questions. Because interviewing can be a time-consuming and costly method of data collection, managers and job analysts may prefer to use the interview as a means to get answers to specific questions generated from observations and questionnaires.

- The use of *structured questionnaires* and *checklists* is most efficient because it is a quick and inexpensive way to collect information about a job. If possible, it is desirable to have several knowledgeable employees complete the questionnaire for verification. Such survey data often can be quantified and processed by computer. Follow-up observations and interviews are not uncommon if a questionnaire or checklist is chosen as the primary means of collecting information. The questionnaire must be extremely detailed and comprehensive so that valuable data are not missed. Compared to other methods, questionnaires are cheaper and easier to administer but are more time consuming and expensive to develop. Management must decide whether the benefits of a simplified method of data collection outweigh the costs of its construction.

Strategically, managers favor methods of data collection that do not require a lot of work and up-front costs if the content of the job changes frequently. Another option may be to adopt an existing structured questionnaire. Among the more widely used structured questionnaires are the Position Analysis Questionnaire, the Management Position Description Questionnaire, and the Functional Job Analysis. Regardless of whether the questionnaire is developed in-house or purchased from a commercial source, rapport between analyst and respondent is not possible unless the analyst is available to explain items and to clarify misunderstandings. Without such rapport, such an impersonal approach may have adverse effects on the respondent's cooperation and motivation.

- The job analyst can *perform the job* in question. This approach allows exposure to the actual job tasks as well as the job's physical, environmental, and social demands. This method is appropriate for jobs that can be learned in a relatively short period of time. However, it is inappropriate for jobs that require extensive training and/or are hazardous to perform.

- The *diary method* requires jobholders to record their daily activities. Diaries are filled out at specific times during the workday and maintained for a period of two to four weeks. This method is the most time consuming of all job analysis approaches, which adds to its cost.

- The *technical conference method* relies on supervisors who have an extensive knowledge of the job (frequently called "subject matter experts"). Job attributes are obtained from these experts. Although a good data-gathering method, it overlooks incumbent workers' perceptions of what their jobs actually entail (Truxillo et al. 2004).

- The *competency model technique* is a popular form of job analysis today. A competency is an underlying characteristic of a person that results in effective and/or superior performance on the job. It is also a cluster of related knowledge, skills, and attitudes that affects one's job performance (Athey and Orth 1999). Competencies are focused on strategic goals and organizational outcome measures. Approximately 75 percent of healthcare organizations have developed some form of competency-based job analysis (Livens, Sanchez, and Décorte 2004). One popular two-level competency model distinguishes "can do" competencies (skills and knowledge derived from education and experience) from "will do" competencies (personality and attitudinal characteristics that reflect an individual's willingness to perform) (Schippmann 1999).

- The *Occupational Information Network (O*NET)* of the U.S. Department of Labor is an Internet database that includes about 20,000 occupations from the earlier printed *Dictionary of Occupational Titles* as well as an update of more than 3,500 additional occupations. The database job descriptions provide employee attributes and job characteristics, such as skills, abilities, knowledge, tasks, work activities, and experience-level requirements. The database is continually updated and is useful for a variety of HR activities, including job analysis, employee selection, career counseling, and employee training.

Figure 7.2 shows the content model for the O*NET, which uses both job-oriented and worker-oriented descriptors. The model also allows occupational information to be applied across jobs, sectors, or industries and within occupations. O*NET's six-domain content model attempts to provide a descriptor framework for describing jobs in greater detail. Not only is O*NET free to any organization, but it also provides comprehensive information on a wide variety of occupations. The website (see www.doleta.gov/programs/onet) also offers downloadable detailed job analysis questionnaires that can be applied to various purposes.

FIGURE 7.2

The Content Model Forming the Foundation of O*NET

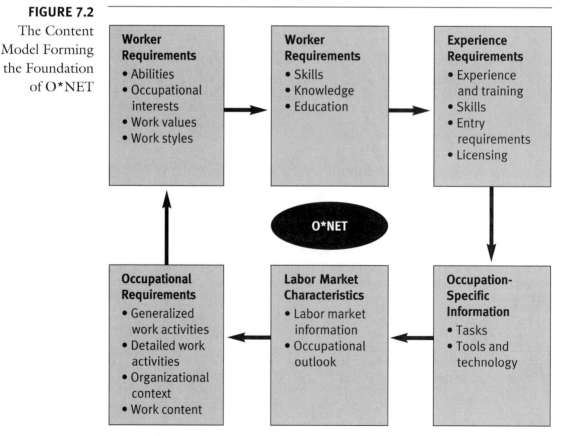

SOURCE: O*NET Resource Center, www.onetcenter.org/content.html

A combination of data-collection methods is often appropriate. The job analyst should employ as many techniques as needed to develop valid and accurate job descriptions and job specifications.

Relation to Other HR Functions

Job analysis provides the basis for tying all the HR functional areas together and for developing a sound HR program. Not surprisingly, job requirements as documented in job descriptions and job specifications influence many of the HR functions that are performed as part of managing employees. When job requirements are modified, corresponding changes must be made in other HR activities. Job analysis is the foundation for forecasting future needs for human resources as well as plans for such activities as recruitment, selection, performance appraisal, compensation, training, transfer, or promotion. Job analysis information is often incorporated into the HR information systems.

Before attempting to attract capable employees, recruiters must know the job specifications for the positions needed to be filled, including the knowledge, skills, and abilities required for successful job performance. The information in the job specifications is used in job-opening notices and as a basis for attracting qualified applicants while discouraging unqualified candidates. Failure to update job specifications can result in a flood of applicants who are unqualified to perform one or more functions of the job. Until 1971, job specifications used in employee selection decisions often were unrelated to the duties to be performed under the job description. In the case of Griggs v. Duke Power Company (401 U.S. 424) (1971), the U.S. Supreme Court ruled that employment practices must be job related. When discrimination charges arise, employers have the burden of proving that job requirements are job related or constitute a business necessity. Today, employers must be able to show that the job specifications used in selecting employees for a job are specifically associated to that job's duties.

Any discrepancies between the knowledge, skills, and abilities demonstrated by the jobholders and the requirements contained in the job description and specification provide clues for training needs. Career development is concerned with preparing employees for advancement to jobs at which their capabilities can be used to the fullest extent possible. The formal qualifications set forth in the job specifications for higher-level jobs serve to indicate how much more training and development are needed for employees to advance. The requirements contained in the job description are the criteria for evaluating the performance of the jobholder. The appraisal may reveal, however, that certain performance criteria established for a particular job are not completely valid. These criteria must be specific and job related. If the criteria used to evaluate employee performance are overly broad, vague, and not job related, employers may be charged with unfair discrimination.

The relative worth of a job is one of the most important factors in determining the compensation for performing a job. This worth is based on what the job demands of an employee in terms of skill, effort, and responsibility as well as the conditions and hazards under which the work is performed. Information derived from a job analysis is also valuable in identifying safety and health considerations. If a job is hazardous (e.g., poses a possibility for contracting AIDS), the job description and specification should reflect this condition. Employers need to provide specific information about such hazards to enable jobholders to perform their jobs safely.

Job analysis information is also important to the employee-relations and labor-relations functions. When employees are considered for promotion, transfer, or demotion, the job description provides a standard for comparison of talent. Regardless of whether the organization is unionized, information obtained through job analysis can often lead to more objective HR decisions. Job analysis can be used in employee selection to determine whether an applicant for a specific job should be required to take a particular kind of test. The performance standards used to judge employee performance for promotion, rewards, discipline, and loyalty should be job related and based on the job description. Job analysis information can also be used to compare the relative worth of each job's contribution to the organization's overall performance. Finally, job analysis can be used to determine training needs by comparing current employee skills to skills identified in the job analysis. Training programs can then be put in place to reduce employees' skill gaps.

Legal Aspects

Although HR managers consider job descriptions a valuable tool for performing HR functions, they encounter the following problems when using these documents (Grant 1988):

1. They are often poorly written and offer little guidance to the jobholder.
2. They are generally not updated as job duties or specifications change.
3. They may violate the law by containing specifications that are not related to job performance.
4. The job duties included are often written in vague, rather than specific, terms.
5. They can limit the scope of activities of the jobholder in a rapidly changing environment.

A major goal of job analysis is to help the organization establish the job relatedness of its selection and performance requirements. Job analysis helps employees to meet their legal duties under equal employment opportunity law. Section 14 C.2 of the "Uniform Guidelines for Employee Selection Procedures" states that "There shall be a job analysis which includes an analysis of the important work behaviors required for successful performance. . . . Any job analysis should focus on work behavior(s) and the tasks associated with them" (EEOC 1978). Today's legal environment has created a need for higher levels of specificity in job analysis and job descriptions. Federal guidelines now require that the specific performance requirements of a job be based on valid job-related criteria (EEOC 1978). Employment decisions that involve either job applicants or employees and that are based on vague and non-job-related criteria are increasingly being challenged, and the challenges have mostly been successful. Managers of small healthcare organizations, where employees may perform many different job tasks, must be particularly concerned about writing specific job descriptions.

When writing job descriptions, employers must use statements that are terse, direct, and worded simply, excluding unnecessary phrases and terms. Typically, the sentences that describe job duties begin with verbs (see Appendix A). The term "may" is used for those duties performed only by some workers on the job. Excellent job descriptions are of value to both the employee and the employer. For the employee, job descriptions help them learn their job duties and remind them of the results they are expected to achieve. For the employer, job descriptions can minimize the misunderstandings that occur between supervisors and subordinates regarding job requirements. Good job descriptions also establish management's right to take corrective action in the event that the duties specified in the document are not performed at all or are performed at an inadequate or inappropriate level.

Job analysis is surrounded by several legal constraints largely because it serves as a basis for selection decisions, compensation, performance appraisals, and training. These constraints have been articulated in the "Uniform Guidelines for Employee Selection Procedures" and in several court decisions. Again, as the guidelines state, "Any job analysis should focus on work behavior(s) and the tasks associated with them." To determine this, organizations should assess job skills, knowledge, and abilities needed to perform the jobs. After this is known, selection procedures can be developed (Thompson and Thompson 1982).

Job analyses that were not performed in organizations have resulted in the successful challenge to the validity of the organizations' selection decisions; see Albermarle Paper Company v. Moody (422 U.S. 405) (1975). Numerous court decisions regarding promotion and job analysis also exist. In Rowe v. General Motors (32 5 U.S. 305) (1972), the court ruled that a company should have written objective standards for promotion to prevent discriminatory practices. In U.S. v. City of Chicago (573 F. 2nd 416 [7th Cir.]) (1978), the court ruled that the standards should describe the job for which the person is being considered for promotion. In both cases, these objective standards can be determined through job analysis (Nobile 1991).

Before the "Uniform Guidelines" and the associated court cases discussed earlier, labor contracts required consistent and equitable treatment of unionized employees. The information provided by job analysis is helpful to both management and unions in contract negotiations and in avoiding or resolving grievances, jurisdictional disputes, and other conflicts. For these reasons, unionized employers have found it advantageous to prepare written job descriptions and job specifications. The passage of the Americans with Disabilities Act (ADA) also had a major impact on job analysis. Managers must now adhere to the legal mandates of the ADA when preparing job descriptions and job specifications (Mitchell, Alliger, and Morfopoalos 1997). The ADA requires that job duties and reasonabilities be essential functions for successful job performance. If the job requires the jobholder to perform certain essential physical and mental tasks, these requirements should be stated in the job description. Section 1630.2 (n) of the ADA provides three guidelines for rendering a job function essential (EEOC 1992):

1. The reason the position exists is to perform a function.
2. A limited number of employees are available among whom performance of the function may be distributed.
3. The function may be highly specialized, requiring needed expertise or abilities to complete the job.

Managers who write job descriptions in terms of essential functions reduce the risk of discriminating on the basis of disability. Once the essential functions of a job are defined, the organization is legally required to make a reasonable accommodation to the disability of the individual.

The job analysis process is the basic method used to identify essential job functions. An *essential job function* is one that is fundamental to successful performance of the job, while a *marginal job function* is incidental to the main function of the job (i.e., it is a matter of convenience and not a necessity). Qualified individuals with disabilities are persons who have a disability but meet the skill, education, and experience of the job requirements and can perform the essential functions with or without reasonable accommodation. *Reasonable accommodation* means the employer may be required to alter the accommodations of a particular job to enable a partially disabled person to perform all essential functions. However, employers cannot be required to make an accommodation that imposes undue hardship.

Other legislation that requires a thorough job analysis includes the following:

- The Fair Labor Standards Act categorizes employees as exempt and non-exempt based on the job analysis.
- The Equal Pay Act requires equal pay for equal work. When pay differentials exist, job descriptions can be used to show whether jobs are substantially different in terms of skill, effort, responsibility, and working conditions.

- The Civil Rights Act often requires the use of job specifications to defend against charges of discrimination, initial selection, promotion, and other HR decisions.
- The Occupational Safety and Health Act requires that job applicants are shown in advance the job descriptions that specify the elements of the job that may endanger employee health or are considered distasteful.

The Changing Environment

The traditional approach to job analysis assumes a static job environment, where jobs remain relatively stable apart from incumbents who hold these jobs. It assumes jobs can be meaningfully defined in terms of tasks, duties, processes, and behaviors necessary for job success. Unfortunately, these assumptions discount technological advances that are often so accelerated that jobs that are defined today may be obsolete tomorrow. In a dynamic environment where job demands change rapidly, job analysis data can quickly become outdated and inaccurate. Obsolete job analysis information can hinder an organization's ability to adapt to change. Several approaches to job analysis may respond to the need for continuous change.

First, adopt a future-oriented approach to job analysis. This strategic analysis of jobs requires managers to have a clear view of how duties and tasks can be restructured to meet organizational requirements in the future. One method to this approach was performed by researchers in one study. They asked experts on a particular job to identify aspects of the job, the organization, and the environment that might change in the next few years and how those changes might affect the nature of the job (Schneider and Konz 1989). The collected data were then used to describe the tasks, knowledge, skills, and abilities needed for doing the job in the future. By including future-oriented information in job descriptions, healthcare organizations can focus employee attention on new strategic directions (Priem, O'Brien, and Gamble 2004).

For example, one organization decided to change its strategic focus to increasing its "customer-consciousness" orientation (George 1990). Job descriptions were then amended to include tasks, knowledge, skills, and abilities related to customer contact and responsibilities. These new job descriptions focused more on what the organization wanted to be doing in the future.

Second, adopt a competency-based approach to job analysis that places emphasis on characteristics of successful performers rather than on standard job duties and tasks (Hunt 1996; Van Wart 2000). These competencies will match the organization's culture and strategy and will include such things as interpersonal communication skills, ability to work as part of a team, decision-making capabilities, conflict resolution know-how, adaptability, and self-motivation (Carson and Stewart 1996; Van Wart 2000). This technique enhances a culture of continuous improvement, as organizational improvement is a constant aim. Both the first and second approaches to change-oriented job analysis have potential impracticalities, including the dependence on the ability of managers to accurately predict future job needs, the uncertainty that the analysis will comply with EEOC guidelines, and the ambiguity in job descriptions as a result of creating them based on estimates.

Third, conduct a generic job analysis. The traditional job analysis approach serves to constrain desired change and flexibility by compartmentalizing and specifically defining presumably static job characteristics. It impedes shifting decision making downward in the organization, cross-training employees, and getting employees involved in quality improvement efforts (Blayney 1992). Reducing the number of job titles and developing more generic job descriptions can provide needed flexibility to manage unanticipated change.

For example, Nissan Motor Company has only one job description for hourly production employees. This description is generic and gives the organization the opportunity to use employees as needed. Cross-training and multiple job assignments are possible with this approach. However, employees may experience more conflict and ambiguity with generic job descriptions. Undoubtedly, most jobs are getting bigger and more complex.

The last item on a typical job description is often "any other duty that may be assigned," and this is increasingly becoming *the* job description. This enlarged, flexible, complex job changes the way virtually every HR function is performed. For example, in recruitment and selection, individuals who possess the technical skills required to perform the job are not viewed as ideal candidates anymore. HR managers are also looking for broader capabilities such as competencies, intelligence, adaptability, and an ability/willingness to work in teams.

The rapid pace of change in healthcare makes the need for accurate job analysis even more important now and in the future. Historically, job analysis was conducted and then set aside for a reasonable time. Today, however, job requirements are in such a constant state of flux that job descriptions and specifications must be constantly reviewed to keep them relevant. By one estimate, people may have to change their entire skill sets three or four times during their careers (Snyder 1996). If this projection is right, the need for accurate and timely job analysis is becoming even more important. Organizations that do not revise or review job descriptions and specifications may recruit new employees who do not possess the needed skills or may not provide necessary training to update employee skills.

Managerial Implications

Several challenges may limit the impact and effectiveness of job analysis in healthcare organizations. Top management support of job analysis may be lukewarm or nonexistent, and updating job descriptions and job specifications may not occur. The reason for these may be a lack of understanding of and appreciation for the job analysis process and its significance in supporting the effective implementation of all HR functions. As a result, job analysis is not performed and job descriptions and specifications are not modified as jobs evolve over time. The organization, in turn, operates with outdated information, which adversely affects employee and organizational outcomes.

These aforementioned situations may create the following challenges (followed by possible strategies):

1. *Only single methods of job analysis may be used.* A combination of methods might provide better and more reliable data. In addition, input from job incumbents, supervisors, and experts may provide more usable and valuable data for job descriptions and job specifications.

2. *The jobholder and supervisor may be excluded from the job analysis process.* Because of their extensive knowledge of the relative importance of various job functions, both jobholder and supervisor should be involved in the process.

3. *Sometimes the employee is involved in the process but is not allowed sufficient time to complete the job analysis with any level of quality.* This often results in a poorly written, insignificant, vague, and nonspecific job description or specification that is of little value to the organization and may create legal liability. Obviously, employees should be allowed sufficient time during work hours to complete their input into the job analysis process.

4. *Because neither managers nor employees are trained or motivated to generate quality data, their data may be distorted.* This could be overcome through training, making employees aware of the importance of the process, and providing desired rewards for good data.

5. *Sometimes job descriptions imply that the job incumbent will only perform those job duties outlined in the description.* This could foster an "it's not my job" philosophy. Consequently, the last duty shown on the job description should be phrased as "any other duty that may be assigned." This is increasingly becoming the job description. Healthcare executives can no longer select individuals who possess narrow skills required to perform a job. They must go deeper, and seek other competencies such as ability to adjust and willingness to work in teams. Such qualities should be incorporated into job specifications.

6. *Many job analyses do not go beyond the initial phase of reporting what the jobholder currently does.* The job should also be critiqued to determine whether it is being done correctly and whether other job functions may enhance the jobholder's contributions to achieving the organization's strategic objectives.

Finally, speed is of the essence. Job requirements are changing so rapidly that they must be constantly reviewed to keep them relevant. Yet the time that can be devoted to job analysis has been diminished. Recently, "job analysis at the speed of reality" has been developed as a shorter version of the interview method. Through this process, a validated job analysis can be completed in between two and three hours (Hartley 2004).

Job Design

Job design is an outgrowth of job analysis and is a process of structuring jobs to help improve organizational efficiency and employee job satisfaction. The process involves changing, eliminating, modifying, and enriching duties and tasks to capture the talents of employees so that they can contribute to the fullest and develop professionally. Job design should simultaneously facilitate the achievement of organizational objectives and recognize the capabilities and needs of those who perform the job.

Job design encompasses the manner in which a given job is defined and how it will be conducted. This involves such decisions as "will the job be handled by an individual or by a team of employees?" and such determinations as "how does the job fit into the overall organization?" Organizing tasks, duties, and responsibilities into a unit of work to achieve a certain objective requires a conscious effort. Each job design process must acknowledge any unique skills possessed by a number of employees of a given profession and must incorporate appropriate professional guidelines or task limitations. In healthcare, most professionals are constrained by which functions and tasks they may legally perform and under what type of supervision. For example, many technical functions require the performance either by a physician or by another professional under the direct supervision of physicians. Such legal constraints obviously reduce the flexibility of healthcare executives in designing jobs.

Specialization in Healthcare

As a result of technological change, increased specialization, and the emergence of the hospital as the central focus of the healthcare system, approximately 700 different job categories exist in the healthcare industry. The most rapid growth in the supply of the healthcare workforce has occurred in new categories: More than two-thirds of all healthcare employees work in nontraditional allied health or support service positions (U.S. Census Bureau 1998).

Researchers have concluded that specialization has inherent limitations and has been taken to extremes in healthcare (Fottler 1992). Because of the inherent disadvantages of specialization, new approaches to organizing work and job design are needed. The foremost criticism is that specialized workers may become bored and dissatisfied because their jobs may not offer enough challenge or stimulation. Boredom and monotony set in and absenteeism rises, bringing in a possibility that the quality of work will suffer. To counter the problems of specialization and to enhance productivity and employee job satisfaction, healthcare executives have implemented a number of job-design and job-redesign options to achieve a better balance between organizational demands for efficiency and productivity and individual needs for creativity and autonomy. Four alternative redesign approaches are (1) job redesign (i.e., enlargement, enrichment, and rotation), (2) employee empowerment, (3) work-group redesign (e.g., employee involvement groups, employee teams), and (4) work-schedule redesign. Each of these approaches is explored below.

Job Enlargement

Job enlargement involves changes in the scope of a job to provide greater variety to the employee. It is a *horizontal expansion* of duties with the same level of autonomy and responsibility. Alternatively, job enrichment adds additional autonomy and responsibility and is a *vertical expansion of duties.* One specific profession that was developed in response to either job enlargement or job enrichment is the *multiskilled health practitioner* (MSHP). The MSHP is a "person cross-trained to provide more than one function, often in more than one discipline" (Vaughan et al. 1991). These combined functions can be found in a broad spectrum of healthcare-related jobs and range in complexity, from the nonprofessional to the professional level. The additional functions (skills) added to the original worker's job may be of a higher, lower, or parallel level.

Most theories of job enrichment stress that unless jobs are both horizontally and vertically enriched, little positive impact is made on motivation, productivity, and job satisfaction (Lawler 1986). Because the MSHP concept may involve horizontal, vertical, or both types of enrichment, whether it should be expected to enhance organizational outcomes is unclear. Research on the concept reveals that the outcomes have been positive in terms of enhanced productivity, job satisfaction, and patient satisfaction (Fottler 1996). However, those positive outcomes depend on many "contingencies," such as whether the "right" employees are chosen for the program (i.e., those with higher-order needs for personal growth), implementation processes, available training opportunities, legal constraints, and continuing top-management commitment.

Employee Empowerment

Various job enlargement/job enrichment approaches, such as the MSHP, are programs by which managers and supervisors formally change the job of employees. A less structured approach is to allow employees to initiate their own job changes through the concept of empowerment. Ann Howard of Development Dimensions International defines empowerment as "pushing down decision-making responsibility to those close to internal and external customers" (Simison 1999). To support empowerment, organizations must share with the workforce information, knowledge, power to act, and rewards.

Empowerment encourages employees to become innovators and managers of their own work and gives them more control and autonomous decision-making capabilities (Ettore 1997).

Empowerment can involve employee control over the job content (i.e., functions and responsibilities), the job context (i.e., the environmental conditions under which the job is performed), or both (Ford and Fottler 1995). Most healthcare organizations are not ready for both and are advised to implement empowerment on an incremental basis. For empowerment to thrive and grow, organizations must encourage participation, innovation, access to information, accountability, and a culture that is open and receptive to change (Garcia 1997). Examples of organizations that have successfully implemented employee empowerment include Cigna Healthcare, the State of Illinois, Mesa (Arizona) Community College, and the State of Kentucky.

Work-Group Redesign

Table 7.1 outlines the six forms of work groups or teams currently being used in healthcare. Teams are groups of employees who assume a greater role in the service process. They provide a forum for employees to contribute to identifying and solving organizational problems. With work teams, managers accept the notion that the group is the logical work unit to resolve organizational problems and concerns.

Regardless of which team structure is employed, several team processes have been identified with successful teams. These include commitment to shared goals, motivated and energetic team members, consensus decision making, open and honest communication, shared leadership, a climate of trust and collaboration, valuing diversity, and acceptance of conflict and its positive resolution. A good team also requires that employee selection partially consider the potential employee's interpersonal skills and that extensive training for team members be provided (Bohlander and McCarthy 1996). The manager must also adapt to the role of leader (rather than supervisor) and not be threatened by the growing power of the team.

Because many teams fail to operate at full potential, organizations must be aware of several obstacles to the effective functions of teams, including overly high expectations, inappropriate compensation, lack of training, and lack of power (Levy 2001). For example, new team members must be retrained to work outside their primary functional area, and compensation systems must be constructed to reward individuals for team achievements. New career paths to general management and/or higher clinical positions must be created from the team's experience. Finally, managers who feel threatened by the growing power of the team and reduced power of management may need further training or incentives to work with teams (Yandrick 2001). Complete training would enhance skills in team leadership, goal setting, conduct of

Type	Description	
Cross-functional team	A group staffed by a mix of specialists (nurses, physicians, and managers) and formed to accomplish a specific objective. Usually, membership on this team is assigned rather than voluntary.	**TABLE 7.1** Types of Employee Teams in Healthcare
Project team	A group formed specifically to design a new service. Members are assigned by management on the basis of their ability to contribute to team success. The group normally dispatches after task completion.	
Self-directed team (or autonomous workgroup)	A group of highly trained individuals who are accountable for a whole work process that provides a service or product to an internal or external customer. Members use consensus decision making to perform job duties, solve problems, or deal with internal or external customers.	
Task force team	A group formed by management to resolve a major problem. This team is responsible for developing a long-term plan for problem resolution that may include a change for implementing the proposed solution.	
Process improvement team (or employee involvement group)	A group made up of experienced employees from different departments or functions and charged with improving quality, decreasing waste, or enhancing productivity in processes that affect all departments. Members are normally appointed by management.	
Virtual team	A group with any of the above purposes that uses advanced competitor and telecommunication technology to link geographically dispersed team members.	

meetings, team decision making, conflict resolution, effective communication, and diversity awareness (Bell and Smith 2003).

Work-Schedule Redesign

The goal of work-schedule redesign is to give employees greater control over their time. Various types of adjustments in work schedules alter the normal workweek of five eight-hour days in which everyone begins and ends their workday at the same time. Such adjustments are made to improve organizational productivity and morale by giving employees increased control over their work schedules. By allowing employees greater flexibility in work scheduling, employers can reduce some of the most common causes of tardiness and absenteeism—that is, the time pressures of life. Employees can adjust their work schedules to accommodate their lifestyles, reduce pressure to meet a rigid schedule, and gain greater satisfaction. Employers can enhance their attractiveness when recruiting and retaining personnel while improving their customer service (poor service is a direct result of low levels of employee satisfaction). Productivity and quality may also be enhanced (Gale 2001a, 2001b).

Under the *compressed workweek* scheme, the number of days in the workweek is shortened by lengthening the number of hours worked per day. The four-day 40-hour week (4/40) is the most common form of compressed workweeks, and the three-day 39-hour week (3/39) schedule is less common. The compressed schedule accommodates the leisure-time activities and personal appointments of employees. Potential barriers to this schedule design are the stringent rules under the Fair Labor Standards Act that require the payment of overtime to nonsupervisory employees who work more than 40 hours a week. Long workdays may also increase the amount of exhaustion and stress for employees and managers. A 2006 survey by the Society for Human Resource Management (SHRM) reported that 35 percent of the employer respondents offered some type of compressed workweek (Thompson 2006).

Flextime, or flexible working hours, allows employees to choose daily starting and quitting times, provided that they work a certain number of hours per day or week. Typically, there is a "core period" during the morning and afternoon when all employees on a given shift are required to be on the job. In healthcare, flextime is most common in clerical or management functions, such as claims processing, health insurance, and human resources. However, flextime is not appropriate for patient care positions, because these functions must be staffed at all times, while communication and coordination are a continuing challenge in other positions. The 2006 SHRM survey found that 57 percent of the employer respondents used some form of flextime (Thompson 2006).

Job sharing is an arrangement whereby two part-time employees share a job that otherwise is held by a full-time employee. Job sharers sometimes work three days a week to create an overlap day for face-to-face conferencing. Job sharing can be scheduled to conform to peaks in the daily or weekly workload. However, more time may be needed to orient, train, and develop two employees who share one role.

Among notable healthcare organizations that have developed a physician job-sharing program is HMO Kaiser Permanente in northern California. This program allows physicians to job share. Job sharing is best suited for employees who wish to work part time and older workers who wish to phase into retirement. Job sharing can reduce absenteeism because it allows employees to have time to accommodate their personal needs even when employed. It also aids retention of valuable employees.

A 2005 survey by the Families and Work Institute found that 46 percent of respondent organizations with 50 or more employees allowed some employees to job share, while only 13 percent of the respondents allowed all employees to do so (*HR Focus* 2006a). A survey of 1,020 employers by Hewitt and Associates showed that slightly more than 25 percent of the respondents offered job sharing (Bach 2006).

Job sharing may pose problems for employers. Among the possible concerns are the time required to orient and train a second employee and prorating of employee benefits between the two job sharers. The key to making this approach work is good communication between partners through phone calls, e-mails, voice mails, or written updates (Schultz, McCain, and Thomas 2003). It also helps if the two partners have worked in the organization together before they decide to share a job.

One of the most significant work-schedule innovations is telecommuting (Conklin 1999). *Telecommuting* is the system of performing work away from the office with the use of computers, networks, telephones, and fax machines. In 2000, an estimated 25 percent of the U.S. workforce were telecommuting either full time or part time. The number of telecommuting employees increased from an estimated 19 million in 2000 to 31.5 million in 2002 (Garvey 2001). The 2006 SHRM survey revealed that 26 percent of the employer respondents offered some type of telecommuting (Thompson 2006).

The most important reasons that employers use telecommuting are to reduce costs (33 percent), improve productivity (16 percent), increase employee retention (16 percent), boost employee morale (15 percent), and enhance customer service (11 percent) (Reilly 1997). It also decreases overhead costs as it eliminates or minimizes the need for office space. The two most important advantages of telecommuting are increased flexibility for employees and improved ability for organizations to attract workers who may not otherwise be available (Wells 2001). Drawbacks of telecommuting include the potential loss of employee creativity because of lower levels of face-to-face interaction, the difficulty of developing appropriate performance standards and evaluation systems, and the challenge of formulating an appropriate technology system for telecommuting (Capowski 1998). Telecommuting may also negatively affect employee–supervisor relationships (Wells 2001; Janove 2004). In addition, if some employees are denied the opportunity to work from home, they may pursue legal action or become dissatisfied employees. Telecommuting is obviously more appropriate for companies that are not engaged in direct patient care. Recent evidence indicates that, when given a choice, employees prefer a mix of working part of the time from home and part of the time at the employer's premises (Garchiek 2006).

Another work-schedule innovation is the use of *contingent workers*. The U.S. Department of Labor separates contingent workers into two groups: (1) independent contractors and on-call workers, who are called to work only when needed, and (2) temporary or short-term workers. Both of these groups have been growing and represent approximately 10.7 percent and 4.1 percent, respectively, of the U.S. workforce (*HR Focus* 2005; *HR Focus* 2006b). The reasons to use contingent workers include seasonal fluctuations in customer demand, project-based work, acquisition of skill sets not available among current employees, hiring freezes, rapid growth, and inadequate supply of certain occupations (e.g, registered nurses). Contingent workers may pose managerial challenges, such as unclear management reporting relationships, lack of accountability for performance, high relative compensation, low retention rates, variable attitudes and work quality, and inadequate orientation and training.

In sum, the healthcare industry can and does use all of the work-schedule design approaches discussed here for positions that do not involve clinical care of patients. Positions that involve direct patient care must be staffed 24 hours a day, seven days a week. A compressed workweek or job sharing are the most appropriate work-schedule adjustments for employees in such positions.

Summary

Job analysis is the collection of information relevant to the preparation of job descriptions and job specifications. An overall written summary of the task requirements for a particular job is called a job description, and an overall written summary of the personal requirements an individual must possess to successfully perform the job is called a job specification. Job analysis information developed in the form of job descriptions and job specifications provides the basic foundation for all human resources management functions.

Some combination of available job analysis methods (i.e., observation, interviews, questionnaires, job performance, diary, technical conference, competency model, and O*NET) should be used because all have advantages and disadvantages. Key considerations regarding the choice of methods should be the fit between the method and the purpose, cost, practicality, and an overall judgment on the appropriateness of the method for the situation in question. The primary purpose of conducting a job analysis should be described clearly to ensure that all relevant information is collected. In addition, time and cost constraints should be specified before choosing one or more of the available data-collection methods.

Healthcare executives should follow these steps when conducting a job analysis: (1) determine purpose, (2) identify jobs to be analyzed, (3) explain the process to employees, (4) collect job analysis information, (5) organize the information into job descriptions and job specifications, and (6) review and update the documents frequently. Job descriptions and job specifications, as derived from job analyses, must be done and their processes must be valid, accurate, and job related. Otherwise, the healthcare organization may face legal repercussions, particularly in the areas of employee selection, promotions, and compensation. The "Uniform Guidelines" and associated court cases provide standards to help executives avoid charges of discrimination when developing documents from job analysis data. In today's rapidly changing healthcare environment, healthcare executives should consider the potential advantage of future-oriented job analyses when change is more predictable and generic job analyses when change is less predictable. Both of these concepts may have legal or practical limitations that must be considered before the concepts are fully adopted.

Various new approaches to job design are required as healthcare organizations strive to overcome the effects of excessive specialization. Among the most significant of these are job redesign approaches such as the multiskilled health practitioners, employee empowerment, various team concepts, and work-schedule redesign.

Discussion Questions

1. Why should healthcare executives conduct a job analysis? What purpose does it serve?

2. What are job descriptions and job specifications? What is their relationship to job analysis? What will happen if a healthcare organization decides not to use any job descriptions at all?

3. Consider the position of the registered nurse in a large hospital. Which of the eight methods of job analysis will you use to collect data on this position, and why?

4. Describe the steps involved in the job analysis process.

5. How can the existence of a high-quality job analysis make a particular human resources function, such as employee selection, less legally vulnerable?

6. Are healthcare jobs static, or do they change over time? What may cause a job to change over time? What implications does this change have for job analysis?

7. Describe and discuss future-oriented job analysis and generic job analysis. How may each be used to help healthcare executives cope with a rapidly changing and competitive environment? What are some potential pitfalls of each approach?

8. What are the advantages and disadvantages of using multiskilled health practitioners?

9. Access information on work teams at www.workteams.unt.edu. What types

of work teams are most appropriate for achieving which objectives in the healthcare industry? Cite at least one successful team effort in healthcare.

10. Select one healthcare position with which you are familiar. What work-schedule innovations make the most sense for this position? Why?

Experiential Exercises

Exercise 1 Form a team with four fellow students to make a 30-minute class presentation on this topic: the future of job analysis in the healthcare industry. All the work on this challenging project must be done by the entire team; however, your group cannot have any face-to-face meetings. Your virtual team must come up with ways to deal with the following issues:

1. How will you organize the virtual team? Would you select a team leader? If so, based on what criteria?
2. On what bases would you select team members?
3. Without face-to-face encounters, how will you ensure that every member on the team does his or her assigned tasks so that a high-quality presentation is produced?

Exercise 2 Form a team of four or five fellow students. As a group, select one healthcare job (e.g., registered nurse, physical therapist, receptionist) with which all of the team members have some familiarity. Based solely on the group members' understanding of the selected job, outline the methods for conducting an analysis of the job. Draft a job description and a job specification that you believe represent the job. What future changes to the job do you think may affect your job description and job specification?

Exercise 3 You are a student in a master's in health administration program and have recently started your internship in a large, urban health system. Your preceptor has asked you to write a job description for your position, which is titled "Student Intern in Health Services Administration." Review the job analysis data sources and data-collection methods in this chapter. During your review, indicate the process and methods you will use to gather data. After completing those processes, write a model job description and job specification for your position.

References

Anthony, W. P., P. L. Perrewe, and K. M. Kacmar. 1993. *Strategic Human Resource Management.* Fort Worth, TX: Dryden Press.

Ash, R. A. 1988. "Job Analysis in the World of Work." In *The Job Analysis Handbook for Business,* edited by S. Grael, 3–23. New York: Wiley.

Athey, T. R., and M. S. Orth. 1999. "Emerging Competency Models for the Future." *Human Resource Management* 38: 215–26.

Bach, P. 2006. "Job Sharing Can Make for a Balanced Life." *Knight Ridder Tribune Business News* (January 31): A1.

Bell, A. H., and D. M. Smith. 2003. *Learning Team Skills.* Upper Saddle River, NJ: Prentice-Hall.

Blayney, K. D. (ed.). 1992. *Healing Hands: Customizing Your Health Team for Institutional Survival.* Battle Creek, MI: W. K. Kellogg Foundation.

Bohlander, G. W., and K. M. McCarthy. 1996. "How to Get the Most from Team Training." *National Productivity Review* 20 (3): 25–35.

Capowski, G. 1998. "Telecommuting: The New Frontier." *HR Focus* 75 (4): 2.

Carson, K. P., and G. L. Stewart. 1996. "Job Analysis and the Sociotechnical Approach to Quality: A Critical Explanation." *Journal of Quality Management* 1 (1): 49–56.

Clifford, J. P. 1994. "Job Analysis: Why Do It and How Should It Be Done?" *Public Personnel Management* 23 (3): 321–40.

Conklin, M. 1999. "9 to 5 Isn't Working Anymore." *Business Week* (September 20): 94–98.

Equal Employment Opportunity Commission (EEOC). 1978. "Uniform Guidelines for Employee Selection Procedures." *Federal Register* 43 (166): 38290–315.

———. 1992. *A Technical Assistance Manual on the Employment Provisions (Title 1) of the Americans with Disabilities Act.* Washington, DC: EEOC.

Ettore, B. 1997. "The Empowerment Gap: Hope vs. Reality." *HR Focus* 74 (7): 1–6.

Ford, R. L., and M. D. Fottler. 1995. "Empowerment: A Matter of Degree." *Academy of Management Executive* 4 (31): 21–29.

Fottler, M. D. 1992. "The Evolution of Health Manpower Utilization Pattern in Health Services and American Industry: Implications for Implementing the Multiskilled Concept." In *Healthy Hands: Customizing Your Health Team for Industrial Survival,* edited by K. D. Blayney, 1–23. Battle Creek, MI: W. K. Kellogg Foundation.

———. 1996. "The Role and Impact of Multiskilled Health Practitioners in the Health Services Industry." *Hospital & Health Services Administration* 41 (1): 55–75.

Gale, S. F. 2001a. "Expert Wisdom in Launching Flexed Programs." *Workforce* 80 (6): 64–71.

———. 2001b. "Formalized Flex Time: The Perk that Brings Productivity." *Workforce* 80 (2): 39–42.

Garchiek, K. 2006. "Workers Pick Office Over Telecommuting." *HR Magazine* 51 (9): 28–29.

Garcia, J. 1997. "How's Your Organizational Commitment?" *HR Focus* 74 (1): 22–34.

Garvey, C. 2001. "Teleworking HR." *HR Magazine* 46 (8): 56–60.

George, W. 1990. "Internal Marketing and Organizational Behavior: A Partnership in Developing Customer-Conscious Employees at Every Level." *Journal of Business Research* 20 (1): 63–70.

Grant, P. C. 1988. "Why Job Descriptions Don't Work." *Personnel Journal* 67 (1): 53–59.

Hartley, D. E. 2004. "Job Analysis at the Speed of Reality." *Training and Development* 58 (9): 20–22.

HR Focus. 2005. "Contingent Workforce Brings More Questions than Answers." *HR Focus* 82 (7): 6–7.

———. 2006a. "Have You Considered Job Sharing as a Retention Tool?" *HR Focus* 83 (9): 10–11.

———. 2006b. "More Contingent Workers Are a Blessing and Sometimes a Challenge for HR." *HR Focus* 83 (1): 51–54.

Hunt, S. T. 1996. "Generic Work Behavior: An Investigation into the Dimensions of Entry-level Hourly Job Performance." *Personnel Psychology* 49 (1): 51–83.

Janove, J. W. 2004. "Managing by Remote Control." *HR Magazine* 49 (3): 119–24.

Johnson, C. 2001. "Refocusing Job Descriptions." *HR Magazine* 48 (8): 66–72.

Lawler, E. E. 1986. *High Involvement Management.* San Francisco: Jossey-Bass.

Leonard, S. 2000. "The Demise of the Job Description." *HR Magazine* 45 (1): 184.

Levy, P. F. 2001. "When Teams Go Wrong." *Harvard Business Review* 79 (3): 51–67.

Livens, F., J. I. Sanchez, and W. D. Décorte. 2004. "Easing the Inferential Leap in Competency Modeling: The Effects of Task-Related Information and Subject Matter Expertise." *Personnel Psychology* 57: 881–904.

Mathis, R. L., and J. H. Jackson. 1985. *Personnel/Human Resources Management.* St. Paul, MN: West Publishing.

Mitchell, K. E., G. M. Alliger, and R. Morfopoalos. 1997. "Toward an ADA-Appropriate Job Analysis." *Human Resource Management Review* 7 (1): 5–26.

Nobile, R. J. 1991. "The Law of Performance Appraisals." *Personnel* 35 (1): 1.

Priem, E. P., K. O'Brien, and L. G. Gamble. 2004. "Perspectives on Non-Conventional Job Analysis Methodologies." *Journal of Business and Psychology* 18 (3): 337–52.

Reilly, E. M. 1997. "Telecommuting: Putting Policy into Practice." *HR Focus* 74 (9): 5–6.

Schippmann, J. J. 1999. *Strategic Job Modeling: Working at the Core of Integrated Human Resources.* Mahwah, NJ: Erlbaum.

Schneider, B., and A. M. Konz. 1989. "Strategic Job Analysis." *Human Resource Management* 28 (1): 51–63.

Schultz, K. L., J. O. McCain, and L. J. Thomas. 2003. "Overcoming the Dark Side of Worker Flexibility." *Journal of Operations Management* 21 (1): 81–94.

Simison, R. L. 1999. "Ford Rolls Out New Model of Corporate Culture." *Wall Street Journal* (January 13): A–1.

Snyder, D. 1996. "The Revolution in the Workplace: What's Happening to Our Jobs?" *Futurist* 30: 8.

Thompson, D. E., and T. A. Thompson. 1982. "Court Standards for Job Analysis in Test Validation." *Personnel Psychology* 35: 865–74.

Thompson, S. 2006. "Working Mothers Flex Their Scheduling Muscle." *Advertising Age* (November): 72–80.

Truxillo, D. M., M. E. Paronto, M. Collins, and J. L. Sulzer. 2004. "Effects of Subject Matter Expert Viewpoint on Job Analysis Results." *Public Personnel Management* 33 (1): 33–46.

U.S. Census Bureau. 1998. *Statistical Abstract of the United States.* Washington, DC: U.S. Government Printing Office.

Van Wart, M. 2000. "The Return to Simpler Strategies in Job Analysis." *Review of Public Personnel Administration* 20 (3): 5–23.

Vaughan, D. G., M. D. Fottler, R. W. Bamberg, and K. D. Blayney. 1991. "Utilization of Multiskilled Health Practitioners in U.S. Hospitals." *Hospital & Health Services Administration* 36 (3): 397–419.

Wells, S. J. 2001. "Making Telecommuting Work." *HR Magazine* 46 (10): 34–45.

Yandrick, R. M. 2001. "A Team Effort." *HR Magazine* 46 (6): 136–41.

APPENDIX A
An Example
of a Combined
Job Description/
Job Specification
Document

ST. VINCENT'S HOSPITAL
Birmingham, Alabama

JOB TITLE   Staff Nurse

DEPARTMENT   Nursing—Labor and Delivery

DATE   8/17/92   JOB CODE   2339   FLSA STATUS   Nonexempt

DEPARTMENT APPROVAL:_____

PERSONNEL APPROVAL:_____

ADMINISTRATIVE APPROVAL:_____

JOB SUMMARY

Assesses, prescribes, delegates, coordinates, and evaluates the nursing care provided. Ensures provision of quality care for selected groups of patients through utilization of nursing process, established standards of care, and policies and procedures.

SUPERVISION

A. SUPERVISED BY: Unit Manager, indirectly by Charge Nurse

B. SUPERVISES: No one

C. LEADS/GUIDES: Unit Associates/Ancillary Associates in the delivery of direct patient care

JOB SPECIFICATIONS

A. EDUCATION

— Required: Graduate of an accredited school of professional nursing
— Desired:

B. EXPERIENCE

— Required: None
— Desired: Previous clinical experience

C. LICENSES, CERTIFICATIONS, AND/OR REGISTRATIONS: Current R.N. license in the State of Alabama; BCLS and certifications specific to areas of clinical specialty preferred.

D. EQUIPMENT/TOOLS/WORK AIDS: POA infusors, infusion pumps and other medical equipment, computer terminal and printer, facsimile machine, photocopier, and patient charts

E. SPECIALIZED KNOWLEDGE AND SKILLS: Ability to work with female patients of child-bearing age and new-born patients in all specialty and subspecialty categories, both urgent and nonurgent in nature.

(Continued)

APPENDIX A

Continued

F. <u>PERSONAL TRAITS, QUALITIES, AND APTITUDES:</u> Must be able to: 1) perform a variety of duties often changing from one task to another of a different nature without loss of efficiency or composure; 2) accept responsibility for the direction, control, and planning of an activity; 3) make evaluations and decisions based on measurable or verifiable criteria; 4) work independently; 5) recognize the rights and responsibilities of patient confidentiality; 6) convey empathy and compassion to those experiencing pain or grief; 7) relate to others in a manner that creates a sense of teamwork and cooperation; and 8) communicate effectively with people from every socioeconomic background.

G. <u>WORKING CONDITIONS:</u> Inside environment, protected from the weather but not necessarily temperature changes. Subject to frequent exposure to infection, contagious disease, combative patients, and potentially hazardous materials and equipment. Variable noise levels. Also subject to rapid pace, multiple stimuli, unpredictable environment, and critical situations.

H. <u>PHYSICAL DEMANDS/TRAITS:</u> Must be able to: 1) perceive the nature of sounds by the ear; 2) express or exchange ideas by means of the spoken word; 3) perceive characteristics of objects through the eyes; 4) extend arms and hands in any direction; 5) seize, hold, grasp, turn, or otherwise work with hands; 6) pick, pinch, or otherwise work with the fingers; 7) perceive such attributes of objects or materials as size, shape, temperature, or texture; and 8) stoop, kneel, crouch, and crawl. Must be able to lift 50 pounds maximum with frequent lifting, carrying, pushing, and pulling of objects weighing up to 25 pounds. Continuous walking and standing. Must be able to identify, match, and distinguish colors. Rare lifting of greater than 100 pounds.

JOB RESPONSIBILITIES AND PERFORMANCE STANDARDS

Assigned

Weight

10% 1. UTILIZES THE NURSING PROCESS (i.e., ASSESSMENT, PLANNING, IMPLEMENTATION, AND EVALUATION) IN THE PROVISION OF PATIENT CARE IN ACCORDANCE WITH THE STANDARDS OF CARE AND POLICIES AS WRITTEN

Assessment
— Admission assessment includes at least the following:
  • Patient identification
  • Current medical history
  • Current obstetrical history
  • Reason for admission
  • Relevant physical, psychological, and sociological status
    Allergies
    Drug use

      Disabilities impairment
      Surgical Consent Form Medical Consent Form
      Pediatrician's Consent Form

— Assessments performed in accordance with the patient care standard, S-2-7010-VI:
- Admission physical assessment
- Affected system each shift
- Labor patients:
  Maternal temperature q 4 hours
  Maternal pulse q 4 hours
  Maternal blood pressure q 1 hour
  Pitocin order
  Vaginal exam prior to Pitocin
  Epidural level of anesthesia hourly
  FHR q 30 minutes during 1st stage
  FHR q 15 minutes during 2nd stage

— Plan of care
- Conceptualized plan of care is developed for each patient:
  Identify one nursing diagnosis pertinent to this patient's care.
  Identify one nursing intervention related to this diagnosis.
  Identify to whom this plan of care should be communicated.
- Nursing intervention(s) relative to the identified nursing diagnosis is documented.
- Written plan of care is initiated on patients whose stay in Labor and Delivery exceeds 24 hours (exception: patients in labor).
- Plan of care mutually developed with patient and/or SO.
- Written plan of care updated in response to changes in patient care needs.
- Plan of care consistent with medical plan of care.
- All components of the written plan of care are included:
  Date
  Problem number
  Nursing diagnosis
  Nursing orders
  Patient goal(s)
  Projected resolution date
- Patient goals stated are:
  Realistic
  Measurable
- Patient's response to care given is documented.
- Changes in patient's condition are documented.

10% 2. DETERMINES CONDITION OF PATIENTS AND CLASSIFIES APPROPRIATELY

— Appropriate acuity level is determined based on care provided to the patient/SO.
— All asterisk (*) items have narrative documentation.

(Continued)

APPENDIX A

Continued

5%   3. DEMONSTRATES KNOWLEDGE OF DISCHARGE PLANNING, REHABILITATIVE MEASURES, AND COMMUNITY RESOURCES BY MAKING APPROPRIATE AND TIMELY REFERRALS

— Initial assessment of discharge needs is accomplished through a complete patient/family history on admission.

5%   4. DEMONSTRATES KNOWLEDGE AND UNDERSTANDING OF TEACHING/LEARNING PROCESS AND IMPLEMENTS PATIENT TEACHING TO MEET LEARNING NEEDS OF PATIENT AND/OR SIGNIFICANT OTHER

— Patient and/or significant other are involved in the identification of learning needs for short-term teaching/counseling during labor.

— Patient teaching during labor is evidenced by anticipatory guidance relative to all procedures and events.

5%   5. ASSUMES RESPONSIBILITY FOR ASSIGNING, DIRECTING, AND PROVIDING CARE FOR GROUPS OF PATIENTS

— Demonstrates necessary skills and knowledge to make appropriate assignments and considers the following factors when making patient care assignments:
  • The patient's status
  • The environment in which nursing care is provided
  • The competence of the nursing staff members who are to provide the care
  • The degree of supervision required by and available to the associates
  • The complexity of the assessment required by the patient
  • The type of technology employed in providing nursing care
  • Relevant infection control and safety issues
— Demonstrates the necessary skills and knowledge to provide care for patients in accordance with the Nursing Department and unit specific required skills and competencies
— Compassionately gives personal patient care to provide comfort and well-being to the patient, acknowledging psychological needs
— Delegates aspects of care to other nursing staff members as appropriate
— Appropriately documents and communicates pertinent observations and care provided

10% 6. ADMINISTERS MEDICATIONS, INTRAVASCULAR FLUIDS, AND TREATMENTS IN ACCORDANCE WITH HOSPITAL STANDARDS AND FEDERAL REGULATIONS

— Demonstrates or obtains knowledge of drugs and fluids to be administered
— Accurately administers medications and intravascular fluids as ordered and scheduled
— Accurately and completely documents administration and patient's response to drugs and intravascular fluids

— Demonstrates ability and appropriate technical skills and procedures in accordance with physician's orders and nursing policies and procedures:
  - Procedures and treatments performed in a timely manner
  - Makes adequate preparation for performance of procedures and/or treatments
  - Completes appropriate documentation

10% 7. MAINTAINS EFFECTIVE COMMUNICATION WITH SUPERVISORS, HOSPITAL ASSOCIATES, MEDICAL STAFF, PATIENTS, FAMILIES, AND VISITORS

— Enhances cohesiveness of unit staff group through effective interpersonal communication
— Communicates with all persons involved in a patient's care in a manner that facilitates timely meeting of stated goals
— Utilizes approved lines of authority and channels of communication in sharing concerns
— Actively participates in a minimum of four (4) interdepartmental meetings annually
— Interacts effectively with patients, families, and/or significant others
— Supports problem-solving approach to both unit and patient needs
— Follows through on problems that may compromise patient care by using the appropriate chain-of-command
— Gives a thorough concise change of shift report

5% 8. RESPONDS APPROPRIATELY TO ENVIRONMENTAL AND SAFETY HAZARDS AND FUNCTIONS EFFECTIVELY IN EMERGENCY SITUATIONS

— Recognizes, takes action, and reports unsafe acts or situations involving patients, visitors, or staff
— Responds promptly and appropriately to environmental and safety hazards
— Promptly removes unsafe equipment from patient care areas and notifies the appropriate department
— Functions promptly and effectively in codes, emergencies, or other stressful patient situations
— Identifies high-risk patients and monitors accordingly
— Complies with hospital and departmental policies and procedures concerning infection control
— Demonstrates correct and safe technique in the use of equipment according to specific product information and policy and procedure manuals
— Maintains a clean, neat, and safe environment for patients, visitors, and staff according to hospital and unit policies

5% 9. UTILIZES HOSPITAL SYSTEMS EFFECTIVELY TO ENSURE ECONOMICAL USE OF EQUIPMENT AND SUPPLIES

— Effectively utilizes unit dose, classification, pneumatic tube, beepers, emergency checks, and services of other hospital departments
— Demonstrates appropriate economical use of supplies and equipment

(Continued)

— Ensures appropriate handling of charges
— Accurately utilizes the computer system
— Correctly initiates and discontinues daily charges when indicated
— Ensures that supplies and equipment necessary for patient care are stored in an organized and efficient manner
— Follows appropriate procedure for obtaining and returning or cleaning and/or disposing of equipment and supplies

5%   10. DEMONSTRATES THROUGH ACTIONS THE ACCEPTANCE OF LEGAL AND ETHICAL RESPONSIBILITIES OF THE PROFESSIONAL NURSE

— Documents effectively, accurately, and in a timely manner, on the patient's medical record according to hospital and department standards and policies
— Adheres to drug handling regulations
— Exhibits knowledge of reportable incidents, appropriate documentation, and follow-up
— Maintains current State R.N. license
— Protects patients' rights to privacy and confidentiality
— Demonstrates professional responsibility for nonprofessional group members
— Accurately transcribes or verifies accuracy of physician orders

5%   11. ASSUMES RESPONSIBILITY FOR KEEPING SKILLS CURRENT AND KNOWLEDGE UPDATED THROUGH STAFF DEVELOPMENT AND CONTINUING EDUCATION PROGRAMS

— Actively seeks learning experiences
— Appropriately verbalizes learning needs
— Attends a minimum of eight (8) hours or eight classes of relevant continuing education/staff development programs annually
— Maintains current Educational Profile

10%   12. COMPLETES A VOLUME OF WORK THAT ENSURES OPTIMUM PRODUCTIVITY WHILE MAINTAINING QUALITY PATIENT CARE

— Completes care of assigned patients in a timely manner
— Assists other associates in completing their assignments in a timely manner. Supports cost-effective methods for improving patient care
— Willingly accepts adjustment of posted schedule to meet unit emergencies and patient care needs as requested
— Demonstrates an ongoing awareness of, and participation in, the Quality Review (QR) program
— Is alert to potential OR problems and actively participates in solving such problems. Responds with improved performance to results obtained from OR monitors. Does not incur excessive unscheduled overtime

5%   13. PARTICIPATES IN ASSIGNED COMMITTEES, CONFERENCES, PROJECTS, STAFF DEVELOPMENT PROGRAMS, AND STAFF MEETINGS
  — Attends and actively contributes to assigned committees, projects, and so forth
  — Assists immediate supervisor in the orientation and performance evaluation of associates
  — Actively supports departmental projects
  — Effectively implements approved departmental changes
  — Adapts to changes in a positive, professional manner
  — Attends staff meeting or reads and signs all minutes of staff meetings not attended

The associate is expected to perform this job in a manner consistent with the values, mission, and philosophy of St. Vincent's Hospital and the Daughters of Charity National Health System.

Reviewed/Revised By:

_____   Date_____

_____   Date_____

_____

_____

This job description is meant to be only a representative summary of the major duties and responsibilities performed by incumbents of this job. The incumbents may be requested to perform job-related tasks other than those stated in this description.

_____

_____

SOURCE: Reprinted with permission from St. Vincent's Hospital, Birmingham, Alabama.

RECRUITMENT, SELECTION, AND RETENTION

Bruce J. Fried, PhD, and Michael Gates, PhD

Learning Objectives

After completing this chapter, the reader should be able to

- understand the major steps and decisions involved in designing and implementing a recruitment effort,
- discuss the factors considered by people in deciding to accept a job offer,
- describe the relationship of job requirements (as developed through job analyses, job descriptions, and job specifications) to other human resources management functions,
- design a recruitment and selection effort for a particular job,
- address the advantages and disadvantages of internal and external recruitment and other sources of job applicants,
- explain the concepts of person–organization fit and its relevance to recruitment and selection,
- offer alternative selection tools and how they can be used in the selection process,
- articulate the concept of validity in the use of selection tools, and
- identify the most important factors related to turnover and retention and strategies that can improve retention.

Introduction

In this chapter, attention turns to the processes of recruitment, selection, and retention. We explore these three topics together because they are integrally related not only with each other but also with other human resources management (HRM) functions. For example, the development and stringency of criteria for selecting job applicants depend, to a large degree, on the success of the recruitment effort. An organization can be more selective when a relatively large supply of qualified applicants is available. Similarly, developing a recruitment plan for a particular position depends on the existence of an accurate, current, and comprehensive job description. If we are concerned with retaining valued employees, then we may include in our selection process criteria that increase the probability that employees will stay with the organization. While more difficult than assessing technical readiness for the job, methods exist for assessing employee qualities and commitment, career interests, and adaptability—some of the qualities that may be associated with retention. As with all HRM functions, organizations must be cognizant of legal considerations when developing and implementing recruitment and selection procedures. Each of these functions must be addressed from both strategic and operational perspectives.

Effective recruitment and selection are key to employee retention. An important measure of the effectiveness of these functions is the extent to which the organization is able to attract committed employees who remain with the organization. Many factors affect retention and, as discussed later, recruitment and selection procedures can have an impact on retention. Further, we know that employee retention is tied to the effectiveness of orientation and "on-boarding" procedures; therefore, we should also focus on these practices in our efforts to improve retention.

These three functions are highly interdependent, but we address them separately and sequentially in this chapter. These concepts include the following:

- Recruitment steps
- Sources of job applicants
- Organizational fit, and its importance in the selection process
- Reliability and validity of selection decisions
- Selection instruments
- Types of selection interviews and ways to improve their effectiveness
- Factors and strategies related to employee retention and turnover

Recruitment

The goal of recruitment is to generate a pool of qualified job applicants. Specifically, recruitment refers to the range of processes an organization uses to attract qualified individuals on a timely basis and in sufficient numbers and to encourage them to apply for jobs in the organization. When we think of recruitment strategies, our attention often focuses on a set of key questions:

- Should the organization recruit and promote from within, or should it focus on recruiting external applicants?
- Should the organization consider alternative approaches to filling jobs with full-time employees, such as outsourcing, flexible staffing, and hiring contingent workers?

- Should the organization find applicants who have precisely the right technical qualifications or applicants who best fit the culture of the organization but may require additional training to improve their technical skills?

The success of recruitment is dependent on many factors, including the attractiveness of the organization, the community in which the organization is located, the work climate and culture of the organization, managerial and supervisory attitudes and behavior, workload, and other job-related considerations. Before we explore these aspects, we first address recruitment from the perspective of applicants and potential employees. What factors influence an individual's decision to apply for and accept employment with a particular organization? If we consider applicants and employees as customers, then an understanding of their needs and expectations is central to the development and implementation of effective recruitment strategies.

Factors that Influence Job Choice

What do potential employees look for in a job? Once an individual is offered a position, how does that person make the decision to accept or reject the offer? People consider a number of factors related to the attractiveness of the position and the organization, as well as factors specific to the individual. Applicants consider their own competitiveness in the job market and whether alternative positions that provide better opportunities are available. They are also sensitive to the attitudes and behaviors of the recruiter, or whoever is their first contact with the organization. First impressions are very potent because the issue of "fitting in" with the organization is often decided at this stage, and early negative first impressions may be difficult to reverse. Questions foremost in the applicant's mind are, "Is this the kind of place I can see myself spending 40 or more hours a week?" and "Will I fit in?" They may also be concerned with opportunities for career mobility and promotion.

As discussed later, employers go through a similar process when making selection decisions, determining if the applicant will fit into the organizational culture and ways of working. Applicants are more likely to accept positions in organizations that share their values and style. Organizations engage in a "signaling" process, in which they send out messages about their values in an attempt to attract candidates with similar beliefs (Barber 1998). Consider, for example, the recruitment potential of the following recruitment messages:

- "A power to heal. A passion for care." (WakeMed 2007)
- "Every life deserves world class care." (The Cleveland Clinic 2007)
- "Caring for our patients begins with caring for our people." (North Shore–Long Island Jewish Health System 2007)

Consider the values statement of the world-renowned Mayo Clinic, spoken by Dr. Charles W. Mayo: "There are no inferior jobs in any organization. No matter what the assigned task, if it is done well and with dignity, it contributes to the function of everything around it and should be valued accordingly by all" (Mayo Clinic 2007). Mayo Clinic's website also indicates that it is one of *Fortune*'s "100 Best Companies to Work For" and that it has been a Magnet hospital since 1997. Seeking to attract members of minority groups to its workforce, Kaiser Permanente (2007) devotes a substantial portion of its web-based recruitment efforts to promoting its National Diversity Program and its emphasis on culturally competent care. Similarly, to distinguish itself from other hospitals, the nursing recruitment web page for Johns Hopkins Hospital (2007) states: "Though your choices are vast in today's nursing market, we challenge you to discover for yourself what is different about a nursing career with our world-renowned, Magnet-recognized team and America's #1 hospital."

With these examples in mind, we can see that organizations promote themselves as good places to work by appealing to a variety of potential employee needs and interests. Considerable research has been done on job choice factors (Schwab, Rynes, and Aldag 1987); however, it is difficult to make a generalization about which factors are most important in employment decisions. The relative importance of these factors varies, depending on the individual, the organization, the job, and environmental factors such as the level of unemployment. Understanding the factors that affect job choice is central to developing effective recruitment strategies. A helpful way to think about the reasons for a job choice is to distinguish between vacancy characteristics and individual characteristics.

Individual characteristics are personal considerations that influence a person's job decision. The factors considered by a family physician to accept employment with a rural health center may be quite different from the factors that drive a nurse's decision to accept employment with an urban teaching hospital. Also, one's life stage may affect the salience of these decision factors. *Vacancy characteristics*, on the other hand, are those associated with the job, such as compensation, challenge and responsibility, advancement opportunities, job security, geographic location, and employee benefits; each of these factors is explained below.

The level of compensation and benefits is often considered, on face value, as a key element in an individual's decision to accept a position with an organization. For many positions in healthcare, we have seen the area of compensation further complicated by differential pay rates, hiring (or signing) bonuses, and relocation assistance. Hot-skill premiums, or temporary pay premiums added to base pay to account for temporary market escalations in pay (Heneman and Judge 2003, 588–89), have become particularly common in healthcare, although premiums usually remain in place even after market pressures ease. The importance of compensation, however, is complex. On the one hand, substantial evidence has shown that under certain circumstances employees may leave an organization for another to obtain what amounts to an incremental increase in compensation. However, in other cases, even a relatively generous level of compensation can be outweighed by the presence or absence of other important factors.

The amount of challenge and responsibility inherent in a particular job is frequently cited as an important job choice factor, and this element is likely even more salient in healthcare organizations where professionals seek out positions that maximize use of their professional knowledge, training, and skills. Similarly, many applicants place value on jobs with substantial advancement and professional development opportunities. While the availability of such opportunities is significant to all ranges of applicants, these opportunities are likely to be a particularly important determinant for professionally trained individuals and those in management roles (or aspiring to management roles) (London and Stumpf 1982). Traditionally, advancement opportunities for clinically or technically trained individuals are scarce in healthcare because the only avenue to advancement is often through promotion to supervisory or management responsibilities. For many clinicians, taking on supervisory responsibilities may lead to a feeling of loss of their professional identity. In healthcare (and other industries as well), dual career-path systems have been established to enable highly talented clinicians to move up while not forcing them to abandon their clinical interests and expertise. Such systems provide specialists who are interested in pursuing a technical career with alternative career paths while maintaining an adequate pool of clinical and technical talent within the organization (Roth 1982).

Job security is clearly an important determinant of job choice. The current healthcare and general business environment is characterized by an unprecedented number of mergers, acquisitions, and reorganization, which lead to frequent downsizing and worker displacement. This phenomenon was once limited largely to blue-collar workers, but professionals and employees in middle and senior management roles are also at risk in the current environment. An illustrative manifestation of the importance of job security is evident in union organizing and collective bargaining. Not too long ago, compensation and benefits were the most highly valued issues in labor negotiations. Today, however, job security and restrictions on outsourcing have gained increasing importance in employees' decision to unionize (Mayer 2005; Caudron 1995). In fact, in several instances, unionized employees have made wage concessions in return for higher levels of job security (Henderson 1986).

Geographic location, along with other lifestyle concerns, has become a key player in job decisions, especially for individuals in dual-income families, in which the employment of a spouse may be a significant determinant of job acceptance. In healthcare, location is a particularly acute issue because healthcare organizations are often, by necessity, located in less-than-desirable locales that may not be attractive to applicants. The level and type of employee benefits continue to grow as an important determinant of job acceptance. Particularly in highly competitive industries, many companies have moved beyond traditional benefits, such as health insurance and vacation pay, into more innovative offers, including membership in country/health clubs, on-site day care, and financial counseling. SAS Institute, Inc., the software producer based in Cary, North Carolina, is known worldwide for its extensive and innovative benefits.

Table 8.1 illustrates how different job applicants assess the relative importance of job features. Although the depiction in the table oversimplifies the job choice process, it shows how individuals value different aspects of the job depending on personal preferences and life circumstances. The first column briefly describes each applicant. The second column states each applicant's minimum standards for job acceptance along four dimensions: pay, benefits, advancement opportunities, and travel requirements. These four dimensions are sometimes categorized as noncompensatory standards—that is, no other element of the job can compensate if these standards are not met, or, more simply, these are "deal killers." Thus, Person 3, who does not like to travel, will be unlikely to accept a job that requires substantial travel, regardless of anything else; similarly, for Person 2, health insurance coverage is an absolute requirement for job acceptance. The third column showcases each of the three jobs according to the four noncompensatory standards.

This type of analysis is useful for applicants because it provides a way of narrowing down job choices. Assuming a job applicant is considering several job offers that meet minimum requirements, he or she can engage in a more refined job choice process that allows for comparing job factors (Barber et al. 1994). Using less important job choice factors, an individual can trade off the strengths of one job dimension for the weaknesses in another.

The Recruitment Process

The recruitment process uses the organization's human resources (HR) plan as a foundation. An *HR plan* includes specific information about the organization's strategies, the types of individuals required to achieve organizational goals, recruitment and hiring approaches, and a clear statement of how HR practices support organizational goals. Those involved in recruitment and selection must, of course, have a thorough understanding of the position that needs to be filled, including its relationship with other positions and the job requirements. The recruitment process ideally begins with a job analysis (which addresses questions of job tasks, knowledge, skills, and abilities) and development of specific qualifications required of applicants.

The early stages of the recruitment process involve an examination of the external environment, particularly the supply of potential job applicants

TABLE 8.1

Three Hypothetical Job Applicants

Job Applicant	Minimum Standards for Job Acceptance	Job Description
Person 1: 23 years old, single	*Pay:* at least $40,000 *Benefits:* Health insurance coverage of at least 25 percent *Advancement opportunities:* Very important *Travel requirements:* Unimportant	*Job:* Insurance company provider relations coordinator *Pay:* $45,000 *Benefits:* Health insurance covered at 50 percent *Advancement opportunities:* Recruitment done internally and externally *Travel requirements:* Average 25 percent travel
Person 2: Sole wage earner for large family	*Pay:* at least $50,000 *Benefits:* Health insurance coverage of at least 50 percent *Advancement opportunities:* Very important *Travel requirements:* Cannot travel more than 25 percent of the time	*Job:* Healthcare consultant *Pay:* $55,000 *Benefits:* Health insurance covered at 50 percent *Advancement opportunities:* Strong history of promotions within one year *Travel requirements:* Average 50 percent travel
Person 3: Spouse of high-wage earner	*Pay:* at least $35,000 *Benefits:* Unimportant *Advancement opportunities:* Unimportant *Travel requirements:* Cannot travel more than one week per year	*Job:* Research assistant in academic medical center *Pay:* $37,000 *Benefits:* Health insurance covered at 50 percent *Advancement opportunities:* Generally hires externally for higher-level positions *Travel requirements:* Little or none

TABLE 8.2
Human
Resources
Information
System
Recruitment
Data

HRIS Data	Uses in Recruitment
Skills and knowledge inventory	Identifies potential internal job candidates
Previous applicants	Identifies potential external job candidates
Recruitment source information • Yield ratios • Cost • Cost per applicant • Cost per hire	Helps in the analysis of cost effectiveness of recruitment sources
Employee performance and retention information	Provides information on the success of recruitment sources used in the past

and the relative competitiveness for the position. This analysis should also examine compensation and benefits given to individuals who hold similar jobs in competing organizations. It may also entail an evaluation of external recruitment sources, such as colleges, competing organizations, and professional associations, to determine if these were successful recruitment sources in the past. Other aspects to consider in this assessment are the logistics and timing of a recruitment effort; for some positions, seasonal elements to the recruitment process are at play, such as graduation from nursing school.

The process should then review past recruitment efforts for this and similar positions: Is this a job that will require an international search, or will the local labor market suffice? Optimally, a *human resources information system* (HRIS) will provide useful information during the recruitment process. While the sophistication of an HRIS varies from one organization to the next, many such systems include some or all of the information described in Table 8.2. A *skills inventory* database maintains information on every employee's skills, educational background, training acquired, seminars attended, work history, and other job-development data. This inventory may also include data on applicants who were not hired. A well-managed database broadens the pool of possible applicants from which to draw.

Recruitment and selection can be very costly, and accurate information about costs is essential. Table 8.3 illustrates the variety of measures that may be used to assess the effectiveness and efficiency of the recruitment process. Each of these factors varies depending on the job, but overall having a mechanism in place to assess the cost effectiveness of recruitment methods is important. Again, a good HRIS and cost-accounting system can help the organization understand the major costs associated with recruitment and selection.

Type of Cost	Expenses
Cost per hire	• Advertising, agency fees, employee referral bonuses, recruitment fairs and travel, and sign-on bonuses • Staff time: salary; benefits; and overhead costs for employees to review applications, set up interviews, conduct interviews, check references, and make and confirm an offer • Processing costs: opening a new file, medical examination, drug screening, and credential checking • Travel and lodging for applicants, relocation costs • Orientation and training
Application rate	• Ratio-referral factor: number of candidates to number of openings • Applicants per posting • Qualified applicants per posting • Protected class applicants per posting • Number of internal candidates, number of qualified internal candidates • Number of external candidates, number of qualified external candidates *The measures above can be calculated for all referral sources or by individual referral source.*
Time to hire	• Time between job requisition and first interview • Time between job requisition and offer • Time between job offer and offer acceptance • Time between job requisition and starting work
Recruitment source effectiveness	• Offers by recruitment source • Hires by recruitment source • Employee performance (using performance evaluation information and promotion rates) • Employee retention by recruitment source • Offer acceptance rate (overall and by recruitment source)
Recruiter effectiveness	• Response time, time to fill, cost per hire, acceptance rate, employee performance, and retention
Miscellaneous	• Materials and other special or unplanned expenses, new employee orientation, reference checking, and drug screening

TABLE 8.3

Measures of Recruitment Effectiveness and Efficiency

SOURCE: Adapted from Fitz-enz and Davison (2002)

Recruitment Sources

An initial question in the recruitment process is applicant sourcing, or specifying where qualified job applicants are located. We often distinguish between internal recruitment (which usually entails promotion or transfer from within the organization) and external recruitment (identifying applicants from outside of the organization). Table 8.4 is a summary of the advantages and disadvantages of internal and external recruitment. On the positive side of *internal recruitment,* candidates are generally already known to the organization—the organization is familiar with their past performance and future potential and

TABLE 8.4
Advantages and Disadvantages of Internal and External Recruitment

Advantages	Disadvantages
Recruiting Internal Candidates	
• May improve employee morale and encourage valued employees to stay with the organization	• Possible morale problems among those not selected
• Permits greater assessment of applicant abilities; candidate is a known entity	• May lead to inbreeding
	• May lead to conflict among internal job applicants
• May be faster, and may involve lower cost for certain jobs	• May require strong training and management development activities
• Good motivator for employee performance	• May manifest the Peter Principle
• Applicants have a good understanding of the organization	• May cause ripple effect in vacancies, which need to be filled
• May reinforce employees' sense of job security	
Recruiting External Candidates	
• Brings new ideas into the organization	• May identify candidate who has technical skills but does not fit the culture of the organization
• May be less expensive than training internal candidates	• May cause morale problems for internal candidates who were not selected
• External candidates come without dysfunctional relationships with others and without being involved in organizational politics	• May require longer adjustment and socialization
• May bring new ideas to the organization	• Uncertainty about candidate skills and abilities, and difficulty obtaining reliable information about applicant

is aware of their expectations. Internal candidates also tend to know specific organizational processes and procedures and may not require as much socialization and start-up time. Internal recruitment may also be used as a morale builder and viewed as a career ladder because it encourages highly valued and productive employees to stay with the organization.

On the negative side of internal recruitment, however, is the possible manifestation of the *Peter Principle,* a common phenomenon in which successful employees continue to be promoted until they reach one position above their level of competence (Peter and Hull 1969). With the Peter Principle, employees may be promoted regardless of their aptitude for the new position. This is noteworthy in healthcare, where individuals with strong clinical skills may be promoted into supervisory and management roles without the requisite skills and training for those responsibilities. For example, a world-renowned clinician and researcher may be promoted to vice president of medical affairs even though that person is not the best candidate. Effective organizations seek to prevent this phenomenon by ensuring the accuracy of job descriptions and by requiring internal (and external) candidates to meet the specified job qualifications. If an individual who does not possess all the job qualifications is hired, a manager has to be cognizant of the person's need to be trained in those areas requiring remediation. Internal recruitment may also have the disadvantage of causing disarray in the organization. At times, promotion creates a ripple effect—one individual moves into a different position, leaving a vacancy; this vacancy, in turn, is filled by someone else who causes another vacancy, and so forth.

External recruitment refers to turning to sources of applicants outside the organization, including educational institutions, such as high schools, vocational schools, community colleges, and universities. Depending on the position, external recruitment may also be done through advertising on the Internet and in print media. An advantage of external recruitment is that candidates may bring in new ideas. In addition, the organization may be able to more specifically target candidates with the skills needed rather than to settle for an internal candidate who may know the organization but may lack specific skills and knowledge. External candidates also tend to be unencumbered by political problems and conflict and therefore may be easier to bring into a difficult political environment than an internal applicant. This is often a rationale for selecting a chief executive officer from outside.

Many applicants are not easy to characterize as coming from either an internal or an external source. For example, hiring candidates who have worked for the organization in a contingent or part-time capacity, including contract employees, is not uncommon. This is increasingly the practice in nursing, where traveling or agency nurses may apply or be recruited for a full-time position. As a general rule, obtaining as many qualified job applicants as possible is a good idea. From the organization's perspective, a large number of applicants permits choice and sometimes may even stimulate a rethinking of the job design. For example, an applicant may emerge who has additional skill sets that are not necessarily relevant to the job as currently designed but are useful nonetheless. Successful organizations are flexible enough to take advantage of these opportunities. Note also that it is advisable to design recruitment efforts in such a way that they yield applicants who have at least the minimum qualifications. Processing a large number of unqualified applicants can be expensive as well as a waste of time for both the organization and applicants. To prevent this waste, some organizations scan electronic resumes to identify key words and to screen applicants.

Employee referral is an excellent source because the current employee knows the organization and the applicant and can thus act as the initial screen. A person identified and hired through this mechanism may therefore bring advantages common to both internal and external recruitment. Employee referral can be a powerful recruitment strategy, yielding employees who typically stay longer with the organization and who exhibit higher levels of loyalty and job satisfaction than do employees recruited through other mechanisms (Rynes 1991; Taylor 1994). Some employee referral programs give monetary rewards to employees whose referrals were successful—that is, if the new hire remains with the organization for a defined period of time. Keeping the information of employee-referred applicants who were not hired is advisable because such referrals may be mined for open positions in the future. More and more organizations are using web-based systems to encourage employee referrals for internal and external recruitment (Calandra 2001).

Former employees are also a fruitful source of applicants. Employees who have left under good condition—that is, as a result of other employment opportunities, organizational downsizing and restructuring, relocation, and personal factors—sometimes may seek or be available for reemployment with the organization. Their capabilities and potential are already usually well known to the organization. Returning employees may also send an implicit message to current employees that the work environment is not so bad after all.

Depending on the position involved, employment agencies and executive search firms (both state sponsored and private) may be useful as applicant search and screening vehicles. Agencies may specialize in different types of searches and typically work either on a commission or on a flat-fee basis.

Content of the Recruiting Message

An important objective of recruitment is to maximize the possibility that the right candidate will accept the organization's job offer. What are the appropriate messages to include in recruitment? Four types of information should be communicated to applicants:

1. *Applicant qualifications:* education, experience, credentials, and any other preferences that the employer has within legal constraints
2. *Job basics:* title, responsibilities, compensation, benefits, location, and other pertinent working conditions (e.g., night work, travel, promotion potential)
3. *Application process:* deadline, resume, cover letter, transcripts, references, and contact person and address for the application packet
4. *Organization and department basics:* name and type of organization, department, and other information about the work environment

A *realistic recruitment message* is the most advantageous. This message is a direct statement to the applicant about the organization and the job; it is not a public relations pitch that the employer thinks the applicant wishes to hear (Heneman and Judge 2003). So far, only limited research has been done on the effectiveness of this technique.

Realistic Recruitment Message and Realistic Job Preview

However, considerable research is available on the effectiveness of the *realistic job preview.* The goal of a realistic job preview is to present practical information about job requirements, organizational expectations, and the work environment. The preview should include negative and positive aspects of the job and the organization, and it may be presented to new hires before they start work. The use of realistic job previews is related to higher performance and lower attrition from the recruitment process, lower initial expectations, lower voluntary turnover, and lower turnover overall (Phillips 1998). A realistic job preview can be presented in a number of ways: verbally, in writing, or through the media (Wanous 1992). Certainly the most straightforward approach is for the prospective or new employee to hold frank discussions with coworkers and supervisors. In addition, the new employee may observe the work setting and perhaps shadow an employee who is doing a similar job.

Regardless of the approach used, preventing surprises and providing the employee with an honest assessment of the job and the work environment are key.

Evaluating the Recruitment Function

Assessing the effectiveness of recruitment efforts is critical. Such an evaluation process is dependent on the existence of reliable and comprehensive data on applicants, a well-functioning HRIS, the quality of applicants, the applicants' disposition, and recruitment costs. Common measures of the success of a recruitment function include the following:

- *Quantity of applicants.* The proper use of recruitment methods and sources will yield a substantial number of candidates (depending on the market supply) who meet at least the minimum job requirements.

Having a sufficiently large pool of applicants allows the organization a better chance of identifying the most qualified candidates. However, attracting many applicants is also associated with increased recruitment costs. Therefore, the minimum job requirements need to be established to maintain a balance among the number of candidates, the quality of applicants, and the cost.

- *Quality of applicants.* A well-designed recruitment effort will bring in employees who have the appropriate education, qualifications, skills, and attitudes.
- *Overall recruitment cost and cost per applicant.* A recruitment effort's costs are often unacceptable to the organization. The overall cost per applicant and the cost of the recruiting methods and sources should be examined. This analysis provides the opportunity to determine the cost effectiveness of alternative recruitment methods. The financial impact of using part-time or temporary help while looking for the right applicant should also be considered as these costs can be substantial.
- *Diversity of applicants.* Assuming that one goal of the recruitment program is to identify and hire qualified candidates who represent the diversity of the service population or to address diversity goals, the organization can consider its recruitment goal met if it can show that candidates from diverse cultural and demographic backgrounds have been considered or are holding positions for which they are qualified.
- *Recruitment time or time-to-fill.* The more time spent on proper recruitment, the greater the chance that the ideal candidate will emerge. However, a lengthy recruitment process also results in greater costs, disruption of service or work, and potential dissatisfaction of current employees who end up filling in for the missing jobholder.

Selection

Employee selection is the process of collecting and evaluating applicant information that will help the employer to extend a job offer. To a great extent, the selection process is a matter of predicting which person, among a pool of potentials, is likely to achieve success in the job. Of course, the definition of success is not always straightforward. Job performance may be defined in terms of technical proficiency, but the goals of a selection process may also include longevity in the position or fit with the culture and goals of the organization. Thus, evaluating the effectiveness of a selection process may include not only the time taken to fill the position but also the hired individual's performance and length of service, among other factors.

Selection must be distinguished from simple hiring (Gatewood, Feild, and Barrick 2008). In selection, a careful analysis is performed of an applicant's knowledge, skills, and abilities as well as attitudes and other relevant factors. The applicant who scores highest on the specified selection criteria is then extended an employment offer. Sometimes, however, offers are made with little or no systematic collection and analysis of job-related information. A common example is hiring an individual based on political considerations or based on the applicant's relationship with the owners of or the managers in the organization. In such instances, these non-job-related factors may take precedence over objective measures of job suitability. In circumstances where a position has to be filled in a short period of time, or when there is a labor shortage in a particular area, an organization may simply hire whoever is available, assuming the individual possesses the minimum level of qualifications. This is a frequent occurrence in staffing health centers in remote or otherwise undesirable locations. Applicant availability, rather than the comparative competence of the applicant, is the key criterion for selection in such situations.

The Question of Fit

Traditional selection processes are based on ensuring person–job fit. As noted earlier in this book, an accurate job description, based on sound job analysis, provides the foundation for selecting a candidate who has the required specifications for the job. In current practice, managers tend to be concerned mostly with applicant competencies, assessing whether the person has the knowledge, skills, and abilities to perform the job. Of increasing importance is the idea of *person–organization fit*—the extent to which an applicant's values match the values and culture of the organization. *Value congruence* is perhaps the overriding principle of person–organization fit (Kristof-Brown, Zimmerman, and Johnson 2005, 285). Furthermore, research suggests that sincere applicants are likely to be as concerned as the organization is with person-organization fit (Rynes and Cable 2003). This dramatically changes the dynamic of hiring, from a selection method that is based on concrete and observable indicators of *person–job fit* to a selection approach that seeks to assess person–organization fit. However, selection methods for fit are far from perfect and largely untested. Arthur and colleagues (2006) suggest that if person–organization fit is used as a selection criterion, then measures must be held to the same psychometric and legal standards as are more traditional selection tests.

While the idea of person–organization fit is appealing, among the questions asked by researchers and managers is whether it is actually associated with job performance. That is, while we know that applicants and employers intuitively seek to incorporate person–job fit into selection decisions as a means of reinforcing job satisfaction and organizational culture, does "fit" predict job performance? The evidence shows mixed results. Hoffman and Woehr (2006) found that person–organization fit is weakly to moderately related to job performance, organizational citizenship behavior, and turnover. In their meta-analysis of studies in this area, Kristof-Brown, Zimmerman, and

Johnson (2005) revealed that person–organization fit is strongly associated with job satisfaction and organizational commitment and is moderately correlated with intention to quit, satisfaction, and trust. However, the same study found a low correlation between fit and overall job performance. This evidence should not discourage efforts to achieve person–organization fit, but institutions need to have realistic expectations for higher levels of performance as a result of fit.

What does this line of inquiry imply for healthcare organizations? First, in some cases, considering fit, either person–job or person–organization, is not possible. For example, in difficult-to-fill positions, whoever meets minimum qualifications may need to be hired. Known to some sardonically as the "warm body" approach, this is a situation that Rosse and Levin (2003) defined as when a manager hires "anyone with a warm body and the ability to pass a drug test." Whether this type of hiring is effective in the long run is debatable, and certainly hiring without concern for fit has been shown to lead to poor long-term outcomes. Second, in situations in which fit can be taken into consideration, the extent to which job fit versus organizational fit is determined depends on the nature of the job and work environment. There is no fixed rule for deciding on the appropriate balance between the two types of fit, but this should be discussed explicitly among hiring decision makers. Both person–job and person–organization fit have great importance for hiring a nurse on a psychiatric unit. However, person–organization fit may be less important in hiring a medical data-entry clerk, although an argument could clearly be made for the significance of that fit for this job.

Currently the most widely accepted measure of person–organization fit is the Organizational Culture Profile (OCP) (O'Reilly, Chatman, and Caldwell 1991). However, the main difficulty with the OCP is that it is labor intensive and is thus susceptible to respondent fatigue. Therefore, if person–organization fit is used as a selection criterion, an easy-to-administer, valid measure of person–organization fit needs to be established that can be used parallel to measures that assess technical job competency and person–job fit.

Finally, organizations should avoid "ritual hiring," in which organizations or individuals apply well-worn but possibly obsolete hiring practices without assessing whether these procedures predict performance, or perhaps even favor lower-performing applicants (Rosse and Levin 2003). Organizations and jobs change, and so do job requirements. Thus, selection methods need to be current and consistent with the demands of the job. We must question "tried and true" selection methods to determine if they are in fact useful and helpful, and they deserve serious discussion by those involved in and affected by hiring decisions.

Through such processes as targeted selection and behavior interviews, successful selection based on person–organization fit has been made. For example, Women & Infants Hospital of Rhode Island made an explicit effort to select employees on the basis of their fit with the culture, believing that a "person must be qualified to do the job, but they also require the right personality." After starting a hiring program using behavior-based interviews and in-depth analysis of candidates, the hospital saw patient satisfaction rise from the 71st percentile to the 89th percentile nationally, while turnover was reduced by 8.5 percent. Labor disputes also decreased, while productivity increased (Greengard 2003). The choice between seeking internal or external candidates is not often clear, and it is not at all unusual for organizations to simultaneously pursue both internal and external candidates. UNC Hospitals use the Targeted Selection® (see DDI 2008) approach in which all employees are assessed on core values and attitudes specific to the organization.

Job Requirements and Selection Tools

If the goal of selection is to identify among a group of applicants the person to whom a job offer should be made, then the organization needs to use tools to evaluate each applicant's knowledge, skills, and abilities. Selection tools refer to any procedures or systems used to obtain job-related information about job applicants. A great many selection tools are available, including the job application form, standardized tests, personal interviews, simulations, and references. However, having a clear understanding of job requirements should precede the choosing of tools. While this may seem obvious, it is not uncommon for a selection process to move forward without adequate information about job requirements.

The use of selection tools should be based on a full-range knowledge of the job requirements, such as education, credentials, and experience. Also, the informal and less technical aspects of job performance, such as interpersonal skills, attitude, judgment, values, fit, ability to work in teams, and management abilities, should be specified. Without understanding the job, the organization runs the risk of hiring someone who may not perform successfully. As the organization moves into the hiring process, conducting a job analysis is advisable. The analysis may include seeking out the views of individuals who currently hold the position or who are in a similar position and obtaining the perspectives of supervisors and coworkers.

A *critical incidents analysis* is also useful for discovering the hidden or less formal aspects of job performance. This process is designed to generate a list of good and poor examples of job performance by current or potential jobholders. Once these examples of behaviors are collected, they are grouped into job dimensions. Measures are then developed for each of these job dimensions. The critical incidents approach involves the following steps:

1. *Identify job experts, and select methods for collecting critical incidents.* Incidents can be obtained from the jobholder, coworkers, subordinates, customers, and supervisors. Collection of critical incidents can be done

in a group setting, with individual interviews, or through administration of a questionnaire. Note that different job experts may have varied views of the same job and thus may identify dissimilar critical incidents; this, in fact, is the strength of this method.

2. *Generate critical incidents.* Job experts should be asked to reflect on the job and identify examples of good and poor performance. According to Bowns and Bernardin (1988), each critical incident should be structured such that

   • it is specific and pertains to a specific behavior;
   • it focuses on observable behaviors that have been, or can be, exhibited on the job;
   • it briefly describes the context in which the behavior occurred; and
   • it indicates the positive or negative consequences of the behavior.

3. *Define job dimensions.* Job dimensions are defined by analyzing the critical incidents and extracting common themes. This information may then be used to inform the selection process.

Table 8.5 provides examples of three critical incidents and the job dimensions in which each incident is grouped. This exercise yields a thorough understanding of the job's technical requirements, the job's formal qualifications, and the informal but critical aspects of successful job performance. Not only does a critical incidents analysis provide a solid foundation for selection, but it also provides protection against charges of unfair hiring practices as it specifically identifies aspects of the job related to performance.

Reliability and Validity of Selection Tools

At the most fundamental level, selection tools should elicit information that is predictive of job performance. As such, applicants who "score" better on selection instruments should consistently exhibit higher levels of job performance than individuals who score at lower levels. Therefore, to be useful, selection tools must ultimately be both reliable and valid.

From a measurement perspective, reliability is defined as the repeatability or consistency of a selection tool. Under this definition, a selection tool is deemed reliable if it provides the same result over and over again, assuming that the trait the selection tool is attempting to measure does not change. In other words, a reliable selection tool is one that yields the same findings regardless of who administers the tool or in what context (e.g., time of day, version of the tool) the tool is used. In general, physical and observable traits and skills (such as height and weight, the ability to lift a given weight, and the ability to compute manually) are more reliably measured than are psychological or behavioral traits (such as competitiveness, intelligence, and tolerance). Table 8.6 provides an overview of the relative reliability of measuring different human attributes. *Construct validity* refers to the degree to which the selection tool actually measures the construct it intends to measure, and this

TABLE 8.5
Critical Incidents Approach to Understanding Job Requirements

Job	Critical Incident	Job Dimensions
Physician, Public Health Department	In an administrative staff meeting to review plans for the coming year, this physician exhibited strongly condescending and rude behaviors toward other team members.	• Ability to work in teams • Respect for other professionals
Nurse, Emergency Room	After a school bus accident, the emergency department was overwhelmed with children and frightened parents. This nurse effectively and appropriately managed communication with parents and successfully obtained further assistance from elsewhere in the hospital.	• Creativity and resourcefulness • Leadership • Ability to work effectively under crisis conditions • Strong interpersonal skills
Medical director, Local Public Health Department	The local media reported an outbreak of salmonella that resulted in one child being hospitalized with the effects of this serious condition. The outbreak was traced to a fast-food restaurant that was inspected by health department personnel less than one week ago. The health department was blamed for not preventing the outbreak. This medical director conducted a thorough internal investigation and found that this was an isolated incident caused by mishandling of food on a single occasion. She communicated effectively at a press conference, defending the health department and assuring the public of the safety of local eating establishments.	• Effective crisis manager • Strong communication and media skills • Strong sense of public accountability

TABLE 8.6
Relative
Reliability of
Human
Attributes

Level of Reliability	Human Attributes
High	*Personal*
	Height
	Weight
	Vision
	Hearing
Medium	*Attitudes and Skills*
	Dexterity
	Mathematical skills
	Verbal ability
	Intelligence
	Clerical skills
	Mechanical skills
Medium to low	*Interests*
	Economic
	Scientific
	Mechanical
	Cultural
Low	*Personality*
	Sociability
	Dominance
	Cooperativeness
	Tolerance

SOURCES: Adapted from Albright, L. E., J. R. Glennon, and W. J. Smith. 1963. *The Use of Psychological Tests in Industry.* Cleveland, OH: Howard Allen; Gatewood, R. D., and H. S. Feild. 1998. *Human Resource Selection, 4th Edition.* Fort Worth, TX: Dryden.

ultimately determines the conclusions that can be legitimately drawn from the tools used. Two types of construct validity are commonly considered: criterion-related validity and content validity. *Criterion-related validity* is the extent to which a selection tool is associated with job performance, and this validity can be demonstrated through two strategies. First is *concurrent validity*, whereby a selection tool is administered to a current group of employees. These employees' scores are then correlated with actual job performance. For the selection tool to demonstrate concurrent validity, a strong correlation has to exist between the score on the selection tool and the score on actual job performance. Second is *predictive validity*, whereby the selection tool is administered to a group of job applicants. Because the selection tool has not yet been validated, actual selection decisions are made on the basis of other measures and criteria. Over time, data are obtained on actual job performance, and the two sets of scores—those from the selection tool under study and those from actual performance measures—are correlated and examined for possible relationships.

Content validity is the extent to which a selection tool representatively samples the content of the job for which the measure will be used. Using this strategy, if a selection tool includes a sufficient amount of actual job-related content, it is considered valid. Expert judgment, rather than statistical analysis, is typically used to assess content validity. One may look to content validity in designing a knowledge-based selection tool for laboratory technicians. An exercise that requires applicants to describe procedures associated with the most common laboratory tests is likely to be judged to have content validity.

Most organizations employ a range of selection tools but pay little or no attention to issues of reliability and validity. In the following section, the reliability and validity of some common selection tools are examined and suggestions on how they can be improved are offered.

A study of about 700 HR directors reveals that 87 percent of respondents used reference checks, 69 percent conducted background employment checks, 61 percent checked criminal records, 56 percent checked driving records, and 35 percent did credit checks (BNA 2001). Few studies, however, assess the reliability of using reference checks to gauge performance in previous jobs. In studies that have been conducted, researchers have sought to determine the level of agreement (interrater reliability) between different individuals who provide a reference for the same applicant. Reliability estimates are typically poor, at a level of 0.40 or less. This may be explained by a number of factors, including the reluctance of many referees to provide negative feedback and the real possibility that different raters may be evaluating different aspects of job performance. Studies of the validity of reference checks have found that this tool has low-to-moderate predictive validity (Hunter and Hunter 1984). Several explanations have been suggested for the poor predictive power of reference checks:

Reference Checks

- Many measures used in reference checks have low reliability; where reliability is low, validity must be low as well.
- Individuals who provide references frequently only use a restricted range of scores—typically in the high range—in evaluating job applicants. If virtually all reference checks are positive, they are still unlikely predictors of performance success for all individuals.
- In many instances, job applicants preselect the individuals who will provide the reference, and applicants are highly likely to select only those who will provide a positive reference.

How can the validity of reference checks be improved? Research in this area offers the following conclusions (Gatewood, Feild, and Barrick 2008):

- The most recent employer tends to provide the most accurate evaluation of an individual's work.

- The reference giver has had adequate time to observe the applicant, and the applicant is the same gender, ethnicity, and nationality as the reference giver.
- The old and new jobs are similar in content.

Reference checks have an intuitive appeal and are well institutionalized in virtually all selection processes. The usefulness of references, however, is decreasing as many organizations advise their employees to provide minimal information on former employees, such as job title and dates of employment. This is done to reduce the liability of the referring organization to lawsuits from both the hiring organization (through charges of negligent hiring) and the job applicant (through claims of defamation of character). Figure 8.1 provides some basic guidelines for the appropriate use of references.

Job Interviews   The job interview is used for virtually all positions largely because those involved in hiring simply wish to find out more than can be obtained from the application, references, and other documentation. The result of the interview is often given the greatest weight in hiring decisions. Job interviews, however, typically have low reliability and validity, are often unfair to applicants, and may be at least partially illegal. They are not reliable in that the questions vary

FIGURE 8.1
Guidelines for the Appropriate Use of Reference Checks

1. Ask for and obtain only job-related information.

2. Do not ask for information in an application or personal interview that may be deemed illegal.

3. Applicants should provide written permission to contact references; this may be included in the application form.

4. Individuals who check references should be trained in how to interview references, probe for additional information, and accurately record reference information.

5. Reference information should be recorded in writing.

6. Use the reference-checking process to confirm information provided by the applicant and to identify gaps in the employment record.

7. Use the reference-checking method appropriate to the job.

8. Be aware if the individual who provides a reference is trying to damage a prospective employee by giving a negative reference.

9. Use the references provided by the applicant as a source for additional references or information.

10. Consider using preemployment information services, particularly for sensitive positions.

from interviewer to interviewer, and two applicants vying for the same position are sometimes asked different questions altogether. Similarly, the manner in which answers to interview questions are interpreted and scored by interviewers may vary substantially as well.

The predictive validity of the job interview—that is, does a positive interview actually forecast job success?—has also been questioned. Job interviews present several problems. First, the questions are usually not given in advance and may bear little relationship with the candidate's performance in the future. This may be seen as unfair because candidates are not given the opportunity to prepare answers that would showcase their knowledge, skills, and abilities. Second, the questions are often not standardized, causing applicants to be treated inequitably because each interviewer poses different questions and each applicant is asked a different set of questions. This prevents the interviewer and the organization from obtaining the information necessary to make informed decisions. Third, untrained interviewers have a tendency to pose legally dubious questions that violate the law or compromise ethical principles, such as inquiries about plans for starting a family or for maternity leaves.

Notwithstanding these problems, the job interview can be an effective and efficient method of acquiring job-competency information and assessing the applicant's suitability for a position and fit within the organization. Furthermore, it can be used as a valuable recruitment tool because it allows the interviewer to highlight the positive features of the organization, the department, and the job.

Those involved in selection can choose between unstructured and structured interview techniques. *Unstructured interviews* present few constraints in how interviewers go about gathering information and evaluating applicants. As a result, unstructured interviews may be very subjective and thus tend to be less reliable than structured interviews. However, because of the free rein frequently given to interviewers, unstructured interviews may be more effective than the structured type in screening unsuitable candidates.

In a *structured interview,* the questions are clearly job related and based on the result of a thorough job analysis. A discussion before the interview among the selection team members is advantageous because it provides the team an opportunity to decide on what responses would be considered high and poor quality. This, in turn, allows the team to score applicant responses. Situational, experience-based, job-knowledge, and worker-requirement questions are most commonly posed during a structured interview.

Situational questions relate to how an applicant may handle a hypothetical work scenario, while experience-based questions ask how the candidate previously handled an issue that is similar to an issue that may be encountered on the new job. Following is an example of a scenario and related situational and experience-based questions. The constructs being assessed in this case are the ability to handle a stressful situation, the competency in dealing with the public, and professionalism.

> *Scenario:* Seven pediatricians work in a busy medical practice, and Monday morning is the busiest time of the week at the clinic. The waiting room is overcrowded, and two of the pediatricians are unexpectedly called away from the office—one for a personal situation and the other to attend to a patient in the hospital. Children and their parents now have to wait up to two hours to see the remaining doctors, and their level of anger and frustration increases as they wait. They are taking out their anger on you.

> *Situational questions:* How would you handle this situation? What and how would you communicate with the remaining physicians about this situation?

> *Experience-based questions:* Think about a situation on your last job in which you were faced with angry and upset patients or customers. What was the situation? What did you do? What was the outcome?

Situational questions should be designed in a way that allows alternative, not just expected, responses to be also evaluated or scored. If a panel—two or more people—conducts the interview, each panelist should be able to confirm answers and their meaning with each other.

Job-knowledge questions assess whether the applicant has the knowledge to do the job. These questions and follow-up probes are predetermined and are based on the job description. Similarly, worker-requirement questions seek to determine if the candidate is able and willing to work under the conditions of the job. For example, applicants for a consulting position may be asked if they are able and willing to travel for a designated portion of their work.

Whatever form is used, job interviews must be conducted with the following guidelines in mind:

1. Prepare yourself. For an unstructured interview, learn the job requirements. For a structured interview, become familiar with the questions to be asked. Review materials or information about the applicant as well.
2. Tidy up the physical environment in which the interview will take place.
3. Describe the job, and invite questions about the job.
4. Put the applicant at ease, and convey an interest in the person. A purposely stressful interview is not desirable, as other reliable and ethical methods can be used to assess an applicant's ability to handle stress. Furthermore, a stressful interview reflects poorly on the organization.
5. Do not come to premature conclusions (positive or negative) about the applicant. This is particularly important for unstructured interviews.

6. Listen carefully, and ask for clarity if the applicant's responses are vague.
7. Observe and take notes on relevant aspects of the applicant's dress, mannerisms, and affect.
8. Provide an opportunity for the applicant to ask questions.
9. Do not talk excessively. Remember that this is an opportunity to hear from the applicant.
10. Do not ask questions that are unethical or that put the organization in a legally vulnerable position (see Figure 8.2).
11. Explain the selection process that comes after the interview.
12. Evaluate the applicant as soon as possible after the interview.

Applications and Resumes

Application forms and resumes usually contain useful information about job applicants. The major drawback to these tools is that they may misrepresent qualifications. Several methods can be used to improve the usefulness of application forms. First, create an addendum to the application that asks applicants to provide information that is specific to the open position. This way, particular knowledge, skills, and abilities can be targeted for different jobs. Second, include a statement on the application form that allows the applicant to indicate that all the information he or she reported is accurate; the applicant should then be required to sign or initial this statement. Third, ensure that illegal inquiries about personal information (e.g., marital status, height, weight) are excluded from the form.

Ability and Aptitude Tests

Various ability and aptitude tests (including personality, honesty, integrity, cognitive reasoning, and fine motor coordination tests) are available, and many of them demonstrate reliability and validity. A number of firms specialize in developing and assessing tests; see, for example, Walden Personnel Testing and Consulting at www.waldentesting.com. Debate is currently brewing about the issue of situational validity—the notion that the nature of job performance differs across work settings and that the validity of tests may vary according to the setting. In general, studies tend to conclude that results of a test on basic abilities are generalizable across work settings, assuming that the test itself is valid and reliable. The key is to ensure that such tests are actually representative of the work involved in a particular job.

Assessment Centers

The use of assessment centers is a highly sophisticated and multidimensional method of evaluating applicants. Assessment centers may be the physical location where testing is done, but they may also refer to a series of assessment procedures that are administered, professionally scored, and reported to hiring personnel. Traditionally, assessment centers have been used to test an applicant's managerial skills, but today they are also employed for a variety of hiring situations. Typical assessment formats include paper-and-pencil tests, leaderless group discussions, role-playing intelligence tests, personality tests,

FIGURE 8.2

Inappropriate
and
Appropriate
Job Interview
Questions

Personal and Marital Status

Inappropriate: How tall are you?

How much do you weigh? (acceptable if these are safety requirements)

What is your maiden name?

Are you married?

Is this your maiden or married name?

With whom do you live?

Do you smoke?

Appropriate: After hiring, inquire about marital status for tax and insurance forms purposes.

Are you able to lift 50 pounds and carry it 20 yards? (acceptable if this is part of the job)

Parental Status and Family Responsibilities

Inappropriate: How many kids do you have?

Do you plan to have children?

What are your childcare arrangements?

Are you pregnant?

Appropriate: Would you be willing to relocate if necessary?

Travel is an important part of this job. Would you be willing to travel as needed by the job?

This job requires overtime occasionally. Would you be able and willing to work overtime as necessary?

After hiring, inquire about dependent information for tax and insurance forms purposes.

Age

Inappropriate: How old are you?

What year were you born?

When did you graduate from high school and college?

Appropriate: Before hiring, asking if the applicant is above the legal minimum age for the hours or working conditions is appropriate, as this is in compliance with state or federal labor laws. After hiring, verifying legal minimum age with a birth certificate or other ID and asking for age on insurance forms are permissible.

National Origin

Inappropriate: Where were you born?

Where are your parents from?

What is your heritage?

What is your native tongue?

What languages do you read, speak, or write fluently? (acceptable if this is relevant to the job)

Appropriate: Are you authorized to work in the United States?

May we verify that you are a legal U.S. resident, or may we have a copy of your work visa status?

FIGURE 8.2

Continued

Race or Skin Color

Inappropriate: What is your racial background?

Are you a member of a minority group?

Appropriate: This organization is an equal opportunity employer. Race is required information only for affirmative-action programs.

Religion or Creed

Inappropriate: What religion do you follow?

Which religious holidays will you be taking off from work?

Do you attend church regularly?

Appropriate: May we contact religious or other organizations related to your beliefs to provide us with references, per your list of employers and references?

Criminal Record

Inappropriate: Have you ever been arrested?

Have you ever spent a night in jail?

Appropriate: Questions about convictions by civil or military courts are appropriate if accompanied by a disclaimer that the answers will not necessarily cause loss of job opportunity. Generally, employers can ask only about convictions and not arrests (except for jobs in law-enforcement and security-clearance agencies) when the answers are relevant to the job performance.

Disability

Inappropriate: Do you have any disabilities?

What is your medical history?

How does your condition affect your abilities?

Please fill out this medical history document.

Have you had recent illnesses or hospitalizations?

When was your last physical exam?

Are you HIV-positive?

Appropriate: Can you perform specific physical tasks? (such as lifting heavy objects, bending, kneeling that are required for the job)

After hiring, asking about the person's medical history on insurance forms is appropriate.

Are you able to perform the essential functions of this job with or without reasonable accommodations?

Affiliations

Inappropriate: To what clubs or associations do you belong?

Appropriate: Do you belong to any professional or trade groups or other organizations that you consider relevant to your ability to perform this job?

NOTE: Questions listed here are not necessarily illegal. For example, it is not illegal to ask an applicant's date of birth, but it is illegal to deny employment to an applicant solely because he or she is 40 years of age or older. In this case, the question is not illegal, but a discriminatory motive for asking is illegal. Unknown or ambiguous motive is what makes any question with discriminatory implications inappropriate. If an individual is denied employment, having asked this and similar questions can lead to the applicant claiming that the selection decision was made on the basis of age, gender, or other characteristic for which it is illegal to discriminate.

interest measures, work-task simulations, in-basket exercises, interviews, and situational exercises. Evidence indicates that positive statistical relationships exist between the use of assessment centers and a high level of job performance (Gaugler et al. 1997).

Turnover and Retention

Among the most important healthcare workforce challenges is staff shortage, and associated with this issue are employee turnover and retention. Larger environmental and systemic pressures contribute to the chronic shortages in healthcare. Although turnover is not appreciably increasing in healthcare, rates are higher in this industry than in others. A number of factors affect the high demand for healthcare workers, including population growth, the aging of the population, improved diagnostic techniques that enable earlier detection of disease and increase patient loads, and heightened consumer demand for a full range of diagnostic and therapeutic technologies (HCAB 2001).

Growth in demand for nurses will outpace the supply, and, together with changing demographic patterns in the nursing workforce, a nursing shortage will be experienced in the foreseeable future. This shortage does not appear to be cyclical, as have past shortages, but is chronic in nature (Ponte 2004; Mee and Robinson 2003). The aging of the nurse workforce is a key factor. In 2005, the average age of the registered nurse (RN) workforce was 43.5; the largest age group comprised RNs in their 40s. By 2012, the average RN age is expected to increase to 44.7 years, with RNs in their 50s representing the largest age group (Auerbach, Buerhaus, and Staiger 2007). Although estimates of the future nurse shortage vary, the most recent analysis estimates a shortfall of about 340,000 nurses by the year 2020 (Auerbach, Buerhaus, and Staiger 2007).

These broad societal factors are largely out of the control of healthcare organizations, and they substantially influence the worker vacancy rates in hospitals. These vacancy rates, in turn, highlight the need for organizations to do a better job at recruiting, selecting, and retaining staff. In this section, we explain our concern with turnover, enumerate the costs associated with turnover, discuss the factors that contribute to turnover, and explore the methods proven to improve retention. Although we use the nursing shortage as a basis to explore the turnover and retention issue, we are aware also of the shortages in other healthcare professions, such as among radiologic technicians and pharmacists. The lessons in our discussion, however, are applicable to other professions as well.

A distinction has to be made between the separate, although related, concepts of turnover and retention. Many organizations view retention as the inverse of turnover and, as a result, cause them to miss out on critical trends that are happening within their systems. According to Waldman and Arora (2004), a *turnover rate* is a simple ratio that provides only a summary of the gross movement in and out of the organization during a specific time frame (usually one year). *Retention rate*, on the other hand, is the number of specific individuals or cohorts that enter and exit the organization. The key distinction is that retention views an individual or a group as an entity; therefore, retention allows for a more thorough examination of how the loss of one individual or cohort influences retention strategies and productivity.

For example, an organization that experiences a slight decline in turnover (say, from 20 percent to 18 percent) over a five-year period may think that it is doing well in addressing its retention problem. However, during that same five-year time span, the retention rate of individuals who have 5 to 15 years of service declined (say, from 70 percent to 35 percent). These rates indicate that the organization has difficulty with retaining experienced employees and needs to explore and implement new retention strategies. Overall, organizations need to thoroughly examine both turnover and retention rates to successfully deal with the challenge of staff shortages.

Studies on Nursing Turnover

The demand for healthcare workers has increased, but the quality of their work life has decreased. The average annual turnover rate for hospital workers is about 20 percent, with substantially higher percentages for particular professional groups. At any one time, approximately 126,000 nursing positions in U.S. hospitals are unfilled (Joint Commission 2004). Generally, nurse turnover in hospitals ranges between 10 percent and 25 percent, and in certain sectors, vacancy rates are even higher. Ninety percent of nursing homes lack sufficient nursing staff to provide even basic care (CMS 2002). Recently, the turnover rate in nursing homes for RNs, licensed practical nurses, and nursing directors was a staggering 50 percent (AHCA 2003).

Nurse dissatisfaction has been cited as a key reason for turnover and even departure from the profession. In a worldwide study of nurses, those surveyed in the United States had the highest rate of job dissatisfaction at 41 percent, which is four times higher than the satisfaction score of the professional workforce in general (Albaugh 2003; Aiken et al. 2001). Multiple studies have examined reasons for nurse dissatisfaction and its consequences. McFarland, Leonard, and Morris (1984) cite lack of involvement in decision making, problems with supervisors, poor working conditions, inadequate compensation, and lack of job security. Swansburg (1990) identifies compensation, poor recognition, lack of flexible scheduling, and increased stress as dissatisfiers. The Maryland Nurses Association (2000) articulates the top five reasons for poor nurse retention: (1) absence of advancement opportunities, (2) stress and burnout related to mandatory overtime, (3) unrealistic workloads, (4) increased paperwork, and (5) nurse perception of lack of respect and recognition in the workplace. The Joint Commission (2004) finds that required overtime is a major source of dissatisfaction.

Turnover has an adverse effect on organizational performance, and study data increasingly point to the impact of turnover and shortages on healthcare quality. A survey conducted by the American Nurses Association (ANA 2001) reveals that 75 percent of respondent nurses felt that the quality of nursing care has declined. Among respondents who claimed that quality has suffered, more than 92 percent cited inadequate staffing as the reason and 80 percent indicated nurse dissatisfaction. The ANA survey also reports that more than 54 percent of respondents would not recommend the profession to their children or friends. A study conducted by the Voluntary Hospitals Association of America finds a correlation between nurse turnover and quality measures. Hospitals with nurse turnover rates under 12 percent had lower risk-adjusted mortality scores and lower severity-adjusted lengths of stay than hospitals whose nurse turnover was above 22 percent. Confirming evidence from earlier studies, Aiken and colleagues (2001) argue that nurse-patient ratios are strongly related to higher levels of dissatisfaction and emotional exhaustion. These studies present the connection among nurse dissatisfaction, turnover, and quality of care.

In addition to the effect on quality, shortages and turnover also have significant financial implications. The costs associated with employee termination, recruitment, selection, hiring, and training represent a substantial non-value-adding element in the organizational budget. A 2004 study of turnover estimates the various costs associated with turnover in an academic medical center (Waldman and Arora 2004). Depending on assumptions made in the analysis, the total cost of turnover reduced the annual operating budget of the medical center between $7 million and $19 million, or between 3.4 percent and 5.8 percent. This research indicates that, at this medical center, more than one-fourth of the total turnover costs were attributable to nurse turnover. Several studies have focused specifically on the cost of nursing turnover. While difficult to measure, both the Advisory Board Company (1999) and Jones (2005) have attempted to capture not only the direct costs of nurse turnover but the hidden costs of reduced productivity (i.e., predeparture, vacancy, and new employee on-boarding) as well. The estimated cost of a single nurse leaving is $42,000 (per the Advisory Board) and $64,000 (per Jones), and these estimates support the claim that nursing turnover has significant financial implications for all healthcare organizations. The following example reiterates this point: Assuming a turnover rate of 20 percent and the cost of nurse turnover ranging between $42,000 and $64,000 per nurse, a hospital that employs 600 nurses would face yearly estimated nursing staff-replacement costs of between $5 million and $7 million per year.

Turnover can be viewed as costly in terms of patient care, financial stability, and staff morale. Nurse turnover affects communication among nurses and between nurses and other healthcare professionals, the quality of care, and care continuity. The work of teams is disturbed as well, as team composition and skills change when a member comes or goes, and members who are left behind often feel low morale and a sense of rejection.

Retention Strategies

Many of the factors associated with effective recruitment are also applicable to retention, because a person's reasons for accepting an employment offer are basically the same reasons for staying with that employer. As such, retention strategies are a necessary follow-up to recruitment. With the opportunities available to nurses in other organizations and professions, viewing retention as an essential HRM function, like compensation and training, is critical.

One study examined the strategies used by nurse managers who have succeeded in achieving low turnover rates and high satisfaction among patients, employees, and providers; good patient outcomes; and positive working relationships (Manion 2004). The study finds that these nurse managers were able to develop a "culture of retention." Through their daily work, these managers created an environment where people want to stay because they enjoy their work and where staff contribute to this sense of attachment. These managers emphasized sincere caring for the welfare of their staff, forging authentic connections with each staff member and focusing on results and problem solving. Note that these strategies are not likely to succeed without a culture of retention.

In today's healthcare environment, much of the turnover that occurs is beyond the control of a single organization. Employee commitment to employers has virtually evaporated. Except in rare instances, the market profoundly affects the movement of employees. Organizations can still control turnover, but their influence is becoming limited. Retention strategies have simply not achieved the type of consistent success once anticipated. Furthermore, each organization needs to develop its own retention strategies and tailor them to the particular circumstances of the institution (Cappelli 2000).

Several generic retention strategies have been shown to work. First, offer competitive compensation. Compensation comes in many forms, including signing bonuses, premium and differential pay, forgivable loans, bonuses, and extensive benefits. Second, structure jobs so that they are more appealing and satisfying. This can be done by carefully assigning and grouping tasks, providing employees with sufficient autonomy, allowing flexible work hours and scheduling, enhancing the collegiality of the work environment, and instituting work policies that are respectful of individual needs. In the nursing environment, job design encompasses elements such as the nurse–patient staffing ratios and mandatory overtime. Third, put in place a superb management and supervisory team. The idea that people quit their supervisors, not their jobs, is true in nursing, as nurses sometimes leave because of poor working relationships with their managers or other healthcare professionals. Fourth, make opportunities for career growth available. Providing career ladders is increasingly difficult, as organizations become flatter and widen their spans of control. Alternatives to promotions need to be developed and implemented.

The American Nurses Credentialing Center established the Magnet Recognition Program to acknowledge and reward healthcare organizations that exhibit and provide excellent nursing care. Designated Magnet hospitals are characterized by fewer hierarchical structures, decentralized decision making, flexibility in scheduling, positive nurse–physician relationships, and nursing leadership that supports and invests in nurses' career development (Cameron et al. 2004). Magnet hospitals have been found to have better patient outcomes and higher levels of patient satisfaction (Scott, Sochalski, and Aiken 1999). Compared to other hospitals, Magnet institutions have lower turnover and higher job satisfaction among nurses (Huerta 2003; Upenieks 2002). Based on these findings, becoming a Magnet healthcare organization seems to be another retention strategy.

The Healthcare Advisory Board (HCAB 2002) conducted an extensive review of recruitment and retention strategies and identified each strategy's relative effectiveness. Much of the discussion in the literature about retention focuses on improving job satisfaction. The HCAB, however, distinguishes between strategies that boost morale and those that enhance retention, and it categorizes retention strategies into four types:

1. *Strategies that neither increase morale nor improve retention.* Examples are providing individualized benefits, concierge services, and employee lounge areas.
2. *Strategies that increase morale but do not improve retention.* Examples include forming morale committees, offering on-site childcare, creating recognition programs, and providing educational benefits.
3. *Strategies that do not increase morale but improve retention.* Examples are improving screening of applicants, monitoring turnover in key areas, and tracking turnover of key employees.
4. *Strategies that increase morale and improve retention.* Examples include establishing staffing ratios, providing career ladders, implementing buddy programs, and allowing flexible scheduling.

The HCAB's review yields five effective retention strategies: (1) selecting the right employees; (2) improving orientation and on-boarding processes by creating a buddy program and other opportunities that help new employees establish professional and personal relationships with colleagues; (3) monitoring turnover to identify specific root causes, including identifying managers whose departments have high turnover rates; (4) developing and implementing ways to retain valued employees; and (5) although marginal in its effectiveness, systematically attempting to reverse turnover decisions.

Every organization faces different challenges in its efforts to retain valued employees. The success of a retention program depends on the ability of the organization to correctly determine the causes of turnover and to enact strategies that appropriately target these causes. Also, the organization must recognize the advantages and usefulness of alternative retention strategies.

Summary

Recruiting, selecting, and retaining employees continue to be important HRM functions, especially in a competitive, pressurized environment like healthcare. Healthcare organizations and their human resources departments face enormous challenges. From a recruitment and selection standpoint, they need to seek employees who (1) have specialized skills but are flexible to fill in for other positions, (2) bring in expertise and are able to work in groups whose members are not experts, (3) are strongly motivated yet are comfortable with relatively flat organizational structures in which traditional upward mobility may be difficult, and (4) represent diversity yet also fit into the organizational culture. From a retention standpoint, they need to identify factors related to retention and develop innovative strategies to improve retention. By doing so, healthcare organizations will be better able to meet various challenges in the coming decades.

Discussion Questions

1. Given two equally qualified job applicants—one from inside and one from outside the organization—how would you go about deciding which one to hire?

2. For various reasons, some healthcare organizations are unable to pay market rates for certain positions. What advice do you give such an organization about possible recruitment and retention strategies?

3. The use of work references is increasingly viewed as unreliable. How can employers legally and ethically obtain information about an applicant's past performance? What measures can be taken to verify information contained in a job application or resume?

4. What are the advantages and disadvantages of recruiting through the Internet? What advice do you give to a hospital that is considering using the Internet for recruitment?

Experiential Exercises

Case Note: This case was developed in collaboration with Caroline LeGarde, Operations Project Administrator, Johns Hopkins Medicine, Baltimore, Maryland

Grayson County Regional Health Center is a private, not-for-profit, 225-bed acute care hospital located in a rural community in a southeastern state. The hospital provides a broad range of inpatient and outpatient services, including cardiology, obstetrics, gynecology, general surgery, internal medicine, urology, family medicine, dermatology, pediatrics, psychiatry, radiology, nephrology, ophthalmology, occupational medicine, and rehabilitation services. The Center offers 24-hour emergency care. The Center is built on a 96-acre site, and its service area includes Grayson County as well as parts of three neighboring rural counties.

Grayson County's population is 60,879, with African Americans making up 53 percent of the population, Caucasians making up 42 percent, and Hispanics and other groups making up 5 percent. Agriculture is the main industry in the area, with cotton as the major crop. Fifteen percent of the labor force works in manufacturing, which includes molded plastics, metal fabrication, paper and wood products, textiles, rubber materials, and clothing. In the last 20 years, the region has suffered severe economic setbacks. Most of the textile industry has moved out of the region because of outsourcing, and the town itself has fallen into disrepair. An increasing proportion of the population—33 percent of children and 22 percent of the elderly—lives below the

poverty line. The county has a civilian labor force of 27,568 and currently has an unemployment rate of 13 percent. The county's infant mortality rate is 12 percent, and 24 percent of the population does not have health insurance.

The Center has approximately 85 physicians, representing 29 subspecialties, on staff. It has affiliation relationships with two academic health centers—one is located about 90 miles away, and the other is located 100 miles from Grayson. The Center currently employs more than 800 employees, is fully certified by the Joint Commission, and is certified to participate in CMS programs. The Center is governed by an 18-member board of trustees, which includes the chief of the medical staff, the immediate past chief of the medical staff, the chief executive officer, and 13 members selected by the board from the community at large. Criteria for board election, as specified in the corporation's charter, include an interest in healthcare, aptitude in business, and evidence of a strong moral and ethical background. The board is required by the corporation's charter to reflect the economic, racial, and ethnic diversity of the service area. The Center has strong community ties and is active in the community. Its staff participate in such activities as community health screenings, health education programs, and health fairs. It serves as the meeting place for many support groups. Although it has been under financial stress for the last five years, it continues to have strong support in the community.

The employee turnover rate at the Center is 40 percent. Over the last few years, the turnover rate for nurses has ranged from 15 percent to 50 percent. Physician recruitment and retention are also major concerns. Currently, only one radiologist is practicing in Grayson County, and there is a shortage of physicians in all specialties. The Center relies heavily on Medicaid and Medicare revenue, leaving the hospital in a difficult financial condition. It is unable to pay market rates for nurses and other professionals. As a result, nursing units are understaffed, and nurses have expressed concerns about being overworked and underpaid. This has also resulted in concerns about the quality of patient care. A local newspaper article reported that patients at the Center were often left on stretchers in the hallway for long periods of time, that staff were unresponsive to patient and family concerns, and that hearing crying in the hallways is not unusual.

Nurses and other professional groups report poor communication between senior management and employees. Poor relation-ships between middle managers and front-line staff are also a problem in some departments. This situation became particularly difficult two years ago when the Center embarked on a large building project. Employees could not understand how the Center could afford to build new facilities but was unable to pay market rates to its staff. The nursing turnover problem at the Center has reached crisis proportions. Recent exit interview surveys indicate that financial concerns are the major reason for leaving. The Center has tried numerous strategies, including improving the work environment by adding amenities (such as lowering prices in the cafeteria) and training middle managers. For a short time 18 months ago, nurse salaries matched market rates, but the Center fell behind again shortly thereafter. The RN vacancy rate currently is 18 percent.

Case Exercises As a consultant to the Center, you are expected to make recommendations to address the nursing shortage. Specifically, you have been asked to develop short-term strategies to cope with the current crisis as well as long-term strategies to improve the overall recruitment and retention picture.

1. How will you go about identifying the most important reasons for the current shortage?
2. How will you proceed with developing short-term and long-term strategies?

Project Chronic and worsening healthcare workforce shortages are likely in the foreseeable future. The objective of this project is for readers to learn about how hospitals and other healthcare organizations are coping with healthcare workforce shortages. Specifically, how do organizations perceive the causes of turnover, and what strategies have they found successful in improving both their recruitment and retention?

1. Identify one professional group (e.g., nurses, laboratory technicians, radiologic technicians, information technology personnel) that is known to be experiencing recruitment and retention problems.

2. Choose two healthcare organizations that employ this professional group.

3. Locate the individual or individuals most directly accountable for recruiting and retaining professionals in this group. This person may be a staff in the HR department, a nurse recruiter, or another employee.

4. Find the approximate number of professionals in this group needed by the organization.

5. Obtain the following information on this group:
   a. Current vacancy rate
   b. Turnover and retention rates for the last five years

6. Discuss with the appropriate individuals their perception of the causes of recruitment challenges and of turnover and the reasons people choose to stay with their organizations. If possible, interview front-line staff in this professional group to obtain their perceptions on these issues.

7. If possible, explore the costs associated with recruitment, retention, and turnover at the facilities you have selected. Do the organizations keep track of these costs? If not, why? If so, do they use this information to make decisions concerning future recruitment and retention efforts?

8. In your discussions, explore the strategies both organizations have used to increase the success rate of their recruitment and retention efforts. Do the organizations know which strategies have been successful and unsuccessful? If so, which strategies have proven successful? Which strategies have not been effective? What strategies may be effective but are difficult to implement?

9. Summarize your findings in a five-page paper.

References

Advisory Board Company. 1999. "A Misplaced Focus: Reexamining the Recruiting/Retention Trade-off." *Nursing Watch* 11: 1–14.

Aiken, L. H., S. P. Clarke, D. M. Sloane, J. A. Sochalski, R. Busse, H. Clarke, P. Giovannetti, J. Hunt, A. M. Rafferty, and J. Shamian. 2001. "Nurses' Report on Hospital Care in Five Countries." *Health Affairs* 20 (3): 43–53.

Albaugh, J. 2003. "Keeping Nurses in Nursing: The Profession's Challenge for Today." *Urologic Nursing* 23 (3): 193–99.

American Health Care Association (AHCA). 2003. *Results of the 2002 AHCA Survey of Nursing Staff Vacancy and Turnover in Nursing Homes.* Chesterfield, MO: Health Services Research and Evaluation, American Health Care Association.

American Nurses Association (ANA). 2001. *Analysis of American Nurses Association Staffing Survey.* Silver Spring, MD: American Nurses Association.

Arthur, W., S. T. Bell, A. J. Villado, and D. Doverspike. 2006. "The Use of Person-Organization Fit in Employment Decision Making: An Assessment of Its Criterion-Related Validity." *Journal of Applied Psychology* 91 (4): 786–801.

Auerbach, D. I., P. I. Buerhaus, and D. O. Staiger. 2007. "Better Late than Never: Workforce Supply Implications of Later Entry into Nursing." *Health Affairs* 26 (1): 178–85.

Barber, A. 1998. *Recruiting Employees: Individual and Organizational Perspectives.* Thousand Oaks, CA: Sage Publishing.

Barber, A. E., C. L. Daly, C. M. Giannantonio, and J. M. Phillips. 1994. "Job Search Activities: An Examination of Changes Over Time." *Personnel Psychology* 47 (4): 739–65.

BNA. 2001. "Internet, E-mail Monitoring Common at Most Workplaces." *BNA—Bulletin to Management* (February 1).

Bowns, D. A., and H. J. Bernardin. 1988. "Critical Incident Technique." In *The Job Analysis Handbook for Business, Industry, and Government,* edited by S. Gael, 1120–37. New York: Wiley.

Calandra, B. 2001. "You've Got Friends." *HR Magazine* 46 (8): 49–55.

Cameron, S., M. Armstrong-Stassen, S. Bergeron, and J. Out. 2004. "Recruitment and Retention of Nurses: Challenges Facing Hospital and Community Employers." *Nursing Leadership* 17 (3): 79–92.

Cappelli, P. 2000. "A Market-Driven Approach to Retaining Talent." *Harvard Business Review* (January–February): 103–11.

Caudron, S. 1995. "The Changing Union Agenda." *Personnel Journal* 74 (3): 42–49.

Centers for Medicare & Medicaid Services (CMS). 2002. *Minimum Nurse Staffing Ratios in Nursing Homes.* Washington, DC: CMS.

The Cleveland Clinic. 2007. [Online information; retrieved 11/07.] http://cms.cleveland-clinic.org/hospitalist.

DDI. 2008. Targeted Selection®. [Online information; retrieved 3/08.] www.ddiworld.com/products_services/targetedselection.asp.

Fitz-enz, J., and B. Davison. 2002. *How to Measure Human Resources Management.* New York: McGraw-Hill.

Gatewood, R. D., H. S. Feild, and M. Barrick. 2008. *Human Resource Selection,* 6th Ed. Mason, OH: Southwestern College Publishing.

Gaugler, B. B., D. B. Rosenthal, G. C. Thornton, and C. Bentson. 1997. "Meta-Analysis of Assessment Center Validity." *Journal of Applied Psychology* 72 (3): 493–511.

Greengard, S. 2003. "Gimme Attitude." *Workforce Management* 81 (7): 56–60.

The Healthcare Advisory Board (HCAB). 2001. *Competing for Talent: Recovering America's Hospital Workforce.* Washington, DC: The Advisory Board Company.

———. 2002. *Hardwiring for Right Retention: Best Practices for Retaining a High Performance Workforce.* Washington, DC: The Advisory Board Company.

Henderson, R. I. 1986. "Contract Concessions: Is the Past Prologue?" *Compensation and Benefits Review* 18 (5): 17–30.

Heneman, H. G., and T. A. Judge. 2003. *Staffing Organizations.* Middleton, WI: Mendota House.

Hoffman, B. J., and D. J. Woehr. 2006. "A Quantitative Review of the Relationship Between Person-Organization Fit and Behavioral Outcomes." *Journal of Vocational Behavior* 68 (3): 389–99.

Huerta, S. 2003. "Recruitment and Retention: The Magnet Perspective." Chart. *Journal of Illinois Nursing* 100 (4): 4–6.

Hunter, J., and R. Hunter. 1984. "The Validity and Utility of Alternative Predictors of Job Performance." *Psychological Bulletin* 96 (1): 72–98.

The Johns Hopkins Hospital. 2007. [Online information; retrieved 11/07.] www.hopkinsnursing.org.

Joint Commission. 2004. "Health Care at the Crossroads: Strategies for Addressing the Evolving Nursing Crisis." [Online information; retrieved 11/07.] www.jointcommission.org/NR/rdonlyres/5C138711-ED76-4D6F-909F-B06E0309F36D/0/health_care_at_the_crossroads.pdf.

Jones, C. B. 2005. "The Costs of Nursing Turnover, Part 2: Application of the Nursing Turnover Cost Calculation Methodology." *Journal of Nursing Administration* 35 (1): 41–49.

Kaiser Permanente. 2007. "Diversity and Inclusion." [Online information; retrieved 11/07.] www.kaiserpermanentejobs.org/workhere_diversity.asp.

Kristof-Brown, A. L., R. D. Zimmerman, and E. C. Johnson. 2005. "Consequences of Individuals' Fit at Work: A Meta-Analysis of Person-Job, Person-Organization, Person-Group, and Person-Supervisor Fit." *Personnel Psychology* 58 (2): 281–342.

London, M., and S. A. Stumpf. 1982. *Managing Careers.* Reading, MA: Addison-Wesley.

Manion, J. 2004. "Nurture a Culture of Retention." *Nursing Management* 35 (4): 28–39.

Maryland Nurses Association. 2000. "Commission on the Crisis in Nursing Summit 2000." *Maryland Nurse* 3 (2): 1–10.

Mayer, K. M. 2005. "Demands for Labor Givebacks Grow More Aggressive." *Wall Street Journal* (October 27).

Mayo Clinic. 2007. "Jobs at Mayo Clinic." [Online information; retrieved 11/07.] www.mayoclinic.org/jobs.

McFarland, G. K., H. S. Leonard, and M. M. Morris. 1984. *Nursing Leadership and Management: Contemporary Strategies.* New York: John Wiley & Sons.

Mee, C. L., and E. Robinson. 2003. "Nursing: What's Different About this Nursing Shortage?" *Nursing* 33 (1): 51–55.

North Shore–Long Island Jewish Health System. 2007. [Online information; retrieved 11/07.] www.northshorelij.com/body.cfm?id=10&oTopID=0.

O'Reilly, C. A., J. Chatman, and D. F. Caldwell. 1991. "People and Organizational Culture: A Profile Comparison Approach to Assessing Person-Organization Fit." *Academy of Management Journal* 34 (3): 487–516.

Peter, L. J., and R. Hull. 1969. *The Peter Principle.* New York: William Morrow.

Phillips, J. M. 1998. "Effects of Realistic Job Previews on Multiple Organizational Outcomes." *Academy of Management Journal* 41 (6): 673–90.

Ponte, R. P. 2004. "The American Healthcare System at a Crossroads: An Overview of the American Organization of Nurse Executives Monograph." [*Online Journal of Issues in Nursing* 9 (2); retrieved 3/08.] http://nursingworld.org/MainMenuCategories/ANAMarketplace/ANAPeriodicals/OJIN/TableofContents/Volume92004/No2May04/NurseExecutivesMonograph.aspx.

Rosse, J. G., and R. A. Levin. 2003. *The Jossey-Bass Academic Administrator's Guide to Hiring.* San Francisco: Jossey-Bass.

Roth, L. M. 1982. *A Critical Examination of the Dual Ladder Approach to Career Advancement.* New York: Center for Research in Career Development, Columbia University Graduate School of Business.

Rynes, S. L. 1991. "Recruitment, Job Choice, and Post-Hire Consequences: A Call for New Research Directions." In *Handbook of Industrial and Organizational Psychology,* 2nd Ed., edited by M. D. Dunnette and L. M. Hough, 399–444. Palo Alto, CA: Consulting Psychologists Press, Inc.

Rynes, S. L., and D. M. Cable. 2003. "Recruitment Research in the Twenty-First Century." In *Handbook of Psychology: Industrial and Organizational Psychology,* Vol. 12, edited by W. C. Borman, D. R. Ilgen, and R. J. Klimoski, 55–76. Hoboken, NJ: John Wiley & Sons Inc.

Schwab, D. P., S. L. Rynes, and R. J. Aldag. 1987. "Theories and Research on Job Search and Choice." In *Research in Personnel and Human Resources Management,* edited by G. Ferris and T. R. Mitchell. Greenwich, CT: JAI Press.

Scott, J. G., J. Sochalski, and L. Aiken. 1999. "Review of Magnet Hospital Research: Findings and Implications for Professional Nursing." *Journal of Nursing Administration* 29 (1): 9–19.

Swansburg, R. C. 1990. *Management and Leadership for Nurse Managers.* Boston: Jones & Bartlett.

Taylor, G. S. 1994. "The Relationship Between Sources of New Employees and Attitudes Toward the Job." *Journal of Social Psychology* 134 (1): 99–110.

Upenieks, V. 2002. "Assessing Differences in Job Satisfaction of Nurses in Magnet and Nonmagnet Hospitals." *Journal of Nursing Administration* 32 (11): 564–76.

WakeMed. 2007. [Online information; retrieved 11/07] http://wakemed.org.

Waldman, J. D., and S. Arora. 2004. "Measuring Retention Rather than Turnover: A Different and Complementary HR Calculus." *Human Resource Planning* 27 (3): 6–9.

Wanous, J. P. 1992. *Recruitment, Selection, Orientation, and Socialization of Newcomers,* 2nd Ed. Reading, MA: Addison-Wesley.

ORGANIZATIONAL DEVELOPMENT AND TRAINING

Rita Quinton, SPHR

Learning Objectives

After completing this chapter, readers should be able to

- discuss the role of organizational development and training and its contribution to the bottom line;
- understand the impact of the centralization and decentralization of education or training;
- define the process of training development;
- distinguish between training and facilitation, and articulate how this difference affects the transferability of new skills into the workplace;
- conduct a training needs assessment;
- express the difference between on-the-job and off-the-job training methods;
- recognize the importance of formal and informal socialization;
- develop a meaningful new-employee orientation;
- explain the process of succession planning development and management; and
- describe the trends in training.

Introduction

One thing is certain in today's global workplace: It will change. With change comes the need to run interference to ensure that the organization continues to meet its goals. *Organizational development* (OD) can assist an organization in achieving homeostasis or balance in the face of change's continual impact on processes and people. The OD department may have different functions in each organization, but its primary function, according to the Society for Human Resource Management (SHRM 2007), is to "increase an organization's effectiveness through planned interventions related to the organization's processes . . . resulting in improvements in productivity, return on investment and employee satisfaction." *Training*—whether as a response to an intervention or as a method for achieving goals—is a large component of what the OD department does. Training can be a strategic tool for organizational success, because it can diagnose the ills of the organization as well as point out the elements that are working well, using employees as the measurement. Ultimately, the OD department is the environmental barometer that gauges the human side of the organization, and it seeks to mold that environment into one that allows sound evaluation methodology and objective data. The OD department can present "before and after" data to show the effects of change.

The activities of the OD department are largely manifested through training, and usually these interventions are directed either by management based on organizational needs or by the analysis process and employee feedback, which may reveal gaps in performance, knowledge, awareness, service, and safety. The scope of training is highly varied. The OD department carries out the learning organization theory that Peter Senge (1994) explored in his book *The Fifth Discipline*. A core function today for many organizations, OD is a complex process that responds to organizational growth and individual needs. Organizational learning, however, is more involved than the simple view that it is the sum of all the training, lessons, and knowledge in an organization. Understanding the key constructs of effective learning is therefore crucial to the success of OD (Dodgeson 1993).

Many organizations have some mandatory or required training for all employees as well as specified training requirements for particular positions that may involve licensing or certification and annual or periodic renewals. Healthcare personnel, for example, may need to obtain a certain amount of training hours per year in their field to maintain professional licensure. Healthcare organizations also undergo an accreditation process every few years to ensure patient safety and quality of services. The Joint Commission (2007) is the major accrediting organization in the healthcare industry, and its qualifying process requires healthcare professionals and staff to have education and training. OD is at the heart of that process, as Joint Commission standards for compliance and patient safety must be met, including tracking and documentation. Documentation at the very minimum includes the name of the training or intervention, the participant's name, and the date of training completion.

Outsourcing the OD function may be appropriate on some occasions—for example, if the staff size is small or if subject-matter expertise does not exist in the department or the organization. Because of the variety of training subjects related to the operations of a healthcare organization (see Table 9.1), it is easy to see how outsourcing may be necessary. However, employees who have experience and knowledge in the topic may be able to serve as effective facilitators or instructors, in place of a staff of the OD department.

Having a central area through which OD and training services are offered is ideal. However, in a number of hospitals and health systems, the training/

Management-Mandated Topics	Position-Specific Topics	Intervention Topics
Antiharassment	Patient safety	Customer service
Diversity	Leadership	Building high-performing teams
Disaster preparedness	Understanding organ donation	Dealing with difficult people
Quality improvement	Patient-centered care	Coaching for excellence
New-employee orientation	In-service	Embracing change

TABLE 9.1
Topics and Dimensions of Training

education function is administered by a cadre of educators located in unrelated departments across the facility. In this case, the organization should at least assign a coordinator of all educational services to ensure that training and other instructional programs are not duplicated; that the offerings are necessary; and that the educational process is consistent throughout, including the design, facilitation, and participant-tracking elements.

Designing Training for Sustainability

To ensure that organizational learning is effective, a systematic approach is prescribed as a best practice. The consistency of planning, execution, and metrics gives credibility and power to the OD process.

Today, training can come in many formats, including in class, e-learning, online asynchronous/synchronous, self-paced DVD, and even videoconferencing. Training may be defined by its delivery mode (e.g., online, self-directed), but it is also defined by its *training design*—the unifying thread of all training modes. Changes in technology and advances in healthcare influence not only the operation of an organization but also its processes, necessitating new training and education and thus training design. Quality assurance reports may be helpful in identifying areas in which training is needed and in which deficiencies exist. Several models for training design exist, and all these models deliver on the primary necessity of an effective training initiative. After all, who wants to train for the sake of training? In today's business climate, no organization or department can afford to be frivolous—at least not if it wants to survive for any length of time.

Two of the most ubiquitous designs are the *ADDIE model* (analysis, design, development, implementation, and evaluation) and the *ISD model* (instructional system design). Both models are a systems approach to training, ensuring that the how, what, why, where, who, and when of training are addressed. Furthermore, these approaches constantly evaluate the training initiative for compatibility with and proficiency in the changing workplace. Figure 9.1 depicts the five steps in these models that are integral to good training design.

The design plan must be detailed and include updated timelines, but the plan must also be flexible enough to change with organizational requirements as they occur. In dynamic healthcare environments, OD departments must be visionary and respond to the needs for learning experiences that are propagated by constant institutional changes (Mailloux 1998). The organizational structure should facilitate, not detract, the success of a training initiative. Decisions about the training method and the involved personnel should follow a systematic assessment. For example, it may be tempting to decide on who the facilitator will be before even assessing the need for training. This action may jeopardize the effectiveness of the training and may add pressure on the process, reducing the purpose of the training to "make it fit" rather than to provide value. Simply, the needs assessment and design phase should drive the training initiative. Sometimes, a needs assessment will reveal that training is not the proper remedy for the problem. For example, lack of employee motivation or poor staff morale cannot be rectified by offering training. Numerous companies have spent thousands of dollars on a training initiative that did not meet its intended objectives.

Step 1 of the training design process is *analysis,* in which facts are collected to determine the intervention necessary, if any. *Needs assessment* is the heart of this phase, serving as a tool to gather information or clues on whether gaps exist in the desired and actual levels of performance according to organizational requirements or performance standards. DeSilets (2007) examined needs assessments from the healthcare perspective and argued that these assessments explore the areas that parallel Gilbert's (1996) human competence model. Gilbert's model suggests that six facets affect performance and need to be studied before training needs are identified: information, resources, incentive, knowledge, capacity, and motives. Under this human competence model, needs assessment should yield information about each of these six facets that (1) describe the issue or problem, (2) examine expeditious solutions or quick fixes, (3) check for impact, (4) improve competency levels, and (5) formulate resolutions (DeSilets 2007). This methodology is relatively easy to use in formulating needs assessment questions, and it is helpful because it focuses the questions and thus ensures that the instrument is thorough and delivers results related to the assessment goal. This insight presents the training design process in a holistic manner, encouraging the view that a needs assessment has catalytic implications for the workplace. Therefore, developing the needs assessment tool—a questionnaire, for example— is crucial because this instrument will deliver the data that will help the training

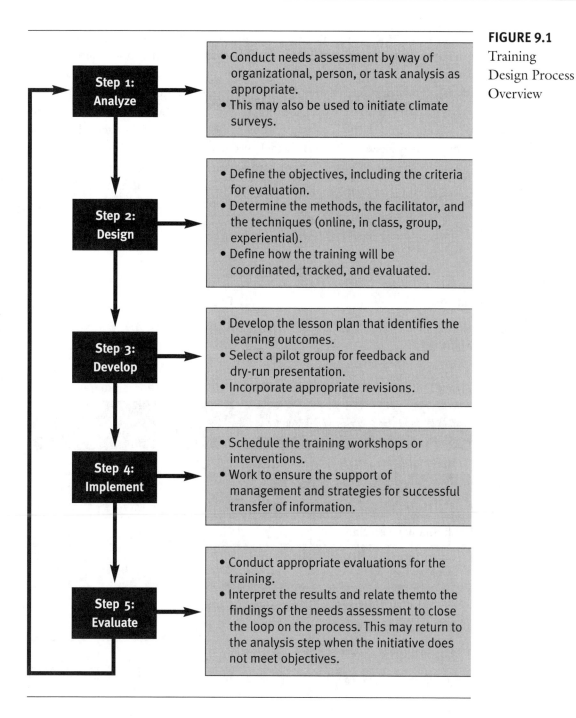

FIGURE 9.1
Training
Design Process
Overview

Step 1:
Analyze
- Conduct needs assessment by way of organizational, person, or task analysis as appropriate.
- This may also be used to initiate climate surveys.

Step 2:
Design
- Define the objectives, including the criteria for evaluation.
- Determine the methods, the facilitator, and the techniques (online, in class, group, experiential).
- Define how the training will be coordinated, tracked, and evaluated.

Step 3:
Develop
- Develop the lesson plan that identifies the learning outcomes.
- Select a pilot group for feedback and dry-run presentation.
- Incorporate appropriate revisions.

Step 4:
Implement
- Schedule the training workshops or interventions.
- Work to ensure the support of management and strategies for successful transfer of information.

Step 5:
Evaluate
- Conduct appropriate evaluations for the training.
- Interpret the results and relate them to the findings of the needs assessment to close the loop on the process. This may return to the analysis step when the initiative does not meet objectives.

designer decide on the best type of intervention. That intervention, in turn, will have an effect on patient safety, personnel issues such as turnover and grievances, or organization-wide productivity and knowledge.

A needs assessment can be performed in many ways. Mailloux (1998) found that nursing educators use various methods to determine learning needs, including reviewing organizational records and reports, supervisors' evaluations and recommendations, and critical incident reports; directly observing; conducting surveys with questionnaires; checking professional standards; brainstorming; testing; reading existing literature; and holding focus groups. Methods that involve the direct feedback of staff, such as a survey, can be administered with an instruction to respondents to either self-identify or anonymously answer. The most widely used and effective method is the survey questionnaire; see Figure 9.2 for a sample self-identification questionnaire.

Step 2 of the design process is *design*, in which the grand plan is established, the time lines are set, and the overall project outline is created. In keeping with good business protocol, developing options to keep the plan flexible

FIGURE 9.2
Sample Needs
Assessment

Name: _____   Department: _____

Shift: _____   Title: _____

Please indicate your interest in the following ideas for in-service programs

Topic	Not Interested	Neutral	Interested	Most Interested
Age-related issues	O	O	O	O
Alcohol/drug abuse—intervention	O	O	O	O
Alternative medicine	O	O	O	O
Anesthesia/conscious sedation procedures	O	O	O	O
Conflict resolution	O	O	O	O
Art of delegation	O	O	O	O
Patient safety	O	O	O	O
Autoimmune disease	O	O	O	O
Basic supervisory training	O	O	O	O
Budget/cost containment	O	O	O	O
Cardiovascular disease	O	O	O	O
Career planning	O	O	O	O

is advisable. The critical tasks in this phase are to accurately outline the objectives, communicate them to all involved, and ensure that they are thoroughly understood. At this point, it is also wise to consider the answer to the number one question of people who attend trainings: What's in it for me? This question must always be at the forefront of training design because it reminds the designer that participants must be kept engaged, and engagement is mostly based on what lessons and experiences participants can take away from the training.

Step 3 of the process is *development,* in which the tangibles take shape. Such deliverables include the curriculum; the learning outcomes; and the dry run, where feedback is crucial to determine whether revisions or mid-course corrections are needed. Training has evolved from the days of the presenter standing in front of a room dumping massive amounts of information on the participants (also known as the "sit and soak" method). Today's trainer serves as the facilitator of ideas and thought, involving the participants so that their transformation can begin even before they walk out the door. During Step 3, the curriculum is molded and sharpened to guide and enhance the facilitation.

Step 4 is *implementation,* in which the roll-out occurs and evaluation data are collected for future analysis. At this time, the flexibility built into the plan earlier helps, as user or participant feedback may dictate design revisions to ensure training quality. Thus, it is prudent to retain this flexibility. To help employees and supervisors manage their time appropriately, make the training schedule available early and hold multiple sessions on different days and times to accommodate individual needs.

Step 5 is *evaluation,* in which the information is reviewed to determine whether objectives were met. Before data can be reviewed, they must be collected, as described later. One of the most common ways to conduct an evaluation is the *pretest and posttest method.* This approach is done before and after training, using a questionnaire that allows respondents to rate certain aspects of the training. The questionnaire may be designed using a Likert-like scale, or it may be a simple yes/no construction. Either way, this method will present information that reveals the differences in knowledge or skills between the two evaluation time frames. Although having a control group who takes the pretest and posttest without going through the training is recommended, this is not possible in every situation. The control group does make the evaluation much clearer and establishes support for training, making arguments for outside influences harder. If the group who has undergone the training shows greater improvement than the control group, the effectiveness and business case of the training can be proven.

If, according to the evaluation, the OD department fell short on the training objectives and the training did not address or improve the situation at hand, then the design process goes back to Step 1. With objectives sometimes shifting with organizational changes, it is not uncommon for the design process to be iterative. Many OD departments often run this cycle on their training programs to maintain quality and to ensure that the objectives continue to be met.

Training Methods

Training methods involve the development of curriculum content and learning outcomes. Although some training occurs on the job and is very effective, most training happens off the job so that learners/employees can concentrate fully on learning. Because the main training objective is for the information to be transferable or applicable to the work of the learner, we examine below the most common methods for accomplishing that goal.

Note that the training method should match a given situation appropriately. Selecting the proper method will optimize the quality and usefulness of the training and will increase the likelihood of accomplishing the objective. Sometimes the best method is a combination of two or three techniques.

Off-the-Job Training

Lecture is usually a verbal presentation by an instructor, and it is effective with large groups and when the dissemination of information is the goal. On the other hand, *group discussion* may also include a lecture, but it affords participants an opportunity to inject their own ideas and thoughts into the training. It is very effective for small groups and where idea generation is needed or is a desired outcome, but the discussions need to be well facilitated to ensure that the group stays on track.

Role playing is very applicable and transferable back to the workplace because it involves creating a realistic scenario, with the learners taking on roles and practicing developing the skill sets necessary to accomplish the task. Although the problem-solving arena is the context in which role playing occurs, it is the development of skills that is the main objective for the learner. The role-playing technique is an excellent way to teach feedback (giving and receiving), coaching, and conflict resolution skills. Use of the case study is another way to build practicality and workplace transferability into the training experience. When a written description of a real-world incident or issue is presented to a group for discussion and formulation of strategies or solutions, the discussion can be lively and engages the learner to think critically. The case study method may demonstrate the viability of many possibilities for resolving the incident as well as serve as a way for group members to practice other skills, including communication, decision making, and even negotiation.

Simulation, like the case study, can be a very efficient mean of providing practical experience to learners. During a simulation, learners are briefed about either a fictitious or real (their own) organization, given information about that organization's culture, and presented with an actual or imagined situation. Learners are then divided into groups to discuss and make a decision about the simulated problem; the work of each group is then evaluated by the other groups. Debriefing by the other groups is a valuable way to demonstrate the practical learning that can be applied or transferred back to the workplace. Simulation is also an excellent teaching tool within departments. For example, a simulation is suitable for training emergency room employees in disaster response and management.

On-the-Job Training

Job shadowing is used to show an employee what a colleague or a supervisor actually does in the position on a daily basis. Common job-shadowing activities include attending meetings, sitting in on decision-making sessions, and virtually following in the footsteps of the person being shadowed. This method works best when a transfer of knowledge (e.g., from the departing employee to the trainee) must occur quickly and when a position is complex. The effectiveness of the method depends on the ability of the person being shadowed and the willingness of the learner.

Coaching is another on-the-job type of training. Although coaching requires patience and an understanding of how to effectively give feedback, it provides timely information or correction that is highly individualized. This method usually demands a high degree of trust between the coach and the learner to ensure that the experience is valuable and that feedback can be freely given.

Employee Socialization

Even before most job candidates arrive for the interview, they have already researched the organization through a website, company literature, or a current or former employee. The interview process, then, adds to the candidates' knowledge, allowing them to piece together an overall picture and to figure out how they will fit into the larger organizational scheme. Therefore, when the new employee reports to the job for the first time, his or her socialization wheel is set in motion.

The formal orientation process provides a huge opportunity to engage the new employee in formulating expectations for a future with the organization. If a formal orientation process is not provided, then the employee will go through an informal process that involves indoctrination by other employees. Certainly an orientation by peers is valuable, but it is not sufficient. When left with only an informal orientation device, the new employee will receive inaccurate, incomplete, and even biased information. This will lead to a cause of frustration for the new employee.

The *new-employee orientation* is a process by which the organization satisfies many employee-centered questions. This is the opportunity for the organization to explain and educate on workplace structure; policies; processes; practices; and related information, standards, and expectations that will assist the newcomers in their development and success with the organization. During the orientation, the employee should be exposed to a balance of job-specific and organization-related information.

Content

Because each organization is unique, the new-employee orientation should be customized, not generic. On the other hand, many topics are resident in every organization's orientation program, such as compensation, benefits, work hours, and career planning. Table 9.2 lists the areas that are commonly covered in new-employee orientations.

Logistics

As today's world continues to expose us to huge amounts of knowledge, and as we try to accommodate all or much of that information in our busy lives, we have developed fast-paced ways to learn. This trend in short-length learning

TABLE 9.2
Types of Information Conveyed in an Orientation

Employee-Centered Information	Organization-Specific Information
Compensation, including pay rates, deductions, overtime, and holiday pay	Overview of organization, including introduction, history, and customs/traditions
Benefits, including insurance, holidays, leave, and retirement	Safety, including precautions and accident-reporting procedures
Facilities, including food services/cafeteria, parking, restrooms, security, first aid, security, and badges/name tags	Employee relations, including reporting sick leave, length of probationary period and limitations of activities associated with that, expectations and disciplinary practices, and grievance process
Details of job duties, including work hours, job description, and performance criteria	
Department tour, including work space/office, entrances/exits, supervisor's location, water fountains, and smoking areas	Policies and procedures
	Where to find resources and who to call to report discrimination or illegal activities
Career planning, including development opportunities and resources for growth	Community activities and sponsored events

has been adopted in orientation programs as well. The usual healthcare workplace situation is this: The supervisor is feeling the pinch of an unfilled position. The usual management response to the situation is this: Get the new hire initiated quickly so that person can attack the learning curve.

One of the best approaches to orienting a new employee is the "eating of the apple" method—one bite at a time. In the workplace, this method translates into breaking up the orientation into brief sessions over a period of days or weeks. The employee remembers much more because the integration of information takes place as he or she adjusts into the new work surroundings, with the information presented in "bites" that the employee can digest thoroughly. This translates into a win for the organization as well, because the employee is given a chance to stay connected to the process, and this in turn may lead to the employee's satisfaction with work and possibly to a greater probability of retention.

Best-Practice Ideas

There are many success stories of organizations that have revamped or renewed their new-employee orientation process. The Mayo Clinic in Rochester, Minnesota, welcomes new employees with balloons, upbeat music, and breakfast. The organization strives to provide a positive, lasting first impression and to keep that momentum going through the orientation process (Hicks, Peters, and Smith 2006). King's Daughters Medical Center, based in Ashland, Kentucky, developed its orientation session around an "interactive sports-themed orientation called New Team Member Training Camp" (Finkel 2005). When new employees arrive for the orientation, music is playing, pennants with inspirational quotes are posted everywhere in the room, and the facilitator is wearing a referee uniform. How do the new employees like the theme? One hundred percent of employees said they felt welcomed, an increase from the 92 percent survey results in 2003, before the change (Finkel 2005).

Succession Planning

The term "succession" contains the word "success." In that sense, succession planning may be explained as a strategy for the organization to succeed. To some degree, succession planning has been occurring in organizations for many years. People have been groomed to take over positions through mentoring and even job-shadowing processes, but most organizations have failed to put in place a formalized structure for recognizing this tradition.

Succession planning is a process for ensuring that the vitality of an organization continues by developing potential successors for the positions identified as critical to operations. (The overall process of succession planning is outlined in Figure 9.3.) With the fluidity of positions and people in

FIGURE 9.3

The Succession
Planning
Process

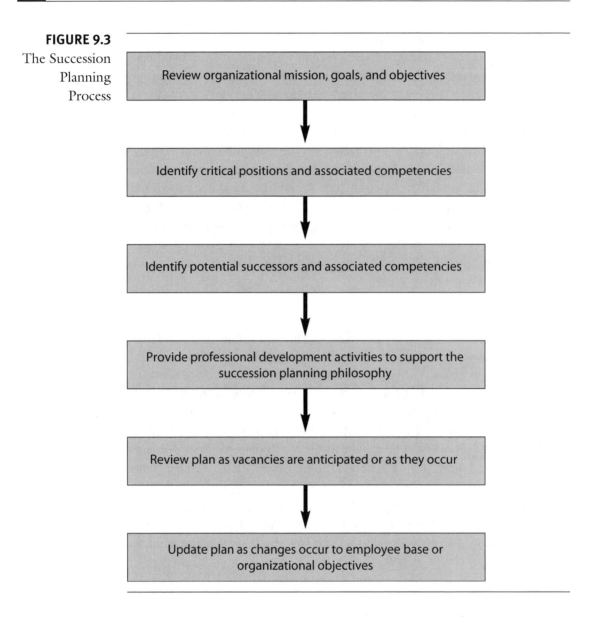

organizations, however, it is important to understand that such planning must be reviewed and revised frequently. A critical step in the succession planning model is to forecast demand and skills gaps for key positions (Blouin et al. 2006). What is critical today is no indication of what will be critical in the future, as evidenced by the rapid changes in technology and other medical advances.

In many organizations, the succession planning process is done only for the top executive position. That line of thinking comes with the philosophy that only "high potential" individuals will benefit from the leadership development that is offered to support the succession planning program (Pintar, Capuano, and Rosser 2007). This mind-set is dysfunctional. Imagine an organization facing a huge wave of employees who are near retirement. No one is in line to fill the positions that these future retirees will leave vacant, because the organization's succession planning is designed exclusively for the top executives. That scenario will cripple the organization. Moreover, it is important to recognize the value of exposing every employee, not just the "high potentials," to the training and workshops targeted to support the development of those who were identified as successors. It is good practice to keep a list of candidates who are eligible to fill a critical position that someone will vacate or already left either through retirement or other means of attrition. Doing so ensures workplace sustainability and signifies the presence of effective leadership. The candidate list may include the names of potential successors; information related to their professional preparation, including the number of years it would take for them to be position-ready; and the competencies necessary for the position. This list can be as simple or as sophisticated as the organization requires.

Succession planning is a vehicle for social responsibility. It can be used by an organization to give an opportunity to or advance underrepresented or protected groups (Workforce Management 2005). Healthcare still lags behind other industries in terms of growing leaders within the organization—a practice that was almost nonexistent in healthcare in the past. According to a study by the American College of Healthcare Executives, the "overall promotion rate for managerial positions hovers around 64 percent," while only 21 percent of the more than 722 healthcare institutions surveyed routinely practiced succession planning (Wilson 2005a). Health First, located in Brevard County, Florida, addressed its succession planning needs in 2007. The organization initiated a formal mentoring process, pairing up senior executives with junior managers and directors from across the organization. To make the mentoring relationships more comfortable for participants, each person comes from different business units, avoiding the conflict that can arise with direct-report relationships and allowing participants to freely express themselves (DeMarco 2007). Similarly, Martin Memorial Health Systems in Stuart, Florida, made a commitment to grow its leadership from within the organization. Martin Memorial instituted a leadership development program that uses career mapping (Wilson 2005b).

In the future, the bench strength of an organization will continue to play an important part in organizational vitality.

Trends in Organizational Development and Training

What will the future bring for OD and training? Will instructor-led, in-class workshops be just a memory in the next few years? How will workplace learning look in the ever-shifting business climate?

For now, organizational learning is at the "head of the table." In this time of extreme competition and globalization, organizations rely on workplace learning strategies to develop highly skilled workers, who are then expected to drive productivity and quality. This practice will likely remain constant. In the past, OD departments have been the first to march to the chopping block, but that has become less common as organizations have increasingly relied on strategic training to drive performance. According to the American Society for Training and Development, the trend shows an acceleration of initiatives toward employee learning, capitalizing on the development of knowledge and skills that are at the heart of organizational impact (Ketter 2006).

The trends in learning delivery are pointing to more use of electronic media, a benefit of prior investments in technology-based delivery such as online learning or e-learning. A fast-growing technological innovation is *m-learning* or mobile learning. With this delivery medium, learning can take place through MP3 players and personal digital assistants. As such, learning becomes easy to access and flexible enough to accommodate just about any schedule. M-learning expansion is just beginning.

Other available technology-based learning methods include videoconferencing, instant messaging, online meeting, and webinar. *Webinars*—a term that combines "web" and "seminars"—have proliferated quickly within the business-to-business sales area because they are able to deliver on-demand training through a live or videotaped broadcast on the Internet. This medium allows both the presenters and the training participants to sit in their own offices or be in different cities or even countries. More and more in-house training departments and organizations with employees at different or remote sites are relying on webinars, which help prevent the high costs of training a widely dispersed staff in a single location. Instant messaging (IM) holds promise as an avenue for training in real time, offering quick responses to real-time on-the-job needs by employees. With slow response times, e-mail does not offer promptness of information. The IM, on the other hand, leaps into the world of constant and instant accessibility. A trainer can establish a schedule for IM accessibility as a way to enhance or as an adjunct to a general workshop, a coaching session, or nurse education.

It is prudent to look at the cost to exclusively deliver training in electronic format. Because so much of the training content is customized according to the need of an organization, relying fully on electronic delivery may not be practical because the costs multiply when customization is involved. These costs are not solely monetary. The most important cost may be that the quality of training in some areas (e.g., interpersonal skills) is not high. This then manifests in the workplace through conflict or poor service, which certainly adversely affects the bottom line. For example, "soft skills" training—team building, conflict resolution, coaching, giving feedback—are based on interaction with others. As such, training in this area is very difficult to deliver effectively outside of a physical classroom. However, with so much business conducted in the virtual world, the development of soft-skills training for the online environment is surely on the horizon.

Summary

Organizational development is part of the changing healthcare landscape. The OD challenge is to remain flexible enough to respond to the educational and training needs of the organization and its employees while stable enough to deliver learning that will power up the enterprise as a whole. Sustained organizational learning depends on the ability of OD departments to facilitate, coach, and guide training toward the desired goals and objectives. Finding the proper training methods that will help toward building a productive, highly functioning workforce is not easy, but adaptability, innovation, and continual pursuit of best practices are some ways to ensure sustainable results. An OD department that serves as a strategic partner to executive management allows the organization to adapt to the constantly shifting environment. Together, this partnership creates a systematic perspective that yields positive responses to organizational development needs.

   This chapter provides an overview for understanding the important role of organizational development and practical applications for development of a successful training initiative, from understanding how needs assessments are conducted to the actual program delivery and evaluation. It serves to bring focus to important organizational processes that begin as the new employees are hired and socialized, and then managed through career and performance development. One method of organizational sustainability is examined through discussion of the succession planning process. The process of training development as it exists today as well as future trends are also presented.

Discussion Questions

1. Using the ADDIE model discussed in this chapter, design a training program that addresses the customer service expectations of walk-in patients in the emergency department. Include an evaluation process that answers the following questions:

   a. What method will you use to evaluate the knowledge transfer?
   b. How will you know whether or not you met your training objective?

2. Your healthcare facility assigned you to explore succession planning as a possible strategy for organizational sustainability.

What will you do? To help you with this assignment,

a. research two other organizations that have adopted a succession planning strategy, and

b. compare and contrast their programs and the outcomes.

3. Describe an example of a successful new-employee orientation. Why are both employee needs and organizational needs important to consider?

4. Why is it important to engage senior management early on in the process when preparing for a learning initiative?

Experiential Exercises

Case 1   Argosy Medical Center, a 400-bed critical care facility located in the Northeast, has been in operation for more than 18 years. Its mission statement is to provide quality healthcare services with the highest standard of excellence from employees who are dedicated to caring and patient satisfaction.

At one time, staff were really excited to be part of the Argosy family, and the patients noticed this attitude and enthusiasm. Argosy became the hospital of choice because the patients felt that the staff really cared about them, which made the patient experience positive regardless of their health status. Patient exit surveys were excellent, and patients frequently wrote glowing comments about the staff's genuine concern and about what a wonderful employer the hospital must be to have such a dedicated workforce.

In the last couple of years, however, the employees seem to have lost their passion. This has resulted in higher patient complaints of poor customer service. Management has attributed this deteriorated employee attitude to higher workloads and burnout. Training was instituted. Employees are required to at-

tend a refresher course, every year, in an effort to keep them motivated and in tune with the hospital mission and to reenergize them about the workplace. The course includes a review of the hospital values, mission, and standards of service that everyone is expected to follow. Because the course is only for one hour, participants do not get to interact, ask questions, or give feedback afterward. In fact, since the refresher course was implemented, employees have not been surveyed to get their feedback or insights. Because the staff are constantly busy, they have had no opportunity to talk among themselves, with their managers, or in focus groups about the decline in employee morale and the poor customer service. Everyone knows the problem is there, but no time has been put aside to address it, other than an organizational reminder to give good customer service regardless of the situation.

Argosy's chief executive officer (CEO) has summoned you, the director of the OD department, to come up with a way to address the problem that is affecting the hospital bottom line, not to mention the increased employee turnover and absenteeism.

Case Study Questions

1. What interventions would you recommend? Come up with two options.

2. Defend your preferred option to the CEO and include a timeline for your plan.

Case 2   Health Valley Hospital provides comprehensive services, including cancer, heart, trauma, and emergency services. It has 2,300 full-time employees. For eight years, Health Valley has had a decentralized philosophy for training and organizational development. In fact, almost every department has its own trainer/educator. The human resources department also has an education component, called Education Services, that provides training in general topics, including new-employee orientation, customer service, leadership/management, and staff development. Education Services does not provide training in topics such as nursing education, patient safety, emergency medical services, and disaster preparedness. Because so many training units exist at Health Valley, and all of them separate from each other, tracking of educational information is handled by each training unit. With constant interruptions and emergencies inherent in the hospital environment, it is understandable that this tracking function sometimes gets pushed down to the low end of daily priorities.

Health Valley's CEO has heard so much about all of the education that occurs within the organization that he wants to highlight it to the hospital's board of directors. The CEO immediately sends a memo to the human resources department asking for all sorts of education-related information, including a listing of all education/training activities, under which should be the details of each training such as the title, objectives, how it meets organizational objectives, the outcomes, the name of the educator or facilitator, and the names of the employees who attended and completed.

Because the training information throughout the organization is not housed in a central location, this CEO request is a major undertaking. Furthermore, each training unit tracks the information (when tracking is done, that is) in many different ways and formats, including spreadsheets, handwritten lists, electronic databases, and file folders. The only way for this request to be handled successfully is for all of the involved units to work together collaboratively and quickly.

Following are some strategies that may help if you were in a similar situation:

1. Contact the education/training/OD department in a local hospital or healthcare facility. Interview the head of the department to gain insight into how the training and tracking function is handled (centralized or decentralized, for example). Ask what works well and not so well, and listen for improvements they would like to make.

2. Formulate a short-term plan for responding to the CEO's primary request.

3. Design a long-term plan for addressing the problem and preventing it from

happening again. How should the information be gathered and stored so that it is readily available next time?

How is having a centralized recording system valuable to the organization and the employees?

Case 3

This case was adapted from Giangregorio, L., P. Fisher, A. Papaioannou, and J. D. Adachi. 2007. "Osteoporosis Knowledge and Information Needs in Healthcare Professionals Caring for Patients with Fragility Fractures." *Orthopaedic Nursing* 26 (1): 27–35.

This study was conducted in a multi-site hospital in Canada. The only healthcare providers eligible for the study were those who worked in regions with patients who had osteoporosis or fractures. Some of the staff included were from fracture clinics, rehabilitation and orthopedics districts, and nuclear medicine. The goal of the study was to identify gaps in knowledge about osteoporosis and related concerns.

The samples were taken between November 2005 and February 2006 from the healthcare providers. A local nurse clinician educator selected them by way of invitation and advertisement. As the participants were identified, they were told of the goal of the needs assessment, which was to pinpoint future training needs. To ensure that those needs identified by the outcomes of the study were thorough, the nurse educator also worked to get volunteers from all shifts to complete the assessment. As is common in these studies, each participant was asked to sign a written consent form.

The questionnaire that each participant completed was comprised of four parts. In the first part, there was a demographic profile with related questions, and in the second part, an assessment of their osteoporosis knowledge with a modified version of the Osteoporosis Knowledge Questionnaire (OKQ). The OKQ is a 22-item, multiple choice questionnaire designed to assess knowledge of osteoporosis and associated preventative measures (Berarducci, Lengacher, and Keller 2002). The results showed that there were variances in osteoporosis knowledge among those health professionals working with clients who were either at risk of fracture or had had a fracture. The primary areas of knowledge deficit were those topics related to the promotion of better health and management of osteoporosis patients. The study participants...surveyed reported using several methods for staying current on the osteoporosis information, with the most widely reported methods being journal or magazine articles, brochures and workshops, or presentations at the workplace. Besides being the most common methods that they used to stay abreast of the topic, those methods were also reported as the most preferred sources of information.

The survey revealed that the participants wanted more information about prevention, nutrition/supplements, what is new on the research horizon, and treatment-related data such as medication risks/benefits. Coincidentally, these same topics were identified as gaps.

Case Study Questions

1. Can you think of another approach to get this information? Focus groups? Would that have been appropriate in this

circumstance? What were the benefits to this needs assessment?

2. What were the outcomes from knowing the information, and what are some possibilities for improvement?
3. Would this methodology work in your workplace? Why or why not?

Reference

Berarducci, A., C. A. Lengacher, and R. Keller. 2002. "The Impact of Osteoporosis Continuing Education on Nurses' Knowledge and Attitudes." *Journal of Continuing Education in Nursing* 33: 210–16.

Web Resources

1. The Joint Commission is the accreditation body for healthcare organizations. According to its website (see www.jointcommission.org), it "evaluates and accredits more than 15,000 health care organizations in the United States." The website is a rich resource for understanding standards and improvements in healthcare, which often drive training and education for those who seek to meet or maintain certification and who strive for excellence.
2. The Society for Human Resource Management (SHRM) is an association for human resources professionals. Its website (see www.shrm.org) has a very active organizational development and learning area. The site also contains information on student organizations and memberships. SHRM produces *HR Magazine* and various human resources publications.
3. The American Society for Training and Development (ASTD) is an organization dedicated to workplace learning and training professionals. For more information, go to www.astd.org. ASTD publishes *T + D* magazine.
4. The Organizational Development Network (OD Network) is "an international professional association of organization development practitioners" (see www.odnetwork.org). OD Network has a listserv that serves as a forum for dialogue around issues of interest to organizational development professionals in the field of healthcare. The listserv features trends, best practices, and networking opportunities.

References

Blouin, A., K. McDonagh, A. Neistadt, and B. Helfand. 2006. "Leading Tomorrow's Healthcare Organizations: Strategies and Tactics for Effective Succession Planning." *Journal of Nursing Administration* 36 (6): 325-30.

DeMarco, J. M. 2007. "Homegrown Leaders." *Modern Healthcare* 37 (33): 23.

DiSilets, L. D. 2007. "Needs Assessment: An Array of Possibilities." *Journal of Continuing Education in Nursing* 38(3): 107–13.

Dodgeson, M. 1993. "Organizational Learning: A Review of Some Literature." *Organization Studies* 24 (3): 375–94.

Finkel, E. 2005. "Employee Orientation a Whole New Ballgame." *Modern Healthcare* 35 (50): 32.

Gilbert, T. F. 1996. *Human Competence: Engineering Worthy Performance.* San Francisco: Pfeiffer.

Hicks, S., M. Peters, and M. Smith. 2006. "Orientation Redesign." *T + D* 60 (7): 43–47.

Joint Commission. 2007. "Facts About the Joint Commission." [Online information; retrieved 9/12/07.] www.jointcommission.org/AboutUs/joint_commission_facts.htm.

Ketter, P. 2006. "Investing in Learning: Looking for Performance." *T + D* 60 (12): 30–34.

Mailloux, J. P. 1998. "Learning Needs Assessments: Definitions, Techniques, and Self-Perceived Abilities of the Hospital-Based Nurse Educator." *Journal of Continuing Education in Nursing* 29 (1): 40–45.

Pintar, K., T. Capuano, and G. Rosser. 2007. "Developing Clinical Leadership Capability." *Journal of Continuing Education in Nursing* 38 (3): 115–21.

Senge, P. 1994. *The Fifth Discipline.* New York: Doubleday.

Society for Human Resource Management (SHRM). 2007. "Glossary of Human Resources Terms." [Online information; retrieved 9/12/07.] www.shrm.org/hrresources/hrglossary_published.

Wilson, L. 2005a. "Top Performing Hospitals Are Promoting from Within." [Online information; retrieved 9/12/07.] www.workforce.com.

———. 2005b. "Florida's Martin Memorial: Growing Talent from Within." [Online information; retrieved 9/12/07.] www.workforce.com.

Workforce Management. 2005. "A Sample Succession Planning Policy." [Online information; retrieved 9/12/07.] www.workforce.com.

10

PERFORMANCE MANAGEMENT

Bruce J. Fried, PhD

Learning Objectives

After completing this chapter, the reader should be able to

- define performance management, and describe the key components of a performance management system;
- understand the purposes and approach of the annual or periodic performance review;
- discuss the reasons that organizations engage in performance management;
- identify the characteristics of good rating criteria for performance appraisal;
- enumerate various sources of information about job performance, and discuss the strengths and shortcomings of each;
- address the three types of information needed to assess employee performance;
- distinguish between rating errors and political factors as sources of distortion in performance appraisal; and
- conduct a performance appraisal interview with an employee, taking into consideration the techniques that make such an interview successful.

Introduction

A central theme of this book is that the performance of individual employees is central to the long-term success of an organization. The ultimate goal of human resources management (HRM), which includes selection, compensation, supervision, and training, is to foster high levels of performance from individuals and teams. In this chapter, we discuss performance management, which comprises all of the organization's activities involved in managing employees. We often give special attention to performance management because it is this function that seeks to coordinate the efforts of various human resources systems involved in improving performance. Performance management also specifically involves the collection of performance information and using that information to conduct formal and informal improvement efforts. While we can think of performance management as a tool for evaluating and improving individual performance, we can also use the performance management system to assess the success of other human resources functions. A well-functioning performance management system can provide insight into the effectiveness of our selection processes, whether training programs are effective, and whether an incentive compensation system is successful in meeting its performance goals. Table 10.1 provides examples of how performance management is related to other human resources functions.

Performance management is a set of tools and practices that comprises setting performance goals with employees, designing strategies with employees to make and sustain improvement, monitoring employee progress toward achieving goals, ongoing feedback and coaching by supervisors and perhaps peers, and measuring individual performance. The term *performance appraisal* is often used to describe this process, but that term tends to limit the process to measurement, which is a necessary but an insufficient part of

TABLE 10.1
Relationship of Performance Management to Other Human Resources Management Functions

HRM Function	Effects of Performance Management	Effects on Performance Management
Job analysis	Performance information may lead to redesign of jobs	Accurate information about jobs is key to develop criteria for performance appraisal
Recruitment and selection	Performance information lets managers know about the effectiveness of alternative sources of recruitment and the effectiveness of their selection criteria and procedures	Ability to recruit and select employees may affect the types of criteria and standards developed for performance appraisal
Training and development	Performance management systems provide information on employees' training and development needs; information on the performance appraisal systems assesses the effectiveness of training	Performance appraisal tools may be designed to assess the impact of training programs
Compensation	Compensation systems may be designed such that performance appraisal information has an impact on employee compensation	A fair and equitable compensation system may lead to higher levels of employee performance

performance management. As discussed in this chapter, performance management is more encompassing than collecting performance information, but it is a data-informed system for improving performance. In this chapter, the term "performance appraisal" is sometimes used to refer to aspects of the process that deal with obtaining performance information.

Issues of employee performance and productivity are at the forefront in healthcare organizations. The Joint Commission (2007) requires accredited healthcare organizations to assess, track, and improve the competence of all employees. The 2008 Joint Commission standards include such phrasing as: "Staff is competent to perform their responsibilities" (3.10) and "The organization evaluates staff performance" (3.20). In addition, the requirements for healthcare organizations of the prestigious Baldrige National Quality Program (2007, 18) include specific criteria related to employee engagement and performance management:

> How does your workforce performance management system support high-performance work and workforce engagement? How does your workforce performance management system consider workforce compensation, reward, recognition, and incentive practices? How does your workforce performance management system reinforce a patient and other customer and health care service focus and achievement of [your] action plans?

Performance management makes sense. The adage "you can't manage what you can't measure" is applicable to performance management. However, performance management has a well-deserved reputation for being very poorly implemented. It is perhaps the most misunderstood and misused human resources function. Measuring and improving employee performance is also among the most highly examined aspects of management, both in scholarly works and in the popular press. Perhaps because it has met with so much failure, it is also one of the areas of management most prone to passing fads, which have been widely adopted in popular management literature and by countless consulting firms that seek to identify and promote the quick fix to improve employee productivity.

In this chapter, we describe the essential components of performance management and present the countless pitfalls that may be faced in virtually every aspect of the process. To the extent possible, we avoid the jargon and fashions that come and go and maintain a focus on those processes found to have the highest likelihood of leading to improved and sustained employee performance. Specifically, we explore the following:

- Reasons that organizations develop and implement performance management systems
- Content of the annual or periodic performance review
- The terms performance criteria, criterion deficiency, criterion contamination, reliability, and validity

- Sources of information about employee performance
- Applicability of multisource or 360-degree performance management approaches
- Performance information based on individual traits, behaviors, and outcomes
- Advantages and disadvantages of common formats for collecting and summarizing performance information
- Common sources of errors and other problems in performance appraisal
- Guidelines for conducting effective performance management interviews

Every manager seeks to have employees who are highly motivated and productive. This is a challenging goal for a number of reasons. First, employee motivation is in itself a complex phenomenon and is influenced by many things outside of the manager's control. Second, whether or not managerial interventions are effective in improving performance is unclear. For instance, compensation clearly has some motivational potential for most employees, but money is not an effective motivator in all circumstances. In healthcare organizations with very small margins, the availability of performance-based rewards tends to be very limited. Third, employee performance is often difficult to observe and measure in a reliable manner. This, of course, varies by job. For example, it is relatively easy to assess the performance of an employee doing medical equipment sales, but evaluating the performance of a case manager for individuals with chronic mental illness is much more challenging. As with all human resources functions, performance management activities are carried out within a legal context, and performance management procedures must abide by relevant employment laws.

Some people believe that performance management is intended mainly for lower-level employees and that the higher one moves in the organization, the less important performance management becomes. This mistaken view is perhaps based on the perception that performance management is something of a punitive process, and if not punitive, it is often carried out in a condescending or demeaning manner. One of the benefits of moving up is that the person no longer has to be subjected to such insulting procedures. This view may also be based on the assumption that higher-level employees *do not need* supervision in the same manner as lower-level employees. Indeed, evidence in the literature indicates that the higher the position, the less likely that a performance appraisal is conducted. Appraisals of senior-level employees are usually poorly and haphazardly done. However, much evidence also suggests that executive-level employees have a strong desire to obtain information about their performance (Longenecker and Gioia 1992).

The bottom line is that performance appraisal and performance management are for everyone in the organization. Further, the process need not be demeaning to any employee, whether at lower level or at executive level. Of course, the types of performance information used may vary according to an employee's level and role in the organization.

The Role of Performance Management

Performance management is a system that integrates the performance appraisal function with other human resources systems to help align employees' work behaviors with the organization's goals (Fisher, Schoenfeldt, and Shaw 2003). One of the most common performance evaluation mistakes is to focus on the annual review, which typically includes paperwork and an interview, both of which are often unpleasant for all parties. Without stretching the analogy, this approach is similar to the focus that most of us give to the annual physical, the one time in the year we think about our health. This is not to say that an annual performance review is not necessary, but this yearly event has a defined and often misunderstood purpose.

Annual appraisals are necessary, but performance management is ideally carried out on a daily basis. An effective supervisor provides feedback continuously and addresses and manages performance problems when they occur. In other words, if a child is experiencing an earache, it is unlikely that a parent will wait to address this until the child's next scheduled physical. Performance management is an ongoing function that includes the following managerial responsibilities and activities:

- Setting performance goals, and making development plans with the employee
- Monitoring employee progress toward the goals
- Providing continual coaching, training, and education as necessary
- Conducting annual performance appraisal against goals and development plan activities
- Establishing a development plan for next year (or another review cycle)

The Annual or Periodic Performance Review
The annual or periodic performance review is only one part of the performance management process, but it is an important part that requires attention. The periodic performance review provides an opportunity for a supervisor and an employee to reflect and plan. The review may include discussions about personnel decisions, such as a promotion, change in compensation, disciplinary action, transfer, or recommendation for training. The review is *not* a time to deliver surprises to employees. Supervisors should continually provide employees with feedback on their performance, and supervisors and employees should come into the annual appraisal with a view toward developing

improvement strategies and problem solving. The performance review should be reserved for the following:

- Giving employees the opportunity to discuss performance and performance standards
- Addressing employee strengths and weaknesses
- Identifying and recommending strategies for improving employee performance
- Discussing personnel decisions, such as compensation, promotion, and termination
- Defining a variety of regulatory requirements that deal with employee performance, and discussing compliance methods

The periodic performance review has both administrative and developmental purposes. Administrative purposes commonly refer to using performance information to make decisions about promotion, termination, and compensation. To defend against charges of discrimination, organizations attempt to maintain accurate and current performance appraisal information on employees. Developmental purposes typically relate to using performance information to improve employee performance; appraisal information identifies employee strengths and weaknesses, which then become the basis for developing improvement strategies. Organizations can, of course, use appraisals for both administrative and developmental purposes. However, there is considerable debate about whether or not a manager or supervisor can actually conduct an honest developmental appraisal, considering that the content of the evaluation has an impact on the employee's income, promotion potential, and other bread-and-butter issues. It is difficult and sometimes unrealistic to expect an employee to focus on his or her development while also waiting for the all-important information about compensation. A common practice is to separate the periodic performance review from the process of informing employees about compensation decisions, perhaps providing the latter information several weeks after the formal review.

Establishing Appraisal Criteria

As is the case with many other human resources activities, an effective performance management system must begin with clear job expectations and performance standards. Of particular importance is the need for managers and employees to agree on the content of the job description and to have a shared understanding of job expectations. Once an agreement is reached, employees and managers together must identify the specific measurable criteria by which performance will be evaluated. These criteria need to be job related and relevant to the needs of the organization. Developing criteria is a challenging task and requires employee–manager collaboration. Criteria must be agreed on well in advance of a formal performance appraisal interview. How should performance criteria be defined? What are useful criteria?

First, criteria should have strategic relevance to the organization as a whole. For example, if patient satisfaction is an important organizational concern, then it makes sense to include patient-relations criteria for employees who interact with these customers. Criteria for individual performance appraisal are in many ways an extension of criteria used to evaluate organizational performance.

Second, criteria should be comprehensive and take into consideration the full range of an employee's major functions as defined in the job description. Criterion deficiency occurs when performance standards focus on a single criterion to the exclusion of other important, but perhaps less quantifiable, performance dimensions (Barrett 1995; Sherman, Bohlander, and Snell 1998). For example, counting the number of visits made by a home care nurse may be relatively simple, but it is certainly more difficult (but no less important) to assess the quality of care provided during those visits.

Third, criteria should be free from contamination. *Criterion contamination* occurs when factors out of the employee's control have a significant influence on his or her performance. In healthcare, this is a particular problem because of the complexity of patient care and the interdependence of the factors that affect quality and clinical outcomes. Clinicians, for example, may have little control over patient volume or the speed with which laboratory test results are reported. Therefore, appraisal criteria should include only those items over which the employee has control.

Fourth, criteria should be reliable and valid. *Reliability* refers to the consistency with which a manager rates an employee in successive ratings (assuming consistent performance) or the consistency with which two or more managers rate performance when they have comparable information. Criteria can be made more reliable by selecting objective criteria and by training managers in applying the criteria. *Validity* is the extent to which appraisal criteria actually measure the performance dimension of interest. For example, if we are interested in measuring a nurse's ability to carry out the nursing responsibilities during emergency medical procedures, is it sufficient to assess knowledge of these responsibilities rather than actual performance under real emergency conditions? Questions of validity are also difficult when measuring attitudes deemed important for a particular job.

Collecting Job Performance Data

Traditional performance appraisal methods involve collecting information from the employee's supervisor. Typically, the supervisor observes the employee's performance using whatever format the organization has designed for performance appraisal (described later in this chapter) and records the appraisal information. Given the complexity of many jobs, however, it is often impossible for one individual to accurately describe each employee's performance. In recent years, various alternative approaches to performance data collection have been developed.

A *self-appraisal* is an evaluation done by the employee on himself or herself; it is generally done in conjunction with the manager's appraisal. This approach is very effective when a manager is seeking to obtain the involvement of the employee in the appraisal process, which is desirable under virtually all circumstances. Because of the obvious potential for bias on the part of the employee, self-appraisals are almost always done for developmental rather than administrative purposes.

Sometimes, managers become concerned with how their performance is perceived by those whom they oversee. In this instance, employees may conduct an evaluation of their boss. This type is also most useful for developmental purposes. *Subordinate appraisal* presents many benefits, among which are identifying the "blind spots" of managers and improving managerial performance. From the subordinate's perspective, this type of appraisal has obvious risks, as not all managers may take kindly to critiques and opinions and may retaliate toward the evaluator. Thus, such appraisals should be done anonymously; where this is not possible, the appraisal is unlikely to yield reliable results.

Team-based appraisal is beneficial in that it explicitly reinforces the importance of teamwork; in other words, measuring team accomplishments sends a message that the organization places a high value on team performance. Organizations may link team performance with pay, although team-based compensation is not a necessary component of team-based appraisal. *Team-based compensation* may exacerbate anxieties and frustrations with the "free-rider" syndrome, where one or more team members benefit from team rewards without putting forth corresponding effort. In using team-based appraisal, with or without compensation, it is critical that team members agree on behavior-based and outcome-based appraisal criteria. Team members may also be involved in assessing the performance of other team members. Again, this approach reinforces to employees the fact that the organization values responsible team behavior and team citizenship, and it has the potential for building team cohesion and enhancing communication. Several questions need to be addressed, including the manner in which team members are involved in appraisals: Are all team members involved in appraising every other team member? Who should provide the feedback to members? While this approach may help build teams, it also presents the risk of alienation and conflict if feedback is provided in a divisive manner. Therefore, whoever is selected to provide the feedback should be trained in interviewing and feedback techniques.

Among the most useful ways to collect job performance information is using multiple sources. *Multisource appraisal*—also known as 360-degree appraisal or multirater assessment—recognizes the fact that for many jobs, relying on one source of performance information is incomplete and inadequate. To obtain a comprehensive assessment of performance, perspectives must be obtained from those within and outside the organization, including the manager or supervisor, peers, subordinates, clients, and other internal and external customers. The advantages of multisource appraisal include the following:

- Emphasis on aspects of performance valued by the organization
- Explicit recognition of the importance of customer focus
- Consistency with team development initiatives
- Contributor to employee involvement and development
- Minimal bias, as it includes multiple perspectives

Typically, multisource appraisal is done for developmental purposes, but it must be designed and administered with great care. Following are some of the limitations and potential pitfalls of multisource appraisal:

- Sources of feedback must have a level of trust in the organization, the managers, and the appraisal process.
- Employees must be assured of anonymity, which is difficult in a small organization or in an environment where a manager has a small span of control.
- Employees may use the appraisal for the purpose of retribution.
- The information obtained may be difficult to integrate or combine.
- The method of feedback must be done by a trained individual in a manner that encourages insight and growth.

Regardless of where performance information comes from (e.g., supervisors, coworkers, external customers), decisions need to be made about the types of information to be obtained in performance appraisals. In general, three types of information are possible:

1. Individual traits
2. Behaviors
3. Results or outcomes

These three types of information can be obtained using the various methods explored in the following section. Each approach has its strengths and shortcomings and is useful for particular types of jobs and circumstances.

Graphic Rating Scale

Graphic rating scale refers to any rating scale that uses points along a continuum and that measures traits or behaviors (Cascui 1991). This method is the most common way to assess performance, largely because it is easy to construct and can be used for many different types of employees. As shown in Figure 10.1, such a scale aims to measure a series of dimensions through anchor points (e.g., 1 through 6) that indicate different levels of performance. As the example in the figure shows, both traits and behaviors of the employee are assessed. Note, however, that many of the items included in the figure, such as "flexible," are prone to subjective judgment.

Please answer the following questions about this employee.

Question	Scale
1. Rate this person's pace of work.	1 2 3 4 5 6 slow fast
2. Assess this person's level of effort.	1 2 3 4 5 6 below full capacity capacity
3. What is the quality of this person's work?	1 2 3 4 5 6 poor good
4. How flexible is this person?	1 2 3 4 5 6 rigid flexible
5. How open is this person to new ideas?	1 2 3 4 5 6 closed open
6. How much supervision does this person need?	1 2 3 4 5 6 a lot a little
7. How readily does this person offer to help out by doing work outside his or her normal scope of work?	1 2 3 4 5 6 seldom often
8. How well does this person get along with peers?	1 2 3 4 5 6 not very well well

One of the drawbacks of a graphic rating scale is that it is quite general, often not representing specific behaviors that indicate positive or negative performance. The scale frequently does not yield information on how any item can be changed because the questions and statements for the behaviors or traits being rated are general. Because of this subjectivity, raters may be uncomfortable using this method, particularly when ratings are linked with compensation. Graphic rating scales can be improved by the use of behaviorally anchored rating scales, where specific observable behaviors are associated with each point on a scale.

Perhaps the most important drawback of graphic rating scales is that they typically do not weight behaviors and traits according to their importance to a particular job. In Figure 10.1, for example, pace of work (item 1) may be extremely relevant to the job of some employees but may be relatively unimportant to others. Thus, certain criteria may be less relevant for particular jobs. Related to this is the common practice of using a one-size-fits-all approach to criteria—sometimes, a scale is borrowed from another organization and, at other times, a scale is adapted for another position, all without giving consideration to how the scale applies to the particular job or organization.

Ranking is a simple method of performance appraisal where managers rank **Ranking** employees simply from best to worst on some overall measure of employee performance. Such a method is typically employed for administrative purposes, such as making personnel decisions (e.g., promotions, layoffs). The major advantages of the ranking method are that it forces supervisors to distinguish among employees, and it does not have many of the problems associated with other appraisal methods. Among the disadvantages of ranking are as follows:

- Focuses only on a single dimension of work effectiveness and may not take into account the complexity of work situations
- Becomes cumbersome with large numbers of employees, forcing appraisers to artificially distinguish among employees
- Simply lists employees in order of their performance but does not indicate the relative differences in employees' effectiveness
- Provides no guidance on specific deficiencies in employee performance and therefore is not useful in helping employees improve

One type of ranking that has come under a great deal of criticism is the process of *forced ranking*, or forced distribution. With forced ranking, employees are evaluated not based on their own set of objectives but based on a comparison to other employees. Managers are instructed to force evaluations of employee performance into a particular distribution, which is similar to grading students "on a curve." For example, managers may be directed to distribute 15 percent of employees as high performers, 20 percent as moderately high, 30 percent as average, 20 percent as low average, and 15 percent as poor. Forced ranking has been rationalized in a number of ways, including (1) to ensure that lenient managers do not systematically inflate appraisals, (2) to push managers to distribute their rankings, and (3) to limit bonuses and other financial payouts. Although these objectives may be met by using forced ranking, they corrupt the entire purpose of performance appraisal, which is to obtain honest information that can be used for employee development and improvement.

The most controversial use of forced ranking is to force out poor performers, sometimes referred to as "rank or yank." This approach was made famous by Jack Welch, former chief executive officer of General Electric (Welch and Byrne 2003). Many variants of this Welch ranking strategy exist, but in essence it works this way: Managers are required to identify the top 20 percent, middle 70 percent, and lowest 10 percent of employees. The bottom 10 percent are told to improve or they will be terminated. The validity of this approach is hotly debated. One study of human resources executives, half of whom worked in organizations that use forced ranking, reported that this approach resulted in lower productivity, inequity, and skepticism and has negatively affected employee engagement, morale, trust in management, and collaboration (Novations Group 2004: Pfeffer and Sutton 2006). In addition, lawsuits have been filed at companies, such as Ford Motor Company and Goodyear, that challenge the legality of forced ranking, claiming that the process discriminates against older workers. Interestingly, Ford abandoned forced distribution in 2001 and settled two class-action cases for about $10.5 million (Bates 2003).

When forced ranking is used, the implicit assumption is that 10 percent of employees (or whatever percentage is selected) are poor employees and therefore perform at a level deemed worthy of dismissal. Finally, the usefulness of this approach in healthcare is limited because of critical staff shortages. That is, a hospital that is facing a nurse shortage would likely not consider a "rank or yank" strategy for its nursing staff.

Behavioral Anchored Rating Scale

Behavioral anchored rating scale (BARS) is a significant improvement over traditional graphic rating scales. This scheme provides specific behavioral descriptions of the different levels of employee performance—that is, poor, good, excellent, and so forth. Table 10.2 is an example of a BARS that measures aspects of the performance of a clinical trials coordinator. Note that the scale assesses the four dimensions of leadership, communications, delivery of results, and teamwork. In some instances, the behavioral measures are relatively easy to observe (e.g., delivery of results), while in other instances, the measures may be a bit more subjective (e.g., teamwork). Using BARS, a manager is able to explain the reason behind the ratings, rather than vaguely state "unacceptable" or "average" on the performance criteria. With BARS, a manager can explicitly state his or her expectations for improved performance.

The advantages of BARS include the following:

- Reduces rating errors because job dimensions are clearly defined for the rater and are relevant to the job being performed
- Clearly defines the response categories available to the rater
- Is more reliable, valid, meaningful, and complete
- Has a higher degree of acceptance and commitment from employees and supervisors
- Minimizes employee defensiveness and conflict with the manager because employees are appraised on the basis of observable behavior
- Improves a manager's ability to identify areas for training and development

Developing a BARS for each job dimension for a particular job is not a trivial task. Among the disadvantages of a BARS is the amount of time, effort, and expense involved in its development. Use of this approach is most justifiable

TABLE 10.2
Behavioral
Anchored
Rating Scale for
a Clinical Trials
Coordinator

Task Dimension	Scale	Definition
Leadership	4	Identifies alternative methods that enhance productivity and quality and that eliminate unnecessary steps
	3	Takes the initiative to bring attention to productivity problems
	2	Has difficulty with change and with providing support for the required change
	1	Uses inappropriate interpersonal skills, and creates unproductive working relationships
Communication	4	Communicates openly, completely, and straightforwardly with management, peers, and coworkers
	3	Listens and seeks intent of communication
	2	Has difficulty with expressing decisions, plans, and actions
	1	Is unable to communicate accurately with team members
Delivery of results	4	Completes 90 percent to 100 percent of all projects within time frame and budget and according to standards
	3	Completes 75 percent to 90 percent of all projects within time frame and budget and according to standards
	2	Completes 50 percent to 75 percent of projects within time frame and budget; sometimes produces substandard work
	1	Completes less than 50 percent of projects within time frame and budget; frequently produces substandard work
Teamwork	4	Contributes positively to problem definition and takes responsibility for outcome
	3	Respects suggestions and viewpoints of others
	2	Has trouble with interactions with others and with understanding individual differences
	1	Does not contribute positively to team functioning

when a large number of jobholders are performing in the same position (e.g., nurses, transporters). BARS is most appropriate for jobs whose major components consist of physically observable behaviors.

A variation of BARS is the *behavioral observation scale* (BOS), a system that asks the rater to indicate the frequency with which the employee exhibits specified highly desirable behaviors. Desirable behaviors are identified through job analysis and discussions with managers and supervisors. Figure 10.2 is an example of a BOS for a patient relations representative. As seen in the figure, six desirable behaviors for this job are identified, and the rater indicates the frequency with which each behavior is observed in the patient relations representative. As with BARS, those who use BOS have a clear understanding of the types of behaviors expected.

Critical Incident

The *critical incident* approach involves keeping a record of unusually favorable or unfavorable occurrences in an employee's work. This record is created and maintained by the employee's manager. A major strength of this method is that it provides a factual record of an employee's performance and can be very useful in subsequent discussions with the employee. The approach does require that the manager closely and continuously monitor employee performance, which is not always feasible, although linking a critical incident method with 360-degree feedback raises the possibility that incidents may be observed and recorded by a number of different individuals in the organization.

Documentation of critical incidents need not be very lengthy, but it should be tied to an important performance dimension. An example of a critical incident for a mental health case manager is given on the next page. This incident illustrates the employee's creativity and negotiation skills, an important performance dimension.

FIGURE 10.2
Behavioral Observation Scale for a Patient Relations Representative

	Almost Never				Almost Always
1. Responds to patient or family concerns within 24 hours	1	2	3	4	5
2. Conducts investigations into complaints effectively	1	2	3	4	5
3. Communicates results of investigations to relevant parties	1	2	3	4	5
4. Follows up with patient or family after investigation	1	2	3	4	5
5. Identifies and analyzes both immediate and distant causes of patient complaints	1	2	3	4	5
6. Makes useful and practical recommendations for improvement based on results of investigation	1	2	3	4	5

In speaking with her client—an individual with severe mental disorder—the case manager discovered that the client was about to be evicted from her apartment for nonpayment of rent. She was able to work with the client and the landlord to work out a payment plan and to negotiate successfully with the landlord to have much-needed repairs in the apartment done. She followed up with the client weekly regarding payment to the landlord and the home repairs, and positive outcomes have been achieved in both areas.

Management by objectives (MBO) refers to a specific technique that has enjoyed substantial popularity. The basic premise of MBO is threefold: (1) the organization defines its strategic goals for the year, (2) these goals are then communicated throughout the organization, and (3) each employee in turn defines his or her goals for the year based on the organizational goals. Achievement of these goals becomes the standard by which each employee's performance is assessed (Carroll and Tosi 1973).

Management by Objectives

MBO has three key characteristics (Odiorne 1986):

1. It establishes specific and objectively measurable goals for employees.
2. It establishes goals in collaboration with employees.
3. It allows managers to provide objective feedback and coaching to improve employee performance.

As with most managerial practices, MBO is most effective when it is supported by and has the commitment of senior management. MBO requires managers to obtain substantial training in goal setting, giving feedback, and coaching. While goal setting is central to MBO, the process by which goals are set is of great importance as well.

Depending on the position of the jobholder, organizations may use a variety of results-oriented methods such as MBO. These approaches are most useful when the work yields objectively measurable outcomes. MBO is most commonly used for senior executives, for whom objectively measurable bottom-line concerns may be paramount; salespeople; and sports teams and individual athletes. The approach may be combined with other performance appraisal methods, particularly for jobs in which both the manner in which work is done and the outcomes are important and measurable.

The Cynicism About Performance Management

Many managers and employees are quite cynical about performance management. This cynicism grows out of a perception that aspects of performance management are distasteful and uncomfortable. Managers are often ill at ease about sitting down and discussing concerns with employees, and employees may resent the paternalism and condescension that often accompany such processes. This cynicism is clearly based in the reality that performance appraisals are traditionally punitive in nature and, particularly when tightly tied to employee compensation, have high emotional content.

Regardless of the type of data used in performance appraisal, what persists are "rating errors," as social psychologists call them. *Rating errors* refer simply to distortions in performance appraisal ratings—whether positive or negative—that reduce the accuracy of appraisals. The most common rating errors are as follows:

- *Distributional.* These errors come from the tendency of raters to use only a small part of the rating scale. They come in three forms:
  1. *Lenient:* Some raters tend to be overly generous with giving positive ratings and, as such, can avoid conflict and confrontation.
  2. *Strict:* Some raters tend to be overly critical of performance and, as such, are deemed unfair when compared with other raters without such a tendency.
  3. *Central:* Some raters tend to rate every employee as average and, as such, can avoid conflict and confrontation.
- *Halo effect.* These errors result from the propensity of some raters to rate employees high (or low) on all evaluation criteria, without distinguishing between different aspects of the employee's work. This leads to evaluations that may be overly critical or overly generous.
- *Personal bias.* These errors arise because of some raters' tendency to rate employees higher or lower than is deserved because of the rater's personal like or dislike of the employee (Wexley and Nemeroff 1974).
- *Similar-to-me bias.* These errors stem from the likelihood of some raters to judge those who are similar to them more highly than they would those who are not like them. Research shows that the strongest impact of similarity occurs when a manager and an employee share demographic characteristics, such as race and age group (Noe et al. 1996).
- *Contrast effect.* These errors are created when raters compare employees with each other rather than use objective standards for job performance.

The most important strategy for overcoming these rating errors is user training in different rating methods. Typically, training helps to increase managers' familiarity with various rating scales and the specific level of performance associated with different points on these scales. The ultimate objective of such training is to increase each manager's consistency in using rating scales and to improve interrater reliability among managers. As a result, error rates are minimized. At a minimum, managers need to be aware of potential rating errors in performance appraisal. Strategies may be offered to help managers both identify their errors and develop strategies to avoid making errors. For example, managers may avoid distributional errors by improving their awareness of the appraisal tool and their understanding of the objective standards used to evaluate performance. Of course, the success of training efforts is contingent on the existence of valid and reliable assessment instruments and clear performance standards.

The reality in organizational life is that, even with well-developed assessment tools and presumably effective management training programs, the process of performance appraisal is often tarnished not because of subtle or unconscious distortions but because of political pressures. Where political pressures are present, distortions are anything but unconscious. Political pressures may cause a manager to inflate, deflate, or completely avoid doing a performance review. One common source of political pressure is the reality that a manager will have to continue working with a particular employee. A mediocre or poor review (although realistic), then, may be perceived as a blemish in the employee–manager relationship and may upset the workplace climate and productivity. In such instances, a manager may inflate an appraisal to avoid the potential negative effects.

A manager may also artificially inflate an appraisal to permit awarding the employee a merit increase or other financial reward. While this destroys the intent of both the performance management and the compensation system, when faced with bread-and-butter issues, managers may choose to err on the side of generosity toward the employee. Managers may also inflate an appraisal to prevent an employee from having a written record of poor performance, to avoid a confrontation with an employee, or to reward an employee's improvement performance. Quoting a manager's observations about performance appraisal, Longenecker, Sims, and Gioia (1987) noted: "The mere fact that you have to write out your assessment and create a permanent record will cause people not to be as honest or as accurate as they should be. . . . We soften the language because our ratings go in the guy's file downstairs [the Personnel Department] and it will follow him around his whole career." As emphasized in this chapter, performance should be assessed using objective criteria. While improved performance may be recognized and discussed during a performance review session with an employee, it is important to stick with the criteria when assigning a rating to an employee's performance. Although somewhat rare, there are instances where a manager inflates an appraisal to enable an employee to be promoted "up and out" of the organization. This strategy obviously has highly questionable legal and ethical aspects. Finally, managers may sometimes give a break to an employee who is having personal problems.

Deflating an appraisal is also sometimes done to "shock" an employee into improving or to teach a rebellious employee a lesson. No evidence exists that such shock treatments are effective, but managers often use strategies with unproven effectiveness. Because careful documentation is usually required for employee termination, managers may also deflate an appraisal to speed up the termination process. Furthermore, providing an overly critical review could be viewed as a way of sending a message to an employee that he or she should think about leaving the organization. Table 10.3 summarizes these and other political

TABLE 10.3

Reasons Managers Inflate or Deflate a Performance Appraisal

Reasons to Inflate	Reasons to Deflate
Maximize merit increases for an employee, particularly when the merit ceiling is considered low	Shock an employee back on to a higher performance track
Avoid hanging dirty laundry out in public if the appraisal information is viewed by outsiders	Teach a rebellious employee a lesson
	Send a message to an employee that he or she should think about leaving the organization
Avoid creating a written record of poor performance that would become a permanent part of the individual's personnel file	Build a strongly documented record of poor performance that may speed up the termination process
Avoid confrontation with an employee with whom the manager recently had difficulties	
Give a break to a subordinate who had shown improvements	
Promote an undesirable employee "up and out" of the organization	

SOURCE: Adapted from Longenecker, Sims, and Gioia (1987)

distortions to the appraisal process. Altering the appraisal process for political purposes is not condoned here, but such tampering has occurred and it is important to recognize the potential for this behavior. An enduring aspect of performance appraisal systems is that implementation is often fraught with problems; as we design performance management systems and train managers in their use, we need to be cognizant of the many opportunities for abuse and misuse.

Conducting Effective Performance Management Interviews

As noted earlier, the ultimate objective of performance management is to improve employee performance. Because performance management has historically focused on the evaluation or measurement aspects, relatively little attention has been given to its improvement aspects.

A key step in the improvement process is to provide performance information to the employee. Many managers are reluctant to provide feedback because of fear of confrontation and conflict. These are real concerns for both managers and employees, given many employees' negative experiences with performance management. In informal surveys that we conduct with our students, we typically learn that the great majority of students either rarely have a performance evaluation or have had a poorly done evaluation. Finding a student who has had a well-implemented appraisal is relatively unusual for us.

The following are techniques for a valuable performance evaluation:

1. *Conduct an appraisal on an ongoing basis.* Checking on how an employee is performing should be a regular occurrence, not just done during the formal appraisal process. Giving continuous feedback is, after all, a key responsibility for managers. By providing ongoing feedback, surprises at the formal appraisal can be avoided.

2. *Evaluate the frequency of a formal performance appraisal.* The frequency of doing a formal appraisal varies to some degree on an employee's performance and longevity in the organization. For a high performer, an annual appraisal (as well as ongoing informal feedback) may be sufficient; such an assessment is usually done to reward good work, to reinforce existing levels of performance, and to discuss employee development and promotion possibilities. For an average performer, more frequent appraisals may be necessary to ensure that improvement goals are on track and will be achieved. For marginal or poor performers, formal appraisals may need to be held monthly (or perhaps more often) to provide an opportunity for closer coaching and, if necessary, disciplinary action.

3. *Prepare for the performance appraisal.* At the appraisal session, the manager should have a set of clear goals for the appraisal, be equipped with data, have a strategy for presenting performance information, be able to anticipate employee reactions, and be prepared to engage the employee in problem solving and planning. An appropriate physical location should be found, and relevant supporting information should be available as a reference.

4. *Use multiple sources of information.* Consistent with multirater or 360-degree appraisal, obtaining performance information from several sources is useful. This is particularly important in situations in which the manager is unable to adequately observe an employee's work, the job is highly complex, or the employee must interact with multiple individuals inside and outside the organization.

5. *Encourage employee participation.* Employee self-appraisal is commonly used as part of the appraisal process. The employee may have greater insight into his or her own performance concerns, and these are often consistent with the manager's assessment. An atmosphere should be created in which the appraisal is structured to benefit the employee, rather than be punitive. This positive environment may be difficult to create given many employees' negative perceptions of the performance appraisal process. Employee participation is also vital because the employee must assume accountability for improvement, and the first step

to being accountable is understanding what needs to be done and being involved in developing strategies toward that effort. Improvement should be viewed as a partnership between the manager and the employee.

6. *Focus on future performance and problem solving.* Reviewing past performance during an appraisal is important, but the emphasis of such a review should be on setting goals for the future and on generating specific strategies for meeting those goals. In many cases, the employee will identify factors outside of his or her control that may contribute to lower-than-expected levels of performance. These are certainly appropriate to discuss during an appraisal session. Follow-up sessions should also be scheduled as appropriate.

7. *Focus on employee behavior and results, not personal traits.* In almost all cases, the purpose of performance feedback is to help employees improve their work, not to change the person. The performance evaluation session is not the time to change an employee's values, personality, motivation, or fit with the organization. If these are true problems, they should have been considered during the selection process. The manager should focus on behaviors and outcomes, not the value of the person. Doling out condescending criticisms and reciting a litany of employee problems are rarely useful and are more likely to generate defensiveness and resentment from the employee.

8. *Reinforce positive performance.* Performance appraisal sessions have gained the reputation for being punitive and negative. One of the most effective ways that a manager can ally oneself with an employee is to ensure that the interview focuses on all aspects of performance, not just the negative. As in other areas of life, rewarding and reinforcing positive performance are essential aspects of productive human relationships.

9. *Ensure that performance management is supported by senior managers.* The best way to destroy any effort at implementing a performance management system is for word to get out that senior management is either unsupportive of or ambivalent about the process. Senior management must assert and communicate that performance management is important to meeting organizational goals and that it must be done at all levels of the workforce. If this message is absent or weak, the performance management system will either fade away or become a meaningless bureaucratic exercise.

10. *Plan follow-up activities and pay attention to expected outcomes and timetables.* Given the complex and hectic nature of organizations, it is easy to lose focus on the "important but not urgent" aspects of work. If plans are put into place, they should be accompanied by timetables, expectations, and concrete plans for follow-up. Without follow-up, the integrity of the performance management process is put into great jeopardy.

Summary

In the past several years, an important transition has taken place: Many organizations have moved from conducting performance appraisals to implementing performance management systems. Historically, performance appraisal focused primarily on judging employee behavior. The process was viewed as negative and punitive in nature and was generally avoided by both managers and employees. Performance management, however, implies an improvement-focused process in which efforts are made not only to assess performance but also to develop specific collaborative strategies to enhance performance. Recognizing that employee performance results from an employee's skills, motivation, and facilitative factors in the work environment, improvement strategies may include training, work process redesign, and other changes that are both internal and external to the employee.

An important aspect of performance management is the development of relevant appraisal criteria for the employee's position and the expectations of the organization. Appraisal data may be gathered through a variety of mechanisms, including self, subordinate, team members, and multisource or 360-degree feedback. Methods for organizing these data may involve a graphic rating scale, ranking, a behavioral anchored rating scale, a behavioral observation scale, a critical incidents record, and achievement of outcomes or objectives. The choice of approach is dependent on the job; the organizational goals; and, perhaps most important, the culture of the organization, particularly its readiness to confront performance issues honestly and openly.

Discussion Questions

1. What is the distinction between performance appraisal and performance management?
2. Why does the Joint Commission now require hospitals and other healthcare organizations to have a performance management system?
3. What is the relationship between performance management and continuous quality improvement?
4. What are the advantages and disadvantages to including discussions of compensation during a performance management interview?
5. What is the difference between performance appraisal rating errors and political factors that influence the accuracy of performance appraisal information?
6. How does a manager decide how often to conduct formal performance management interviews?
7. Why is employee participation in the performance management process important? Under what circumstances is employee participation not necessarily important?

Experiential Exercise

Case

Summit River Nursing Home (SRNH) is a 60-bed nursing home that serves a suburban community in the Midwest. The facility provides a broad range of services to residents, including recreational activities, clinical laboratory, dental services, dietary and housekeeping services, mental health and nursing services, occupational and physical therapies, pharmacy services, social services, and diagnostic x-ray services.

The facility has a good reputation in the community and is well staffed. Licensed practical nurses administer medications and perform certain treatment procedures. Each nursing home resident receives at least two hours of direct nursing care every day. Certified nursing assistants perform most of the direct patient care. A dietary service supervisor manages the daily operations of the food service department along with a registered dietitian. Activity coordinators provide non-medical care designed to improve cognitive and physical capabilities. Two social workers on staff work with residents, families, and other organizations, and an important part of their role is to ease residents and their families' adjustment to the long-term-care environment. They also help to identify residents' specific medical and emotional needs and provide support and referral services. Environmental service workers maintain the facility with a goal of providing a clean and safe facility for the residents. Housekeeping staff also have considerable contact with residents on a day-to-day basis. SRNH has contractual relationships with a dental practice, physical therapists, a pharmacist, a psychologist, and a multispecialty physician practice.

The management team at SRNH consists of an administrator, a finance director, a human resources director, a director of nursing, and administrative support personnel. Recently, concerns about quality have emerged at the nursing home. Several instances of communication breakdown among staff have occurred, and several instances of medication error have also taken place. A resident satisfaction survey also revealed problems, of which management had been unaware. Some of the problems concern contract staff who have not been included in the organization's performance management process.

After discussions with management and employees, it was established that a team atmosphere among staff was lacking. Each member of the management team was asked to develop a strategy to improve the level of teamwork in the facility. The human resources director agreed to take action in three areas:

1. Ensure that all job descriptions addressed teamwork and that these changes are discussed with employees.
2. Develop and implement a team-building training program for all employees, including contract staff.
3. Revise the performance management approach so that it focuses on teamwork as well as individual skills and accomplishments.

The first two strategies were relatively easy to complete. Job descriptions were revised, and supervisors met with employees to discuss these changes. With the assistance of an outside consultant, a training program was implemented to teach employees communication and conflict management skills. Several, but not all, contract employees attended the training program.

The third strategy raised some difficulties. The current performance management system is traditional, using a 12-item graphic rating scale (some with behavioral descriptions) that measures aspects of work such as attitude, quality of performance, productivity, attention to detail, job knowledge, reliability, and availability. The form also provides room for comments by both supervisors and employees. This rating approach, however, was found to be incapable of addressing the team components of the jobs. An additional problem is that several staff members are on contract and are not fully integrated into the organization. These staff members currently do not go through the organization's performance management process.

The human resources director wants to modify the performance management process so that it includes not only the methods to assess and improve team performance but also the contract employees.

Case Exercise

You are a consultant to the human resources director. Your job is to develop a method by which teamwork may be assessed in the performance management process.

1. How would you proceed with the task of modifying the performance management process?
2. What specific strategies do you think should be considered?
3. What obstacles do you see in implementing your approach? How would you overcome these problems?

References

Baldrige National Quality Program. 2007. *Health Care Criteria for Performance Excellence*. Gaithersburg, MD: Baldrige National Quality Program.

Barrett, R. S. 1995. "Employee Selection with the Performance Priority Survey." *Personnel Psychology* 48 (3): 653–62.

Bates, S. 2003. "Forced Rankling." *HR Magazine* 48 (6): 62–68.

Carroll, S., and H. Tosi. 1973. *Management by Objectives*. New York: Macmillan.

Cascui, W. F. 1991. *Applied Psychology in Personnel Management*. Reston, VA: Reston Press.

Fisher, C. D., L. F. Schoenfeldt, and J. B. Shaw. 2003. *Human Resource Management*, 5th Edition. Boston: Houghton Mifflin.

Joint Commission. 2007. *2008 Comprehensive Accreditation Manual for Hospitals*. Oakbrook Terrace, IL: Joint Commission.

Longenecker, C. O., and D. Gioia. 1992. "The Executive Appraisal Paradox." *Academy of Management Executive* 5 (2): 25–35.

Longenecker, C. O., H. P. Sims, and D. A. Gioia. 1987. "Behind the Mask: The Politics of Employee Appraisal." *Academy of Management Executive* 1 (3): 183–93.

Noe, R. A., J. R. Hollenbeck, B. Gerhart, and P. M. Wright. 1996. *Human Resource Management: Gaining a Competitive Advantage*, 2nd Ed. Boston: Irwin McGraw-Hill.

Novations Group. 2004. "Uncovering the Growing Disenchantment with Forced Management Performance Management Systems." White Paper. Boston: Novations Group.

Odiorne, G. 1986. *MBO II: A System of Managerial Leadership for the 80's*. Belmont, CA: Fearon Pitman Publishers.

Pfeffer, J., and R. I. Sutton. 2006. *Hard Facts, Dangerous Half-Truths, and Total Nonsense: Profiting from Evidence-Based Management.* Boston: Harvard Business School Press.

Sherman, A., G. Bohlander, and S. Snell. 1998. *Managing Human Resources,* 11th Edition. Cincinnati, OH: South-Western College Publishing.

Welch, J., and J. A. Byrne. 2003. *Jack: Straight from the Gut.* New York: Warner Business Books.

Wexley, K., and W. Nemeroff. 1974. "Effects of Racial Prejudice, Race of Applicants, and Biographical Similarity on Interview Evaluations of Job Applicants." *Journal of Social and Behavioral Sciences* 20 (1): 66–78.

COMPENSATION PRACTICES, PLANNING, AND CHALLENGES

Howard L. Smith, PhD; Bruce J. Fried, PhD;

Derek van Amerongen, MD; and John D. Laughlin

Learning Objectives

After completing this chapter, the reader should be able to

- describe the purposes of compensation and compensation policy in healthcare organizations;
- distinguish between extrinsic reward and intrinsic reward and the value of each to employees;
- understand the concepts of balancing internal equity and external competitiveness in compensation;
- enumerate the objectives of job evaluation, and discuss the comparative merits of alternative approaches to job evaluation in healthcare settings;
- discuss alternative types of incentive plans;
- articulate the challenges and problems faced in designing and implementing pay-for-performance plans;
- see how different practice settings affect physician income and physician compensation strategies;
- define the conflicts that can arise within different compensation models; and
- have an idea of the future direction of physician compensation.

Introduction

People work for a variety of reasons, although they may not be able to articulate them. These motivators have been studied for many years. Findings from research and practice suggest that several factors lead to job satisfaction and performance, including interest in work, competent supervision, and personal reward. Although "money is not everything," it is a significant motivator and a frequent measure of the value an employer places on jobs and jobholders.

Employees assess their own value in terms of the amount of money they receive for their work and in terms of how their pay compares with that of others. The compensation that people receive also sends a powerful message to employees about what their organizations value. Employees are very focused on whether their compensation is comparable to the rates offered in the general market and the rates given to coworkers who perform the same job. A compensation system must be externally competitive and internally equitable to allow organizations to balance what they value with how they reward employees (Kaplan and Norton 1996).

Across all industries, a compensation system must accomplish several objectives:

- It must fairly reward individuals for labor performed and expertise applied.
- It must align incentives for workers with those for the organization.
- It should reduce or eliminate undesirable behavior—that is, practices that prevent the successful accomplishment of required tasks and achievement of objectives.
- It should be prepared for the evolution of a job or industry, particularly for those involved in a highly technical, complicated, and changing field (like healthcare).
- It should be comparable to or even exceed the compensation systems of similar organizations in the market to give the organization a competitive advantage. This goal is especially critical in healthcare.

Again, although compensation is not the only factor associated with attracting and retaining employees, it is unquestionably important.

Healthcare organizations have a supplementary set of objectives related to improving population health and the processes used to deliver health services. Ideally, the design of compensation systems in healthcare encourages providers to do things that improve health, such as prevention and health promotion activities and compliance with clinical guidelines. This is a primary basis of pay-for-performance plans. Compensation can also facilitate quality and process improvements, such as implementing electronic medical records and use of other appropriate e-tools (electronic tools).

As in many other sectors, in healthcare, compensation is a very significant human resources management (HRM) issue. The healthcare sector, however, presents complexities and nuances that often are not encountered in other service or manufacturing sectors. First, a substantial number of healthcare employees are professionals with advanced education and training who must obtain and maintain licensure. These employees' professional associations exert a strong influence over their compensation. Second, shortages of skilled professionals drive up salaries and wages, allowing healthcare professionals to enjoy both high mobility and lucrative compensation. In some instances, market forces drive up salaries and may create internal inequities and wage compression. Third, healthcare providers cannot always determine the price of services because of third-party payer reimbursement policies. Consequently, third-party payment confounds the need to meet rising wage and salary levels in the marketplace.

In sum, compensation always seems to be at the forefront of HRM in healthcare, requiring continuing vigilant attention from healthcare organizations and managers. Healthcare managers can better respond to this challenge by understanding the basics behind compensation planning and policymaking as well as the unique compensation needs of physicians and other healthcare providers.

This chapter reviews the strategic role of compensation, considers operational issues involved in determining individual compensation, discusses the need for healthcare organizations to establish a process for determining the monetary value of jobs, describes common forms of job evaluation, examines different types of incentive compensation, defines the challenges encountered in developing and implementing compensation plans, and analyzes compensation practices unique to physicians and other healthcare personnel.

The Strategic Role of Compensation Policy

Healthcare work is often extremely stressful. Those who work in the field are attracted by high pay levels commonly associated with high-stress occupations. However, a perception persists about people who work in the field: They do so primarily because of their intrinsic desire to help others. Evidence continues to confirm that nurses and physicians are attracted to their professions because of their altruistic nature (Kingma 2003) and desire to serve the public good, and many jobs in healthcare are intrinsically rewarding. Nevertheless, although most healthcare professionals are driven by the satisfaction they get from their work, they are also influenced to work for and stay with the organization by the financial rewards they receive for their efforts. A good compensation system is particularly important in an industry like healthcare in which professional shortages occur in a cycle, leaving organizations to compete with other providers for the limited supply of employees.

An employee's choice to stay or to leave is complex. Considerable inferential data on how and why this decision is made are documented in the literature (Bartol 1979; Capo 2001; O'Connor et al. 2002) and are discussed in Chapter 8. However, reliably predictive models of employee behavior are elusive. Staff members cite factors such as compensation, match of personal

FIGURE 11.1

Research
Finding:
Professional
Support, Not
Compensation,
Is More
Valuable to
Nurse
Retention

William M. Mercer, one of the world's largest human resources consulting firms, conducted a study with healthcare executives from 185 organizations (93 percent of which were hospitals) to determine factors that contribute to nursing shortages. Their opinions are as follows:

- 30 percent of respondents said RN turnover is a "significant problem."

- 63 percent said RN turnover is "somewhat of a problem."

- 7 percent said RN turnover is not a problem.

- The biggest reason given for turnover problems is "increased market demand."

The results echo the argument that retention of good nurses depends on factors other than compensation: Hospitals that retain more nurses ". . . have fewer patients in their workload, better support services, greater control over their practices, greater participation in policy decisions, and more powerful chief nurse executives. In addition, they [nurses] were less apt to burn out and twice as likely to rate their hospitals as providing excellent care." Although compensation is very important to every person, in healthcare delivery settings professional support is an even more important consideration in people's decision to stay.

SOURCE: Egger (2000)

needs, wants, and expectations from the internal job environment versus external opportunities, job elements (e.g., responsibilities, goals, activities, tasks), organizational culture, and organizational structure as motivators. (See Chapter 8 for a range of factors associated with retention.) Figure 11.1 highlights the main findings of such a study.

In light of studies that confirm the importance but not the criticality of money in healthcare employees' decision to remain with their employers, organizations should develop a compensation policy that aims to enhance other employee motivators. In addition, this policy should align employees' efforts with the objectives, philosophies, and culture of the organization, highlighting and rewarding employees' contributions when organizational goals are achieved. A strategic compensation policy that balances individual needs with organizational interests typically includes the following goals:

- Rewards employee performance
- Achieves internal equity within the organization
- Maintains external competitiveness in relevant labor markets
- Aligns employee behavior and performance with organizational goals
- Attracts and retains high-performing employees

- Maintains the compensation budget within organizational financial constraints
- Complies with legal requirements

The strategic contribution of compensation is apparent in these goals. Compensation directly affects an organization's ability to achieve its fundamental mission and strategic objectives, to maintain fiscal integrity while delivering high-quality services, and to ensure customer satisfaction.

Compensation Decisions and Dilemmas

Strategic compensation goals may come into conflict in certain situations. For example, higher compensation offered to attract certain types of employees can disrupt internal equity. Recruiting physical therapists is a case in point. Physical therapists are in short supply in many parts of the United States; therefore, offering compensation packages that are inconsistent with existing pay rates in the organization may be necessary. The discrepancy between an employee's worth (relative to other employees in the organization) and the amount that employee is paid is often determined by the market. This conflict between the goal of internal equity and external competitiveness is one of the major challenges in establishing an enlightened compensation policy, a conflict that is particularly acute in healthcare because of periodic shortages of professionals. In certain communities where competition for employees is very acute, organizations monitor compensation trends carefully (often on a weekly basis) for key professional groups.

Organizations must make a number of other decisions when developing a compensation policy, which in turn may affect the goals and architecture of their current compensation programs. First, a determination must be made on whether to pay above, below, or at prevailing rates; this decision may be made explicitly or implicitly. Typically, organizations earn a reputation for the amount they pay employees. Second, the types of employee performance, practice, or contribution that are rewarded must be identified. This decision may seem trivial, but the factors chosen to be rewarded usually signal what the organization values. For example, annual raises that are not explicitly tied to performance tend to reward longevity and seniority in an organization, rather than performance. Rewarding longevity seems to contradict the general movement toward a pay-for-performance culture. On the other hand, retaining employees may be as important a goal as providing incentives for high performance. Retention bonuses in fact aim to encourage longevity in the organization.

The trend toward paying for performance is now well established in healthcare. The idea behind a *pay-for-performance system* is not only to compensate employees for their contributions but also to encourage good performance for the sake of maintaining and attracting high-level service reimbursements for the organization. This system is being enacted in the hospital sector and is seriously discussed in seminars and formal education programs. One of the criticisms of organizational "reimbursement" for performance is that payers are possibly rewarding high levels of performance that are attributable more to environmental circumstances rather than to specific strategies undertaken by the organization to motivate high performance. Managers in poorly performing hospitals argue that punishing poorly performing organizations only reinforces historical inequities that may have caused differences in performance in the first place. It is well accepted that organizational performance is affected by factors outside of the institution's control, such as being located in a community with high numbers of uninsured people. The dilemmas that plague organization-level pay for performance parallel those for incentive schemes for employees.

Among the first decisions necessary in designing a pay-for-performance system is establishing the performance criteria to be used in determining compensation. While criteria associated with productivity-oriented pay-for-performance policies are generally established internally, increasingly third-party payers are establishing pay-for-performance programs that tie financial incentives to meeting quality- or outcome-oriented goals using externally established criteria. These sometimes competing criteria can result in unanticipated consequences when certain aspects of performance are rewarded. For example, when excessive emphasis is placed on fiscal concerns, especially cost containment, an imbalance can result in other critical outcomes such as quality, access, and consumer satisfaction. Managers must therefore be especially vigilant about the causal relationship between compensation and outcomes. Careful attention is necessary when defining performance criteria, and caution is also critical when establishing prudent measures and data collection. Additionally, managers must extrapolate from intended policy to desired results and must anticipate dysfunctions associated with policy.

Other concerns are inherent when designing, improving, and implementing compensation programs:

1. The worth of individual jobs must be determined.
2. The value that an employee's education and experience contribute to the position must be assessed.
3. Guidelines on keeping salaries and incentives confidential to the recipient and managers must be formulated and communicated to all concerned.

The point here is sobering: Developing and improving employee compensation policies and practices is a never-ending challenge. Changes in the marketplace, trends within the healthcare professions, redirection of organizational goals and objectives, and other factors suggest that compensation policies and plans are seldom, if ever, stable, reinforcing the fact that compensation is a critical strategic issue in organizations.

Intrinsic Versus Extrinsic Rewards

Compensation should be considered in the context of the overall reward structure of an organization. Rewards can be intrinsic (internal) or extrinsic (external). *Intrinsic compensation* is intangible and may include recognition such as praise from a supervisor for completing an assignment; for meeting established performance objectives; or for having feelings of accomplishment, recognition, or belonging to an organization. *Extrinsic compensation* is tangible (and viewing compensation from a "total compensation" perspective is important) and includes direct monetary compensation (i.e., wages, salaries), benefits, payment for time not worked (e.g., vacation pay), and stock options. In today's environment, potential job applicants are extremely sensitive to the benefit structure offered, in particular health insurance. From the organization's perspective, the cost of indirect compensation is not trivial: As discussed in Chapter 12, the average cost of benefits in healthcare organizations can range between 20 percent to 35 percent of salaries.

Determining which type of reward drives each employee is difficult because in most instances employees are motivated by a combination of intrinsic and extrinsic rewards. In one early approach to defining reward systems and understanding motivation, Herzberg, Mausner, and Snyderman (1959) suggested that employees first must have their basic "hygiene" needs met. Fulfillment of these needs does not produce employee motivation or job satisfaction but is a precondition that ushers in motivation. Thus, extrinsic rewards (most notably remuneration and satisfactory working conditions) are necessary but are insufficient elements for encouraging employees to contribute and subsequently feel a sense of accomplishment. The presence of extrinsic factors may prevent dissatisfaction but does not necessarily lead to satisfaction. This perspective is similar to Maslow's (1970) view that individuals must have their basic needs (biological and safety) met before they are able to achieve high esteem and fulfillment goals that are usually associated with high levels of performance. Managers, therefore, need to be cognizant of these two types of rewards and understand their functions and limitations.

The distinction between intrinsic and extrinsic rewards has substantial implications for managing healthcare professionals and support staff. It is not enough for managers to simply devise a well-orchestrated plan for compensation because pay in and of itself is only part of a complex equation that affects employee satisfaction. Managers must also attend to rewards that may not require fiscal resources. Encouraging employees, establishing a collegial practice environment, consistent setting of performance objectives, and conducting periodic performance assessments are all strategies whose costs tend to be measured more in terms of time and commitment than in terms of direct money expenditures. Assuming a prudent span of management, these are strategies that fiscally challenged healthcare providers can pursue in establishing a fertile

FIGURE 11.2

Balancing Intrinsic and Extrinsic Rewards in Academic Medical Settings

Academic physicians have traditionally been drawn to universities because of opportunities to combine education and research with clinical care. Fiscally strapped academic medical centers and schools of medicine have progressively asked faculty to provide more clinical service as a means to raise revenue. So-called revenue-based compensation (RBC) pays academic physicians according to the clinical revenue they generate, thereby raising faculty members' income as well as that of the medical center and rewarding physicians who generate high revenue.

Richard Gunderman (2004) of the School of Medicine at Indiana University argues that RBC is insidious as far as the intrinsic rewards of academic medicine are concerned. He underscores that RBC can distract faculty members and encourage them to focus on remuneration, eroding their commitment and loyalty to the academic mission. Specifically, there is potential erosion under RBC in the following intrinsic rewards:

1. Institutional prestige

2. Intellectual discourse

3. Opportunities for collaboration

4. Quality of intellectual discourse

5. Infrastructure

The end result is greater potential for faculty to migrate out of academic medicine.

The solution? Gunderman suggests that RBC plans should define revenue in measurable and objective terms, that expectations should be transparent, and that compensation plans should promote the mission of the medical school and the academic departments. These strategies will ensure that compensation is balanced with intrinsic aspects of the academic role.

reward environment. See Figure 11.2 for an example of balancing intrinsic and extrinsic rewards for academic physicians.

Low- or no-cost rewards are particularly of interest to nonprofit and financially stressed healthcare organizations with adverse budgets. In these circumstances, managers should be especially mindful of the potential for using intrinsic rewards to supplement limited extrinsic rewards. This is a delicate balancing point that eventually may result in employees perceiving that their salaries are not comparable to the compensation given in competing organizations. How much imbalance staff members will tolerate is never certain. It behooves fiscally challenged organizations to pursue intrinsic rewards to the greatest extent possible to minimize turnover and its associated costs.

Internal Equity and External Competitiveness

Every organization must maintain a balance between internal equity and external competitiveness in its reward system. Equity theory (Homans 1961;

Adams 1963) is a useful and well-tested framework for understanding the impact of perceived equity and inequity on individual motivation and performance. *Equity* is the perceived fairness of the relationship between what a person contributes to an organization (inputs) and what that person receives in return (outcomes). *Inputs* refer to such things as an individual's education, seniority, skills, effort, loyalty, and experience. *Outcomes* include pay, benefits, job satisfaction, opportunities for growth, and recognition.

According to equity theory, employees calculate the ratio, or balance, between their outcomes and inputs. They then compare their own ratio to the ratio of other people ("referent others") in their organization or another organization. Particularly where professionals are concerned, comparisons may be made to people who hold similar jobs in other organizations. For example, an operating room nurse in a hospital will likely compare his or her ratio with the ratio of other operating room nurses in the same hospital, with other nurses performing different tasks, with other types of staff members (to determine the comparability of their outcomes in relation to their inputs), and with nurses who perform similar work in other organizations. The result of this comparison is a belief by the employee that he or she is either being treated equitably or inequitably. Feelings of inequity create discomfort, and people naturally seek to restore a sense of equity or leave the organization (or field) for a more equitable situation.

Perceived inequity comes in two types. *Overpayment inequity* is a person's belief that his or her ratio is greater than that of the referent. Depending on the person's predisposition, overpayment inequity may lead to feelings of guilt, which can result in efforts to restore equity such as putting in greater effort. The more common phenomenon of *underpayment inequity* is a perception that occurs when an employee finds that his or her ratio is smaller than the referent's. In such a situation, an employee is likely to attempt to restore a sense of equity either by decreasing inputs or by increasing outcomes received from work. With a perception of underpayment, employee motivation, morale, and performance are likely to decline.

This comparing feature of equity theory is pervasive in all organizations. Consider, for example, the interest generated when the salaries of senior executives in *Fortune* 500 firms are publicized in the media. Of course, the comparative judgments made by employees may be highly subjective and based on limited or inaccurate information. Regardless of how subjective we think these assessments are, managers must contend with these perceptions because they affect motivation and performance. Managers must be attentive not only to *their own perception* of the fairness of the reward system but also to *employee perceptions* of the fairness or equity of rewards. Perceptions, rather than reality, often affect motivation and behavior.

Healthcare managers face a substantial challenge in addressing pay equity. Salaries and wages in most of the healthcare professions are common knowledge, as they are widely communicated for recruitment purposes. Consequently, some staff will allude to these differentials as a strategy to seek higher compensation. In addition to demonstrating great patience, managers can emphasize and develop the intrinsic rewards offered by their organization. This may help to defuse that differential and encourage staff to focus on the bigger picture, an approach that is especially appropriate to the professions.

Equity issues are particularly troublesome because of shortages in certain healthcare professions. Newly graduated nurses, for example, may be hired at a salary level that approaches the compensation of well-seasoned and experienced nurses. While the experienced employee may have a cognitive understanding of the market-based reasons for this inequity, the impact of this inequity is likely to remain. Such an employee is faced with several choices: accept the situation, seek additional compensation, change jobs within the organization, take on additional responsibilities, or move to another organization to achieve the financial benefits of being newly hired. In some markets, job hopping is a tried-and-true method of increasing one's compensation.

As mentioned earlier, employees who perceive inequity may attempt to equalize the situation in two ways: (1) increase their outcomes or (2) decrease their inputs. The first way can be accomplished by working harder, and perhaps as a result, the employee will obtain additional compensation or a promotion (note that working harder may also increase the inputs side of the ratio); by organizing other employees, possibly in the form of unionization; and by engaging in illegal activities, such as theft or false reporting of hours worked. The second approach, decreasing inputs, can be done through working fewer hours (e.g., coming in late, leaving early, being absent) and putting forth less effort. Employees may also attempt to restore a sense of equity by changing their perceptions of the inputs or outcomes of others. For example, an employee may convince herself that the referent employee has more experience and is therefore entitled to a higher level of rewards. Similarly, an employee may conclude that while his salary may be lower than that of a referent, working conditions are much better at his organization than at the other organization. In other instances, employees may simply change their frame of reference—that is, they may change the person with whom they compare themselves.

While organizations seek to ensure internal equity, they must also pursue external competitiveness to recruit staff. To be externally competitive, organizations must provide compensation that is perceived to be equitable to the salary given to employees who perform similar jobs in other organizations. If an organization is not externally competitive, it is likely to face problems of turnover and staff shortages, particularly in geographic areas where the supply of certain professionals may be scarce. Healthcare employers have traditionally faced tight labor markets for physicians, nurses, and medical technicians, which lead to the difficulty in attracting and retaining these and other clinical providers. This competition results in an ascending spiral of wages, salaries, benefits, and other forms of compensation that the market cannot afford and that inflates organizational cost structures and eats away at margins. In such a situation, emphasizing intrinsic rewards or intangible incentives can contribute to attracting and retaining high-quality staff.

When confronting a tight labor market, organizations should formulate specific strategies to position themselves in the labor market. As far as pay is concerned, these positioning strategies typically follow a quartile strategy. Most employers seek to position themselves in the second quartile (the middle of the market) or higher, a position that is preferred by other employers according to survey data. By choosing this position, organizations can balance employer cost pressures with the need to attract and retain employees. An employer that uses a first-quartile strategy, on the other hand, is choosing to pay below-market compensation. Employers take this position for several reasons. First, shortage of funds or an inability to pay more may converge with the need to continue to meet strategic organizational objectives. Second, if a large number of applicants with lower skills are available in the labor market, this strategy can be used to attract sufficient workers at a lower cost. A major disadvantage of using a first-quartile strategy is high turnover, and, if the labor supply tightens, the organization may have difficulty attracting and retaining workers. Quality-of-care ramifications in nursing homes that operate in the lower quartile are illustrated in Figure 11.3.

FIGURE 11.3
Quality-of-Care Ramifications of a Low-Quartile Position

Mohr and colleagues (2004) studied nursing homes in the lowest tier—that is, facilities that house mainly (>85 percent) Medicaid residents. They note that nursing homes with high proportions of Medicaid patients have correspondingly fewer resources to hire staff and that poor, frail, and minority residents in these facilities tend to receive substandard care. In particular, their analyses suggest that staffing intensity is statistically lower in Medicaid-dominated nursing homes. Fewer registered nurses are found on staff in lower-tier nursing homes, but not fewer licensed practical nurses. This led the authors to conclude that less-expensive and less-qualified staff are used as substitutes for higher-trained staff by fiscally constrained Medicaid facilities. Physician extenders and administrators are also less prevalent in lower-tier nursing homes.

Quality of care indicators suffer in lower tier nursing homes, according to the study. Medicaid-dominated facilities report higher incidences of pressure ulcers, higher use of physical restraints, and higher use of antipsychotic medications. Clearly, poor quality of care is associated with restricted use of registered nurses as well as limited administrative resources and physician extenders. Mohr and colleagues acknowledge that lower staffing intensity is accompanied by fewer resources to hire and train clinical and administrative staff. In sum, economic constraints lead to higher turnover, lower retention, and ultimately lower quality of care.

A third-quartile strategy, in which employees are paid at above market value, is more aggressive. This strategy may be used to ensure that a sufficient number of employees with the required capabilities are attracted and retained; it also allows an organization to be more selective. However, the expectation in most organizations is that those employees who are paid above-market rates must be more productive and must deliver higher-quality services and products.

Determining the Monetary Value of Jobs

Job evaluation is a formal process for determining the value of jobs in monetary terms. Development and maintenance of an intelligent wage-and-salary system begin with accurate job descriptions and job specifications for each position. This information is used to perform a job evaluation and to conduct pay surveys. These activities ensure that a pay system is both internally equitable and externally competitive. Data gathered in the job evaluation process and pay surveys are used to design, or improve, pay structures, including pay grades and pay ranges.

In theory, job evaluation is used to obtain an objective assessment of a job's worth or contribution to the organization. This level of contribution is then translated into monetary terms. After this monetary value is determined, compensation levels may be adjusted to better reflect market compensation levels. However, in tight labor markets, the use of job evaluation information for setting compensation levels may be of limited use. In certain types of jobs, information from wage and salary surveys may be the dominant or sole method used to set compensation levels. Periodic job evaluations may be conducted, but over extended periods (often, several years), salary decisions may be made almost exclusively on market information. Our discussion, therefore, needs to be placed in the context of volatile and unpredictable labor markets.

In a job evaluation, a job is examined and ultimately priced according to each job's relative importance to an organization; the knowledge, skills, and abilities each job requires; and the difficulty of each job. The premise of a job evaluation is that jobs that require greater qualifications, that involve more responsibility, and that assign more complex duties should pay more than jobs with lower requirements or lesser tasks (Martocchio 2001). Job evaluation is also a way of ensuring that employees perceive equity in the compensation system. To motivate staff, a fair pay value must be assigned to each job.

When conducting a job evaluation, benchmark jobs are identified. These benchmarks require similar knowledge, skills, and abilities and are performed by individuals who have been assigned relatively similar duties. Benchmark jobs are used to establish a basis on which other comparable jobs are evaluated.

Methods of Evaluating Job Value

Perhaps the simplest job value assessment technique, the ranking method lists jobs in order of their inherent value to an organization. The entire job, rather than individual components of the job, is considered. Those who rank jobs use their judgment when ranking, and consequently this method is extremely susceptible to subjectivity. Managers may have difficulty explaining why one specific position is ranked higher than another. Additionally, this method is very cumbersome to do in large organizations because of the sizeable number of jobs in such institutions.

Ranking

Job classification systems categorize jobs based on predetermined require-ments. This approach is most common in the public sector, where jobs are classified according to the federal government's General Schedule (GS) of 18 grades. In the GS system, each job is classified into one of these 18 grades based on knowledge requirements, responsibilities, physical effort, and work-ing conditions. Each grade is associated with a salary range, which varies by geographic location. Similar to ranking, job classification is subject to consid-erable subjectivity and is vulnerable to manipulation. Jobs can be misclassified, or perceived as misclassified, because of assumptions made by the job analyst. Job classification is problematic when applied to multisystem organizations because two jobs with the same title may entail very different responsibilities in different settings. For example, a registered nurse in a skilled nursing facil-ity performs roles that are substantially different from those performed by a registered nurse in an outpatient surgery center.

Job Classification

Job classification systems assign jobs to categories known as pay bands. The *broadbanding* approach to compensation is a response to the constraints im-posed by rigid classification systems in which an employee's maximum com-pensation is limited by a very narrow salary band. Traditional classification sys-tems have very narrow ranges of pay for a job classified in a particular category. If we wish to provide additional compensation to an employee who assumes new responsibilities or learns new skills, traditional classification systems pro-vide little flexibility in how this person is compensated; promotion to a new position and reclassifying the position are the main options. Broadbanding in-volves enlarging these pay bands for jobs in such a way that the compensation for a particular job has more flexibility.

Broadbanding

A broadband is a single, large salary range that spans pay opportunities formerly covered by several separate small salary ranges. Numerous jobs and salary levels can be included within a single broadband. A major advantage of broadbanding is that it provides more flexibility when managing an em-ployee's compensation within a particular pay range. Levels of compensation can be changed without the necessity of changing job titles or reclassifying jobs. Individuals can be moved between jobs without concern for dramatic changes in salary. For example, an employee may be reluctant to move into another position because of the possibility of a salary decrease. With broadbanding, both jobs may be in the same salary range, allowing for stability in salary. Employees can also be more easily rewarded within a broad pay grade for taking on new responsibilities or obtaining new skills. For the employee, career growth can be thought of in terms of increased responsibilities rather than promotion (Wagner and Jones 1994).

Broadbanding is becoming a more popular approach to valuing jobs. A recent survey found that about one-quarter of all employers use some type of broadbanding scheme (Mercer Human Resource Consulting 2006). In fact, a growing number of institutions are looking for alternative pay structures to fit new organizational structures driven by competitive environments. Broadbanding is especially appropriate because it is consistent with trends toward flatter, less hierarchical organizations and the use of cross-functional job positions. Cross-functional positions enable organizations to respond quickly to competitive pressures. With broadbanding, employees can more easily shift responsibilities as market and organizational requirements change.

Broadbanding offers other advantages. First, it enables companies to base compensation decisions on characteristics of people who perform jobs rather than on characteristics of the job alone. Second, authority for compensation decisions is largely decentralized to operating managers. Therefore, managers find it easier to gain approval for changes in compensation because broadbanding enables them to reward employees without going through myriad justifications required in a traditional classification system. Additionally, the wider spread between pay grades gives managers more flexibility to recognize and reward different levels of individual contribution. Third, because broadbanding results in fewer pay groupings, job evaluation is potentially simpler because organizations no longer need complex job evaluation schemes. Managers can encourage employees to move into other job areas that may broaden knowledge, skills, and abilities. Finally, broadbanding allows employees to evaluate their own skill acquisition and cross-training opportunities in terms of professional development and personal growth, rather than focus on pay grades.

Broadbanding, however, is not appropriate for every organization and organizational culture. The narrow range of the traditional pay system may serve as an automatic cost-control mechanism that keeps compensation expenses in check. With broadbanding, all employees may potentially float to the maximum pay level within their band, resulting in higher-than-market compensation for many or most employees. New employees who replace those with seniority may discover that they are paid at significantly lower levels, an artifact of time on the job of their more senior counterparts. However, such an explanation may provide little solace. Perceptions of inequity may become an irritant and may lower morale.

The most difficult aspect of implementing broadbanding is helping employees to think differently about how they are paid. Pay grades have long been used to determine status, titles, and eligibility for perquisites. Consequently, employees sometimes have difficulty relinquishing these preconceptions. Broadbanding also implies fewer upward promotion opportunities. With a smaller number of bands, employees recognize that promotions to a higher grade level will occur less frequently than before. Employees must assume significantly greater job responsibilities to warrant placement in a higher band.

The *point* method is the most widely used job valuation tool. A basic assumption behind this method is that organizations do not pay for jobs but for specific aspects of these jobs, known as compensable factors. Examples of compensable factors include knowledge and skill requirements, job experience, accountability, supervisory responsibilities, and working conditions. These compensable factors are determined through job analysis and are then assigned values or weights—points—based on the extent to which each factor is present. Compensation levels and pay ranges are then linked to these points, although actual compensation for a particular job may vary based on market and other factors.

Point

The point method is popular because it is relatively simple, is based on job analysis, may be used for many jobs, and once established is relatively easy to update. However, this method does have several drawbacks, including the amount of time needed to develop the system and the tendency to reinforce traditional organizational structures and job rigidity. Furthermore, as discussed earlier, compensation levels for particular jobs may be based more on salary survey data than on the results of job evaluation. Often, very significant differences exist between compensation levels derived from job evaluation and compensation levels according to market pay rates.

The following are necessary in developing a point system (Hills, Bergmann, and Scarpello 1994):

- Compensable factors must be acceptable to all parties.
- Compensable factors must validly distinguish among jobs.
- Compensable factors must be relevant to the jobs under analysis.
- Jobs must vary on the compensable factors selected so that meaningful differences in jobs can be identified.
- Compensable factors must be measurable.
- Compensable factors must be independent of each other.
- Job evaluation and market pay rates must be reconciled.

The *factor comparison* method is a combination of the ranking and point methods. It differs from point systems in that compensable factors for a job are evaluated against compensable factors in benchmark jobs in the organization.

Factor Comparison

Benchmark jobs are important to employees and the organization, vary in their requirements, have relatively stable content, and are used in salary surveys for wage determination.

Benchmark jobs are typically evaluated against a set of compensable factors, such as skill, mental effort, physical effort, responsibilities, and working conditions. A pay rate is assigned to each compensable factor for each benchmark job. For example, the job of an emergency room (ER) nurse may be identified as a benchmark job. Analysis determines that of the $17 hourly wage paid to an ER nurse, $5 is paid for mental effort, $3 for responsibility, and so forth. Similarly, we may use a hospital medical technologist's job as a benchmark, and we may decide that of the $15 hourly wage paid to this individual, $4 is paid for mental effort, $2.50 for responsibility, and so forth. A factor comparison scale is developed to evaluate other jobs in the organization. Thus, if we are attempting to evaluate the job of an occupational therapist, the mental effort, skill, and other factors of that job are compared to that of the ER nurse and the medical technologist.

Key advantages of the factor comparison approach are that it can be tailored to one organization and it indicates which jobs are worth more and how much more, making factor values more easily converted into monetary wages. Disadvantages of this method include complexity, time required to establish comparable factors, and difficulty explaining the methodology to employees.

Market Pricing

The approaches to valuing jobs discussed in this section focus almost exclusively on ensuring equity within the workplace. However, clearly, the compensation that an organization, particularly in healthcare, offers is often heavily dependent on labor supply and market wages. We learn about market wages largely from salary surveys carried out by organizations, the government, associations, and external consulting firms. Annual surveys are conducted by the Bureau of Labor Statistics on area and industry wages as well as surveys of professional, administrative, technical, and clerical positions. Private consulting firms that conduct salary surveys include The Hay Group, Heidrick & Struggles International, Inc., and Hewitt Associates. The Society for Human Resource Management and Financial Executives International also conduct wage surveys. In the healthcare sector, the American Hospital Association conducts a series of annual wage and salary surveys. The Internet may also be used to obtain market salary information; see, for example, http://salary.com, a website that provides market information for a variety of jobs across various industries.

Limitations of market pricing of jobs include questionable methodologies that may be used to obtain salary information. Relying on the market to set compensation can also lead to wide variations and fluctuations in salary as shortages ebb and flow. Furthermore, using job titles to inform compensation rates may not take into consideration the wide differences in actual job responsibilities across organizations, resulting in misleading information about appropriate salary levels (Fay and Tare 2007).

Variable Compensation

Team-Based Incentive

Healthcare providers increasingly structure service delivery around work teams, causing human resources managers to consider compensation systems that reward team performance. Team-based rewards can be used to boost productivity and performance, improve quality and customer service, and increase retention. Unfortunately, the actual development of team-based compensation systems is often constrained by the need to reward individual performance. Among the challenges faced in team-based incentive compensation is whether to provide the same-size reward for each member or variable-size rewards for different members depending on such factors as contribution, seniority, and skill levels.

For example, a care delivery team made up of an obstetrician, a case manager, a social worker, and a nurse's aide may be rewarded for a productivity outcome of delivering more infants, experiencing minimal adverse cases, and receiving high patient satisfaction. What level of reward should be assigned to the team? What percentage of the respective base salaries of each team member will the reward constitute? Will inequities in rewards cause some team members to work less in achieving team objectives? These are representative questions that must be addressed before implementing a team-based compensation system.

Healthcare organizations that are interested in rewarding team performance need to strike a balance between individual rewards and team rewards. Paying the same amount to everyone on the team regardless of a team member's competencies or contributions may create pay-equity problems. Team incentives are most commonly incorporated as variable pay—that is, a team-based incentive is added to base pay. While base pay is determined by job evaluation and market information, variable pay is added according to team performance.

Skills-Based or Competency-Based Pay

In skills-based compensation systems, employees are paid according to work-related skills and competencies. Typically, the employees begin at a base pay level and are given the opportunity to increase their compensation by acquiring new skills, knowledge, or competencies, thereby making themselves more valuable to the organization (Baca and Starzmann 2006). The reward structure of this approach is based on the range, depth, and types of skills that individual employees possess. Compensation is increased after an employee demonstrates the ability to perform specific, desired skills.

This compensation approach is based on the idea that employees with a broad range of skills allow the organization more flexibility in deploying its staff. Typically, an employee is hired and is provided training for that job. The employee may then join a work team and be given the opportunity to learn new skills through additional training and on-the-job experience. As the employee learns new jobs, his or her compensation is increased. This approach reinforces the concept of the autonomous work group, where members work interdependently.

Skills-based pay can follow a stair-step approach, in which a logical well-defined progression is followed in skills development. Pay is increased as skills are mastered. A job-point accrual model is used when there is a variety of jobs for which an employee may be trained. Jobs are given a point rating that is based on the difficulty of mastering job skills, and compensation is increased in accordance with points earned. A cross-department model is one in which employees may be trained to work in jobs in other parts of the organization, and compensation increases as the employee masters these jobs (Bunning 1992).

A challenge in skills-based pay is the need for appropriate training to facilitate skills acquisition, and, of course, the system needs to be adequately funded. Perhaps the most promising application of skills-based pay is linking the program with career ladder initiatives, particularly among nurses (see, for example, Schmidt, Nelson, and Godfrey 2003).

Pay for Performance

Pay-for-performance systems are built on the principles that good work deserves to be rewarded and that pay based on good work produces improved performance. In a pay-for-performance system, managers evaluate the work of their employees according to preestablished goals, standards, or company values. Based on this judgment, employees are given variable or contingent financial rewards. Individual compensation is directly linked to personal performance and attainment of objectives consistent with the organization's mission. This approach is intended to motivate employees to perform at the highest level regardless of their particular role or specialty (Grib and O'Donnell 1995). Pay-for-performance programs come in two types in healthcare.

Productivity-focused pay for performance seeks to maximize organizational profitability by tying financial incentives to individual employee productivity. In many settings, physicians are under pressure to meet production targets (Berkowitz 2002; Rost 2002), and pay-for-performance programs are used to align physician incentives with these targets. The common use of fee-for-service reimbursements has led to the widespread adoption of productivity-focused pay for performance, and numerous studies suggest that financial incentives do improve work quantity (Gupta and Shaw 1998). Currently, more than 70 percent of physicians in non-solo practice settings have at least some portion of their income tied to meeting productivity targets (Reschovsky and Hadley 2007). These programs may be structured in a variety of ways. *Piece-rate incentives* reward employees for each unit of output produced, whether this unit is a product or service. *Commissions* are most common in sales and are structured so that employees receive a percentage of their gross receipts. *Bonuses* are one-time financial rewards to recognize individual and/or organizational performance. Other incentive systems are based on encouraging team or organizational performance. *Profit-sharing plans* enable employees to share in the organization's profits, and *gain-sharing plans* allocate to employees a portion of the gains made by the organization as a result of increased efficiency or productivity. This sharing approach has manifested itself in a number of forms such as the Scanlon Plan, the Rucker Plan, and Improshare. Regardless of the program structure, with productivity-focused pay for performance, pay is tied to the accomplishment of goals that are established before the performance period for which the jobholder or employee will be evaluated. The focus is on specific actions that the person performed in pursuit of set goals; see Figure 11.4, for example.

The second type of pay for performance in healthcare is quality focused. Seeking to align physician or organization incentives with the delivery of high levels of care, *quality-focused pay for performance* is created by third-party payers. The use of this type has increased greatly since the late 1990s; however, it is still far less common than productivity-focused pay for performance (Reschovsky and Hadley 2007). Pay-for-quality programs reward activities and practices that are likely to improve healthcare outcomes, including increased prevention screenings, ensuring up-to-date patient vaccinations, investing in information technology designed to reduce medical errors, and consistently adhering to evidence-based medical guidelines. By improving outcomes, quality-focused pay-for-performance programs hope to produce healthier and more satisfied patients and ultimately reduce costs.

Implementing quality-focused pay for performance is complicated and can be expensive. Clearly, for such a program to be effective, the magnitude of the incentives must exceed the costs incurred in meeting the program's targets. These costs can be considerable and may include designing new procedures, training employees on their implementation, and collecting data on process and outcome measures necessary to support the program's reporting requirements. The latter often involves substantial investment in information technology development and support. Additionally, the cost of unreimbursed time that physicians, nurses, and other staff must spend with patients to implement new procedures or to carry out necessary administrative tasks must be considered. For this reason, hospitals and large practice settings with extensive management and information technology support are generally in a

FIGURE 11.4

Financial
Incentives for
Physician
Productivity

In 2002, Conrad and colleagues explored the relationship of financial incentives with physician productivity in 102 medical groups and 2,237 physicians in the Medical Group Management Association (MGMA). The sample is admittedly a very small proportion of MGMA's membership of 5,725 practices (there are 19,478 medical groups in the United States); however, the advantage of this study group is the valuable information it supplied on resource-based relative value scale units produced in 1997. Data were derived from MGMA's annual surveys—the Compensation and Production Survey and the Cost Survey.

The conceptual basis underlying this study relates back to a seminal analysis that Gaynor and Pauly (1990) completed on medical group partnerships. These researchers discovered that physician productivity is extremely sensitive to individual compensation. Tying compensation completely to productivity (i.e., productivity determines 100 percent of a physician's total salary) increased productivity by 28 percent. In practical terms, physicians respond very favorably to incentive-based compensation.

Conrad and colleagues' findings reaffirm those of Gaynor and Pauly. Physicians for the medical groups that base pay on individual performance are more productive than individual physicians. Moreover, the results suggest that bonuses heighten the productivity effect. The individual characteristics of the physicians also play a role in responses to incentives, according to further in-depth study. Physician experience is associated with modest increases in productivity. Gender appears to have some impact, although the statistical results in the Conrad study are affected by the fact that female physicians tended to work fewer hours per week than did their male counterparts.

Turning to incentive effects on each group as the unit of analysis, the findings suggest an inverse relationship with group size—that is, as the size of groups becomes larger, the impact of incentives dissipates. The sense of participating in a cohesive, close-knit professional team seems to be adversely affected by a larger number of providers. In effect, physicians may be less motivated psychologically because they are only one provider among many in a large group practice, possibly leading them to remain at the average production capacity rather than strive to exceed this average. These are important findings because they indicate that large, vertically integrated delivery systems can be inimical to high productivity.

Conrad and colleagues' study has very important practical implications for all healthcare providers. It infers that production of services is linked to the availability of incentives. As healthcare costs continue to escalate and healthcare organizations seek higher productivity from clinicians, the scope and depth of incentive compensation plans will likely continue to grow.

better position than smaller physician practices without such resources to successfully implement this type of pay for performance. Another complicating factor is that most physician practices have contracts with multiple third-party payers, each of which places unique demands on the organization.

Little evidence exists to suggest that quality-focused pay for performance that have been implemented to date have been effective at giving physicians or organizations the incentive to improve quality levels (Rosenthal and Frank 2006). However, one recent large demonstration program by the Centers for Medicare & Medicaid Services (CMS) did show moderate quality improvements (Lindenauer et al. 2007). Despite this, pay-for-quality programs remain of great interest to both private and public third-party payers, both of which are expected to continue to experiment with the system to find the formula that will achieve desired outcomes. Notably, CMS is mandated by the Deficit Reduction Act of 2005 to implement value-based pricing in hospitals for Medicare patients by 2009. Therefore, quality-focused pay for performance will continue to merit significant management attention for the foreseeable future. Figure 11.5 highlights the experiences that some practice executives have had in implementing pay-for-performance programs.

Criticisms of Pay for Performance

Some argue that pay-for-performance systems decrease the focus on customer needs, increase the loss of accurate information about defects and improvement opportunities, discourage achievement of stretch goals, and reduce risk taking and innovation. These disadvantages have been cited because pay-for-performance systems may make the supervisor the most important customer; under these circumstances, employees play to their supervisors rather than to external customers or patients.

The system is also said to deprive providers of essential information because managers learn less about defects and changes that need to be made. Under a pay-for-performance plan, employees may be reluctant to report problems because doing so may have a negative impact on their compensation. Pay-for-performance approaches may also encourage employees to set lower goal aspirations. When goals are set in advance, employees may argue for less ambitious goals than for stretch goals to ensure that they receive performance-related rewards. Finally, pay-for-performance systems may hamper change because innovation disrupts tried-and-tested ways of delivering services, thus lowering efficiency and affecting goal accomplishment. This is especially detrimental in healthcare because constant breakthroughs in performance require substantial changes in the way employees do their work (Berwick 1995; Pfeffer 1998). Pay-for-performance plans may discourage risk taking and reduce creativity because the fear of not getting the reward makes people less inclined to take risks or explore alternative approaches to work. Thus, the efficacy of incentive plans is a topic of considerable debate.

In addition, pay for performance may be viewed as inconsistent with the current trend for transparency. Pay-for-performance programs create an arrangement between payer and physician to accomplish some task, such as increasing the rate of generic prescriptions. However, this goal is always hidden from the consumer, who has no idea that the physician is given an

FIGURE 11.5

Practice
Executives'
Experiences
with
Implementing
Pay-for-Quality
Performance
Programs

Although no clear formula has yet emerged for giving healthcare providers an incentive to improve quality of care through pay-for-performance programs, it is instructive to examine the role that practice executives play in the implementation of these programs. Practice executives are administrators responsible for negotiating quality targets and incentives with health plans. They are responsible for implementing pay-for-performance programs in their respective organizations. The implementation decisions they make can affect the success of these programs. To this end, Bokhour and colleagues (2006) conducted a series of qualitative interviews with practice executives from 69 physician organizations in Massachusetts. These practice executives were responsible for implementing pay-for-performance programs that affect more than 5,000 primary care physicians. The findings of this qualitative study outline the careful and detailed consideration that must be given to program implementation:

- Practice executives indicated that physicians find quality-oriented incentives to be better aligned with their inherent desires to provide high-quality care than were productivity- or utilization-oriented incentives.

- Practice executives did not come to a general agreement that the incentives motivated individuals to achieve quality improvement goals.

- Several issues may explain the failure of pay-for-quality programs to achieve their goals:
  — Physicians said that some measures used were outside of their scope of control. For example, measures for achieving a certain level of preventive screenings relied on patient cooperation.
  — Physicians said that data recording and reporting for the programs were inaccurate or did not represent a true measure of quality. Additionally, these measures lagged behind current clinical or state-of-the-art practices, creating a conflict that reduces the power of the incentives.

- The method of distributing rewards affects the power of the incentives to motivate change. For example, distributing rewards equally to all physicians is much less motivating than distributing rewards based on each physician's achievement of goals. The latter method, however, was sometimes found to be unfair in cases where several physicians were involved in the treatment of a particular patient but only one of them "got credit" toward program measures.

- Some organizations recognize that delivery of quality care depends not only on physicians but also on the active participation of all members of the practice. These organizations choose to retain program rewards for reinvestment in infrastructure that facilitates delivery of quality care rather than for distribution to individuals. While reinvestment provides no incentives to the individual, this system is a move toward improving quality through system-level changes. Still, other organizations create a balance by using a hybrid approach to distributing rewards. That is, some of the reward is reinvested and some is given to individuals to motivate provider-level change.

incentive to prescribe generics to meet some predetermined goal. Consumerism in healthcare depends on creating a transparent process—the consumer must have a full understanding of how and why the physician is performing in a certain way. As such, many payers think that pay for performance may actually slow the complete adoption of transparency in healthcare.

Those who support incentive plans point to the fact that most of us are, in reality, motivated by money. In other words, most people would rather have more money than less money; therefore, money can be used to change employee behavior. Supporters of pay for performance assert that behaviors that are rewarded are repeated and behaviors that are not rewarded (or punished) are eliminated. This suggests that, when rewarding behaviors, organizations must ensure that all relevant aspects of behavior are measured. Incomplete measurement may result in incomplete performance, with employees only doing tasks or engaging in behaviors that are rewarded. Rewards also provide an opportunity for management to communicate values to employees.

The Future of Variable Compensation Arrangements

In an effort to achieve greater levels of effectiveness and efficiency, a variety of new compensation arrangements will likely continue to emerge in healthcare. In particular, pay-for-performance programs will evolve as third-party payers develop a formula that provides an incentive to healthcare providers to deliver higher quality. Change can be good, but healthcare managers should proceed cautiously because compensation is a very charged topic. Tampering with compensation arrangements can have disastrous effects, so consequences cannot be overlooked or underestimated. Nonetheless, the difficult constraints that bind healthcare providers call for taking bold action. Perhaps the most important element in ensuring success in this regard is to involve employees at all levels in the design and implementation of compensation plans. In this way, the plan is more effective and meets broader acceptance.

Special Considerations for Compensating Physicians

Before World War II, most physicians were general practitioners who delivered care in independent practices on a fee-for-service basis (Starr 1982). Medicine was considered one of the more successful cottage industries. This practice changed radically after the war, with an explosion of medical subspecialties nurtured by battlefield needs, the rise of care within hospitals instead of at home, and the advent of employer-based medical insurance. Once consumers of care (patients) were no longer directly responsible for the cost of care they received, payers of the services (i.e., employers or government) and providers of care (i.e., physicians) were no longer obliged to justify costs to consumers. The checks and balances that typically exist in any economic interaction were lost. The result was a system that paid physicians whatever they requested, without the system attempting to validate the appropriateness of those services. This series of events led to the managed care movement (Burchell, Smith, and Piland 2002).

With the development of managed care, attention shifted to using payment mechanisms as a means to modify clinical behavior. Analysts have expressed concern that medical evidence is infrequently used in treatment decisions (Winslow 2000). For example, two patients with the same condition may receive vastly different therapies, or two patients with distinct diseases may be treated virtually the same. Allowing for the "art of medicine" does not explain the inconsistent use of clinical practice guidelines that have been shown to improve outcomes. Furthermore, variation in practice is widespread and is not linked to medical differences in populations. Two adjacent communities, with similar populations and demographics, may have dramatically different rates of surgery or use of certain modalities. Scientific justification for such discrepancies usually does not exist, suggesting that variations in care come from physician choice and habit, not medical data.

A key objective of health policy in the early 1990s was to leverage reimbursement mechanisms to address variation in treatment processes and outcomes. However, the track record for reducing practice discrepancies or improving practice behaviors in the last ten years has been disappointing. Modifying physicians' use of various forms of reimbursement has been a notable failure. Capitation was a system that paid a physician a certain amount for each patient assigned to his or her panel or list of patients. The fee was meant to cover professional services required to care for each patient. The challenge for the practitioner was to provide these services within the limits of capitated payment. As an incentive, any funds left over after delivering care reverted to the physician as revenue. Capitation was initially seen as an incentive to physicians to perform the appropriate level of care without generating excess costs.

In contrast, fee-for-service encourages the use of (and reimbursement for) excessive services and the tendency to neglect preventive measures. The argument was that compensating physicians a set amount per patient (a capitated payment) would encourage them to do as much as possible to keep patients healthy, thereby avoiding the need for expensive services. The Achilles' heel of capitation was that it put physicians at risk for patients who had preexisting conditions or medical predispositions over which physicians had no control. Capitation also rendered physicians responsible for patients whom they had never seen before. While many physician groups initially were enthusiastic about accepting risk payment, mainly because of the increased payments it brought, they usually failed to understand the full implications of being responsible for a population, versus caring for individual patients.

Bankruptcies of medical groups were not uncommon because of their inability to manage the very problems with physician behavior that capitation was supposed to solve. As a result, risk payment methods became increasingly unpopular as a payment option. Because of capitation's inability to change practice patterns (Grumbach et al. 1999; *Managed Care Outlook* 1999) and its adverse impact on both physician group viability and the willingness of groups to participate in such plans, other compensation approaches have surfaced.

An important element that affects the potential for compensation models to change behaviors is the continued growth in physician income. In the early 1990s, the general belief was that by putting the brakes on the rise in salaries, physicians could be brought in line with the directions that health plans and employers wanted them to go. This concept is frequently referred to as *aligning incentives*. However, numerous studies have demonstrated the surprising ability of physicians to continue to increase their incomes, albeit at lower rates of growth than in the 1980s (Thompson 2000; Kilborn 1999). Nevertheless, with most specialists making well more than $200,000 per year in 2007, using income as a tool for change has become difficult.

The ability to increase volume even as the cost per unit decreases has largely protected most physicians from experiencing radical shifts in income. Furthermore, unlike other professions, in medicine an increased supply of physicians has actually led to higher levels of health spending. Unlike in other industries in which more suppliers typically result in lower overall costs and revenues, in healthcare, competition has had minimal impact on total costs.

Payment Mechanisms Associated with Practice Settings

Most variations in how doctors are paid come from the settings in which physicians practice or are employed. Each setting offers benefits and drawbacks to compensation, depending on the goals of the particular practice. To help us understand how practice settings will continue to evolve in the future, let us take a look at how they developed.

Three broad categories of office practice are solo, group, and independent practice association (IPA). One practitioner defines a solo practice, and a group practice is composed of two or more physicians who have established a legal entity to deliver care together. The IPA usually consists of a collection of practices, including both solo and group practitioners, that join forces in taking advantage of economies of scale for contracting, business services, or ancillary services (such as laboratory). The IPA may negotiate on behalf of its practitioner members, and typically it has signature authority to establish contracts and distribute reimbursements.

Office Practice

Office-based physician practice is the classic model in which two or more physicians work together in an office setting. The degree of affiliation between the physicians can range from tight to very loose. A closely knit group comprises physicians who have a common philosophy and approach and who may share both business and clinical functions. A loosely connected group is made up of physicians who share office services, such as clerical and billing, but who practice independently in all other regards, especially concerning fiscal matters.

For solo and group practice physicians, the dominant reimbursement mode is pure fee-for-service (FFS) and salary plus incentive. Over the preceding ten years, fee schedules used in determining payments have been significantly reduced by private payers and government payers. An unintended, but not unexpected, consequence has been an increase in utilization of services so that even as the price of each unit of service has declined, the number of units provided has increased. This increase in service has further resulted in higher incomes for many specialties even as fee schedules are driven lower. As fee schedules are lowered, or discounted, physicians have an incentive to increase volume to make up the difference in their income.

IPAs may seek risk contracts from a payer, particularly if the IPA is large and well integrated. This implies a shared philosophy of care among physicians, with a high degree of self-discipline. Such groups actively monitor utilization internally, usually comparing it to national standards and scientifically validated treatment guidelines. Physicians who deviate significantly from these norms are either reeducated by their peers or are asked to leave the group. Frequently, a sophisticated information-gathering system is in place within the group to facilitate monitoring of outcomes and utilization. Information allows a group to control costs and to maximize efficiency. This creates a climate for accepting financial risk.

Few IPAs have the ability to accept significant risk projects and make them work. More typical is the IPA that is paid from a discounted FFS schedule and has some sort of incentive program to add dollars to the total reimbursement for the group. Such incentive plans may award a portion of any savings to physician members if the group achieves targeted utilization in areas such as pharmaceuticals and lab tests. Incentives may consist of simply a bonus, or they may be more complicated. Money may be put aside to be shared if targets are met, or a percentage increase in the fee schedule may occur if the group successfully manages its patients. The key point is that incentives are designed to encourage the group to perform at a higher level, but regardless of the success in reaching these goals, the physicians are still paid for each service provided.

Staff Model   Some medical groups or HMOs (health maintenance organizations) employ physicians on a straight salary basis or staff model—a model common in the late 1970s and early 1980s. Many early HMOs, such as Prudential and Humana, formulated the staff model as their primary method of caring for their members. Under the staff model, physicians employed by a care delivery organization are not distracted by concerns of generating revenue to cover practice expenses. They are able to focus on practicing medicine.

This model presents several drawbacks—one in particular is the difficulty in recruiting physicians who want to be employees. Most physicians enter medicine to practice independently, not to be under an employer's control. Despite having an employed group of doctors who theoretically have personal goals that are aligned with those of an organization, many HMOs found physician utilization to be as high and as variable as use of physicians in private practices. The work ethic of employed physicians was a significant factor in determining the fiscal success of the staff model. Many medical directors of staff-model HMOs were frustrated by the difficulty in motivating salaried physicians to extend themselves beyond prescribed hours and tasks. As a result, the staff model withered. However, the model is still a force in California, Colorado, Georgia, Hawaii, and Ohio because of the strong presence of the Permanente group, the staff-model organization that serves Kaiser HMO. The era of the salary-based physician practice has seen better days, as noted in Figure 11.6.

FIGURE 11.6
Outfall from the Demise of Staff-Model Groups

For several decades, the Group Health Cooperative of Puget Sound, a staff-model HMO based in Seattle, Washington, has participated with several other HMOs in providing managed care data for public health research. The advantages of a defined population and provider group offered by Group Health have enabled health services researchers to suggest policy improvements in care delivery. Breast cancer screening, sexually transmitted disease, adverse pharmaceutical effects, smoking mortality, and periodic health checkups illustrate areas to which health research has contributed to improve service delivery.

The so-called HMO research network has been supported by staff-model groups, including The Meyers Primary Care Institute (Massachusetts), Group Health, Harvard-Pilgrim Health Plan, Health Partners (Minnesota), Henry Ford Health Systems (Michigan), Kaiser (Georgia, Hawaii, Northern California, Rocky Mountain Region, Southern California Region, Northwest Region), and Prudential. These groups have progressively improved their data systems to the point that large-scale collaborative investigations have been facilitated. Research has focused on both quality of care and fiscal issues.

According to Fishman and Wagner (1998) at Group Health Cooperative's Center for Health Studies, desirable research possibilities may soon deteriorate. They cite the growing transition to IPAs—network organizations where loosely affiliated physician groups do not have strong incentives to partake in research. Cost-savings concerns by IPAs further diminish the potential for research as there is less investment in data systems. Thus, the clinical outfall from the demise of staff-model groups is less high-quality data for disease management.

Hospital Based A large cadre of physicians—hospitalists, pathologists, radiologists, and anesthesiologists, among others—practice almost exclusively within the confines of nonacademic hospitals. In the past, many were directly employed by hospitals and received a straight salary. Recently, however, these physicians have formed professional corporations that contract with hospitals for services, often on an exclusive basis. For instance, a hospital may contract to have services provided by a group of emergency medicine physicians. This group will staff the emergency room, be paid on a contractual basis, and may even take over the administration of the unit. The basis for the contract is typically some formula that represents the billings that the unit generates, with an additional amount included for such items as administration and participation on hospital committees. The same model can apply to other specialties as well. The key interaction from a reimbursement perspective occurs between the administrators of the hospital and the physicians' organization. The doctors function as independent contractors within the hospital; they are "in it" but not "of it."

The scenario changes somewhat for physicians in academic, tertiary care medical centers. Several unique aspects of these institutions must be considered. A large percentage of physicians in an academic setting are in training as residents or fellows. Their salaries are paid in large measure from Medicare reimbursements received by the medical center for the purpose of supporting graduate medical education. Thus, their salaries are not linked to their clinical performance, number of patients seen, rate of procedures performed, or other measures of productivity or quality. For staff or faculty physicians, salary is also the rule (because typically these physicians receive a straight salary that is not based on productivity), although the role of clinical activity is often figured into it.

The mission of the academic physician may be summarized as a combination of teaching, research, and patient care. With decreased reimbursements to hospitals, the need for these physicians to perform more clinical work has grown. This may or may not be accompanied by an increase in salary and often depends on whether a "faculty practice plan" exists. A *faculty practice* plan is essentially a group practice that comprises the faculty of the medical center. It was created as a way to leverage the billings generated by faculty into some sort of shared distributions or at least to negotiate a higher salary for those physicians who produce high clinical volumes. The amount of additional income flowing from the faculty practice plan is usually not great except for subspecialties; the principal source of income for an academic physician remains the salary from the institution. These salaries are invariably lower than those in the private-practice sector and reflect the typical differential for salaries between the academic and commercial environments.

Some physicians within the academic setting may see no patients at all and focus entirely on research. Many of them derive the bulk of their salaries from grants they are able to secure from outside agencies; the remainder may come from the university. As a result, the longevity of a researcher in this environment may well depend on his or her skill at preparing grant applications and performing research that is deemed worthy of outside support.

A growing mode of practice for physicians is working in a temporary staffing arrangement, or locum tenens. *Locum tenens* physicians refer to any temporarily employed physician, who is typically paid a fixed amount for services provided. This trend has been linked to the increase in female physicians (Croasdale 2002), the persistence of physician shortages, the growth in the number of partially retired physicians, and the lifestyle considerations favored by new physicians. Physicians move into these arrangements through personal contacts, advertisements, and assignments from a physician staffing agency (Simon and Alonzo 2004). When hiring a physician through a staffing agency, payment for physician services is made directly to the agency, generally on a fee-per-day basis (Lowes 2007). The use of locum tenens physicians is likely to increase because of the flexibility this system affords to both the physician and the organization. This work arrangement is also part of a significant national trend across all industries—the use of contingent workers.

Locum Tenens

Within the last decade, a rise has been observed in the number of physicians who are employed full time as medical directors, consultants, and administrators. Aside from those who work for managed care organizations, health insurers, and large provider groups, many physicians are now employed by organizations that want to better understand and control the resources they devote to employee healthcare benefits. These physicians fill critical roles as internal experts on medical care and health policy. As such, they are attuned to the unique problems of their employer and are able to help benefits coordinators and human resources administrators address complex employee health coverage issues. They also serve as liaisons between the benefits/human resources personnel and external vendors such as health plans, provider groups, and ancillary providers.

Leaders, Administrators, and Experts

Medical directors are also increasingly employed by state and federal agencies. As healthcare costs continue to escalate, this trend in physicians as policy experts and liaisons will likely evolve. Medical directors are typically salaried and are given the same sorts of benefits and incentives offered to executives in most companies.

Difficulties and Conflicts in Compensating Physicians

The most contentious issues that employers face with salaried physicians, whether in an academic medical center, a provider group, or a hospital system, are the same as for any other employees: benefits, perquisites, and salaries. A difficult challenge in determining physician pay is assessing the parameters based on productivity. Even for a medical group of two physicians, the potential exists for disagreements over what constitutes productivity levels. The following illustrate the complex issues behind the arguments:

- If a patient new to the practice is "counted" at a higher value than a returning patient, what defines a new patient? Someone who has never been seen before? Someone who has not been seen within a given time frame? Someone who has not been seen for a nonacute visit?
- For a procedure-based specialty, such as gastroenterology, does the physician who performs the procedure get full credit, or should partial credit go to the physician who has seen the patient most frequently over the past year?
- For an obstetric practice, should the physician who performs more vaginal deliveries (which represent more time) receive more credit than the physician who has a higher rate of cesarean section operations (which produce higher revenue)?

The details or fine points of a case may seem unimportant, but they are worth careful consideration because they are linked to a dollar value. This can make a significant difference in overall compensation for a physician. Add elements as seniority in the group, the number of call days taken, or outside activities such as service on hospital or medical society committees, and one can appreciate the dilemma many practices face in dividing up practice revenues.

Many medical groups have attempted to address these problems by designing formulas that incorporate multiple contributing factors to be considered when calculating compensation. By their nature, these formulas can become extremely complex in that they try to account for unrelated items that are often difficult to accurately measure. For example, a surgical group may try to include the number of cases seen with various weightings based on the severity of procedures performed, coverage in the emergency room, teaching residency at the medical school, and number of holiday calls taken. Such projects take an inordinate amount of time to devise but typically end up affecting only a small fraction of the total income of the physician. A further problem is the inability of any complicated payment scheme to either reinforce behavior desired by the practice or to extinguish undesirable behavior. Problems in defining incentive pay systems are further described in Figure 11.7.

While employed physicians in large medical groups may not be directly affected by such productivity questions, groups are highly dependent on medical staff members for their contributions in attaining efficiency while upholding high quality of care. For many groups that went on a hiring binge in the mid-1990s, as well as hospitals that adopted practices to lock in patient referrals, the assumption often was that employed physicians would maintain the same high productivity rates they delivered when they were self-employed. However, many physicians sold their practices to reduce their workload, leading to a dramatic drop in patient volumes. As a result, healthcare organizations

FIGURE 11.7

Trends in
Physician Pay
Systems

Epstein, Lee, and Hamel (2004) cite the increasing prevalence of pay-for-performance schemes for physicians. They observe that physicians are more likely to experience schemes that encourage them to improve quality of care and patient satisfaction than utilization. Despite the relatively unsophisticated nature of these approaches (often based on questionable patient survey data), the authors conclude that the magnitude of financial incentives for physician performance is growing. They review three examples to illustrate the diversity of physician compensation approaches.

1. *Bridges to Excellence*. General Electric (GE) and other employers in Massachusetts partnered with Tufts Health Plan, the Lahey Clinic, and Partners HealthCare to create an incentive of $55 per patient per year for physician offices that maintain systems for improving care (e.g., registries and electronic medical records). An additional $100 is awarded to physicians who qualify for the American Diabetes Association's Provider Recognition Program. The diabetes module of Bridges to Excellence now exists in several other cities, including Cincinnati and Louisville, with Humana and GE as codevelopers. Close to $80,000 in incentive rewards were distributed in Cincinnati in 2004, with more than 3,000 participating diabetic patients. Of great significance is the fact that the program has been successfully implemented in a community setting, moving beyond the large academic environment.

2. *Integrated Healthcare Association's Physician Payment Program*. Six health plans in California, known as the Integrated Healthcare Association, issue a physician performance scorecard incorporating clinical measures, patient ratings, and information technology. Clinical measures account for 50 percent of the rating, but other measures constitute the remaining 50 percent. This incentive plan was estimated to result in the distribution of $100 million.

3. *Anthem Blue Cross and Blue Shield Plan*. This New Hampshire health plan rewards physicians who provide preventive services linked to HEDIS (Healthcare Effectiveness Data and Information Set) measures. Physicians in the top performance group receive $20 per patient per year. The average award for all levels of performance per practice is $195.

According to Epstein, Lee, and Hamel, current systems for measuring performance are either lacking or need improvement to align incentives with outcomes.

that employ physicians have been faced with large deficits from their staffs of providers, which have led to severe financial strains.

Future Directions for Physician Compensation

The current framework for compensating physicians has not substantially changed medical practice. The advent of capitation and the use of incentives were assumed to initiate a revolution in how physicians treat patients as well as how physicians would be paid for their services. After a decade of change in the healthcare industry, the vast majority of practicing physicians continue to be paid on some sort of fee-for-service basis or salary plus incentive. Rather than this number decreasing as a result of the expansion of managed care, it is actually growing as more health plans move away from risk-based contracts in a tacit acknowledgment of their failure to substantially modify physician behavior (*Managed Care Outlook* 1999). As such, new compensation methods are necessary to transform patterns of medical practice. Proposed changes to medical care delivery cannot be successful unless physicians support them. This support depends on making certain that physicians are fairly and adequately compensated.

In the coming years, more opportunities for innovation will surface as the healthcare field searches for new paths to follow. These include the following:

- *Physicians will become more creative in defining their fee and payment structures.* Leaders in this area have been cosmetic surgeons who have always been paid out-of-pocket for the bulk of the work they do. They were among the first physicians to make payment for services with credit cards possible and to set up payment schedules in advance of surgery. While these payment options were commonplace in the rest of the economy, in medicine they were revolutionary.

- *Reproductive endocrinologists are now asking for up-front fee—say $30,000—to cover three cycles of in vitro fertilization.* If the patient does not conceive at the end of the third cycle, the fee is refunded except for a small amount to cover costs. Patients are thus provided with a quasi money-back guarantee. By seeking flexibility in payment, recognizing that their services are expensive, and making services more accessible to those without insurance coverage, these specialists have found new ways to secure their revenue stream.

- *Americans spend more than $35 billion per year on complementary and alternative medicine modalities, such as acupuncture, massage therapy, homeopathy, and biofeedback, with much of this expenditure being paid out-of-pocket.* The public seems to have an insatiable demand for these therapies, and physicians will seek to capture some of this huge volume of care by offering more alternative medicine options within the context of traditional medical practices. Because this care occurs outside of a fee schedule negotiated with a payer, it may well come to represent a large portion of some doctors' incomes in the future.

- *For physicians who are still paid primarily by third-party payers, reimbursement will be tied to performance.* Tools for assessing outcomes of care tied to such parameters as use of various treatments and revenue generated will increase in number and utilization. However, indications from practice suggest that the complexity of physician compensation systems will moderate. Structures that incorporated patient satisfaction, committee assignments, and governance service proved to be too complex to measure and administer. Instead, report cards on doctors' practice patterns and performance will become more widely available. Just as consumers now go to a variety of sources, especially the Internet, to research the purchase of a new car or house, they will increasingly be able to do the same for selecting their physicians and hospitals. Providers who perform at a high level will be paid at a higher level than those who do not perform as well.

- *Employers will continue to reduce their role as the primary source of health insurance for their employees.* Individual patients/consumers will consequently be increasingly accountable for making the kinds of healthcare choices currently left up to benefits managers at work. Having this freedom to choose will require consumers to become more educated in managing their own health. This will be facilitated by the creation and availability of thousands of websites devoted to medical topics as well as consumer-oriented information regarding physician quality and costs. Additionally, new business models for healthcare delivery (retail health clinics, for example) will arise in response to consumer-driven healthcare. These new business models will bring new competitive pressures to bear on some traditional physician practice settings. To succeed in an environment in which patients are more informed and discriminating consumers of healthcare services, physicians will need to provide a level of service and quality that represents superior value to patients as the ultimate payer. This ability to attract and retain patients will have a direct bearing on physician income. Physicians able to deliver superior value will see their revenues increase, while others will see their practices wither. Price will certainly be part of this value equation, and physicians will need to respond to price in ways they have never contemplated.

- *Physicians have become extremely entrepreneurial.* This has led to an explosion in the number of outpatient and ambulatory centers that provide services that have traditionally been delivered in hospitals. The common scenario is that the physician has an ownership interest in the center and receives not only the professional fee for the service but also a share of the income that the facility generates. The physician also receives income from testing and diagnostics. This trend is occurring in virtually all markets in the United States and across many specialties, and it has greatly enhanced the income of entrepreneurial physicians and shifted much of the delivery of routine and complex care. As a result, for these physicians, income derived directly from patient encounters is decreasing and being replaced by the large revenues from their ambulatory center partnerships and procedures.

Summary

Note that all the options discussed in this chapter revolve around some variation of the FFS model, which will continue to be the primary method for paying for medical services. Ironically, after an intense decade of experimentation with novel methods of reimbursement, we return to the time-tested FFS structure. Yet important differences exist between models prevalent today and those used two decades ago. FFS payment levels will no longer be dictated by "usual and customary" rates that were established by a de facto agreement of practicing physicians. They will instead be based on a market formulation that relates to the value of services as perceived by patients/customers. Therefore, physicians and groups who demonstrate a higher value will command a higher price for their services. This will remake the FFS system into one that more closely resembles the compensation mechanisms we are familiar with in other sectors of the economy.

Discussion Questions

1. Assume you are a manager at a low-budget healthcare setting (e.g., local health department). What will you do to recruit new staff and to motivate current employees when competitors in the area are able to pay 30 percent to 40 percent more than your organization can?

2. Assume that you are a staff nurse in a hospital that uses an incentive compensation system. Do you have an obligation to disclose the nature of the compensation arrangement to patients? If so, how should this information be communicated and by whom?

3. Regardless of your personal feelings about pay for performance, what cautions will you communicate to a team that is designing an incentive system in a healthcare organization?

4. How will you design a team-based compensation system such that free riders (or "loafers") on the team cannot take advantage of the system?

5. How can job evaluation procedures be used to determine if a healthcare organization is undercompensating its female employees?

6. What effect has managed care had on designing physician compensation models?

7. What are the likely roles for capitation and fee-for-service reimbursement in the future?

8. For a four-person surgical group, what kind of formula may be devised to fairly and consistently measure and reward productivity? What changes may be needed if one surgeon decides to perform more office work and less surgery?

Experiential Exercises

Case Mapleton Family Medicine is a physician group practice located in a small city (population 150,000) in the Midwest. Mapleton is an eight-physician practice, consisting of family physicians, internists, and pediatricians. The practice is owned by two of the physicians; the other six physicians are currently salaried. The owners are concerned with productivity and quality in the practice. There is a relatively long waiting time for appointments, and a recent chart review revealed that the percentage of children who are up-to-date with immunizations has dropped. Also, anecdotal evidence suggests that at-risk persons are not routinely receiving flu and pneumonia vaccinations. Many patients have complained about having to wait up to 90 minutes in the waiting room. At this time, however, the practice is not in a position to hire another physician.

Each physician in the practice currently sees an average of 25 patients per day. The owners want this number increased to 30 patients per day without sacrificing quality of care. To reach this goal, they are thinking of moving to an incentive system, whereby physicians have a base salary equivalent to 75 percent of their current salary and have the opportunity to earn up to 125 percent of their base salary if they meet defined volume and quality goals. While the owners have not completely thought this system through, they want to set 30 patients per day as a base and, through the incentive system, encourage physicians to see, on average, up to 35 patients per day.

In terms of quality, the owners have considered three measures:

1. Patient satisfaction surveys
2. Child-immunization audit data
3. Patient waiting times

Quality goals will be set biannually for each physician. The expectation is that physicians who achieve these goals will earn their full salary (assuming volume is adequate), and quality measures above their goals will result in bonuses according to a pay schedule.

Case Questions

1. You have been brought in to advise the owners on their proposed compensation plan, what advice will you give them before they proceed?
2. Do you see any potential negative consequences of this plan based on the information provided? If so, how will you address these concerns?
3. How do you think the physicians in the practice will react to this plan? Should they be involved in developing the plan, and if so, how should they be involved?

Project As noted in the chapter, healthcare organizations are faced with the challenge of balancing internal equity with external competitiveness. In this exercise, compare two organizations' approaches to setting salary levels. Your first task is to identify two healthcare organizations that are similar in mission and size. For example, you may select two medical group practices, two medium-size community hospitals, or two nursing homes of similar size. You may choose two organizations in the same geographic area and labor market or two that are in different markets.

Your second task is to identify the senior human resources management executive or the individual most closely involved in developing and implementing the compensation program in the organization. You will interview this person, so it is therefore important

that this person understand the compensation philosophy, system, design, and decision-making process. The goal of this exercise is to identify the organization's compensation strategy, including its approach to balancing competing compensation objectives.

Your third task is to summarize the compensation philosophy, policy, and practices in each organization and write a report on the similarities and differences between the two compensation systems.

Questions to Guide a Compensation Comparison

1. What is the policy of the organization on compensating employees at market rates? Is there an explicit policy to pay below market, at market, or above market? Does the approach vary by the type of employee and the particular labor market?
2. Does the organization have a specific strategy for attracting, recruiting, and retaining employees in difficult-to-fill positions? If so, for which positions has this been an issue? What strategies have been used in these circumstances? Examples include (but are not limited to) sign-on bonuses, retention bonuses, paying above market rates, and employee referral programs.
3. How does the organization evaluate jobs—that is, how does it "price" jobs?

Does it conduct a formal job evaluation process? If so, how often and under what circumstances? Are there certain jobs where the market dictates salary, rather than the salary being the result of a job evaluation process?
4. Does the organization face any of the following problems? If so, how does the organization address them?
   - Wage compression
   - Employees "topping out" of their salary range
   - High prevalence of employee departures because of compensation-related factors
   - Perceptions among employees that aspects of the compensation system are unfair

References

Adams, J. S. 1963. "Toward an Understanding of Inequity." *Journal of Abnormal and Social Psychology* 67 (5): 422–36.
Baca, C., and G. Starzmann. 2006. "Clarifying Competencies: Powerful Tools for Driving Business Success." *Workspan* 49 (4): 52–55.

Bartol, K. M. 1979. "Professionalism as a Predictor of Organizational Commitment, Role Stress, and Turnover: A Multidimensional Approach." *Academy of Management Journal* 22 (4): 815–21.

Berkowitz, S. M. 2002. "The Development of a Successful Physician Compensation Plan." *Journal of Ambulatory Care Management* 25 (4): 10–25.

Berwick, D. M. 1995. "Toxicity of Pay for Performance." *Quality Management in Healthcare* 4 (1): 27–33.

Bokhour, B. G., J. F. Burgess Jr., J. M. Hook, B. White, D. Berlowitz, M. R. Guldin, M. Meterko, and G. J. Young. 2006. "Incentive Implementation in Physician Practices: A Qualitative Study of Practice Executive Perspectives on Pay for Performance." *Medical Care Research and Review* 63 (1): 73S–95S.

Bunning, R. L. 1992. "Models for Skill-Based Pay Plans." *HR Magazine* 37 (2): 62–64.

Burchell, R. C., H. L. Smith, and N. F. Piland. 2002. *Reinventing Medical Practice: Care Delivery That Satisfies Physicians, Patients and the Bottom-Line.* Denver, CO: Medical Group Management Association.

Capo, J. 2001. "Identifying the Causes of Staff Turnover." *Family Practice Management* 8 (4): 29–33.

Conrad, D. A., A. M. Sales, A. Chaudhuri, S. Liang, C. Maynard, L. Pieper, L. Weinstein, D. Gans, and N. Piland. 2002. "The Impact of Financial Incentives on Physician Productivity in Medical Groups." *Health Services Research* 37 (4): 885–906.

Croasdale, M. 2002. "Practice Must Cope as More Physicians Work Part-Time Hours." *American Medical News* 45 (39): 1–2.

Egger, E. 2000. "Nurse Shortage Worse than You Think, but Sensitivity May Help Retain Nurses." *Healthcare Strategic Management* 18 (5): 16–18.

Epstein, A. M., T. H. Lee, and M. B. Hamel. 2004. "Paying Physicians for High-Quality Care." *New England Journal of Medicine* 350 (4): 406–10.

Fay, C. H., and M. Tare. 2007. "Market Pricing Concerns." *WorldatWork Journal* (Second Quarter): 61–69.

Fishman, P. A., and E. H. Wagner. 1998. "Managed Care Data and Public Health: The Experience of Group Health Cooperative of Puget Sound." *Annual Review of Public Health* (19): 477–91.

Gaynor, M., and M. V. Pauly. 1990. "Compensation and Productive Efficiency in Partnerships: Evidence from Medical Group Practice." *Journal of Political Economy* 98 (3): 544–73.

Grib, G., and S. O'Donnell. 1995. "Pay Plans that Reward Employee Achievement—Competency-based Payment Plans." *HR Magazine* 40 (7): 49–50.

Grumbach, K., J. V. Selby, C. Damberg, A. B. Bindman, C. Quesenberry, A. Truman, and C. Uratsu. 1999. "Solving the Gatekeeper Conundrum: What Patients Value in Primary Care and Referrals to Specialists." *JAMA* 282 (3): 261–66.

Gunderman, R. B. 2004. "The Perils of Paying Academic Physicians According to the Clinical Revenue They Generate." *Medical Science Monitor* 10 (2): 15–20.

Gupta, N., and J. D. Shaw. 1998. "Let the Evidence Speak: Financial Incentives Are Effective." *Compensation and Benefits Review* 30 (2): 26, 28–32.

Herzberg, F., B. Mausner, and B. Snyderman. 1959. *The Motivation to Work.* New York: John Wiley.

Hills, F. S., T. J. Bergmann, and V. G. Scarpello. 1994. *Compensation Decision Making,* 2nd Edition. Forth Worth, TX: Dryden.

Homans, G. C. 1961. *Social Behavior: Its Elementary Forms.* New York: Harcourt, Brace and World.

Kaplan, R. S., and D. P. Norton. 1996. *The Balanced Scorecard*. Boston: Harvard Business School Press.

Kilborn, P. T. 1999. "Doctors' Incomes Rising Again Despite HMOs." *Cincinnati Enquirer* (April 22): A2.

Kingma, M. 2003. "Economic Incentive in Community Nursing: Attraction, Rejection or Indifference?" *Human Resources for Health* [Online publication; retrieved 5/12/05.] www.human-resources-health.com.

Lindenauer, P. K., D. Remus, S. Roman, M. B. Rothberg, E. M. Benjamin, A. Ma, and D. W. Bratzler. 2007. "Public Reporting and Pay for Performance in Hospital Quality Improvement." *New England Journal of Medicine* 356 (5): 486–96.

Lowes, R. 2007. "Locum Tenens: When You Need One, How to Get One: Here's How to Find and Use These Substitute Doctors." *Medical Economics* 84 (9): 38–42.

Managed Care Outlook. 1999. "Florida Blues Ditch Capitation in Favor of Fee-for-Service." *Managed Care Outlook* [Online publication; retrieved 5/21/05.] www.managedcaremag.com.

Martocchio, J. 2001. *Strategic Compensation*. Upper Saddle River, NJ: Prentice Hall.

Maslow, A. 1970. *Motivation and Personality*, 2nd Edition. New York: Harper & Row.

Mercer Human Resource Consulting. 2006. *Compensation Planning Survey*. New York: Mercer Corporation.

Mohr, V., J. Zinn, J. Angelelli, J. M. Teno, and S. C. Miller. 2004. "Driven to Tiers: Socioeconomic and Racial Disparities in the Quality of Nursing Home Care." *Milbank Quarterly* 82 (2): 227–56.

O'Connor, J. P., D. B. Nash, M. L. Buehler, and M. Bard. 2002. "Satisfaction Higher for Physician Executives Who Treat Patients, Survey Says." *Physician Executive* 28 (3): 17–21.

Pfeffer, J. 1998. "Six Dangerous Myths About Pay." *Harvard Business Review* 76 (3): 108–19.

Reschovsky, J., and J. Hadley. 2007. "Physician Financial Incentives: Use of Quality Incentives Inches Up, but Productivity Still Dominates." Issue Brief No. 108. Washington, DC: Center for Studying Health System Change.

Rosenthal, M. B., and R. G. Frank. 2006. "What Is the Empirical Basis for Paying for Quality in Health Care?" *Medical Care Research and Review* 63 (2): 135–57.

Rost, K. T. 2002. "What You Don't Know Can Hurt You: Why Managed Care Organizations Have a Legal Duty to Disclose the Use of Financial Incentives to Limit Medical Care." *Journal of Health Law* 35 (1): 145–69.

Schmidt, L. A., D. Nelson, and L. Godfrey. 2003. "A Clinical Ladder Program Based on Carper's Fundamental Patterns of Knowing in Nursing." *Journal of Nursing Administration* 33 (3): 146–52.

Simon, A. B., and A. A. Alonzo. 2004. "The Demography, Career Pattern, and Motivation of Locum Tenens Physicians in the United States." *Journal of Healthcare Management* 49 (6): 363–75.

Starr, P. 1982. *The Social Transformation of American Medicine*, 198–235. New York: Basic Books.

Thompson, E. 2000. "Physician Compensation Report: Docs' Income Growth Stabilizes." *Modern Healthcare* (August 7): 37–41.

Wagner, F. H., and M. B. Jones. 1994. "Broadbanding in Practice: Hard Facts and Real Data." *Journal of Compensation and Benefits* 10 (1): 27–34.

Winslow, R. 2000. "A Type of Heart Drug Wins Wide Use Owing to Small Firm's Efforts." *Wall Street Journal* (November 17): A1.

12

EMPLOYEE BENEFITS

Dolores G. Clement, DrPH, FACHE; Maria A. Curran;
and Sharon L. Jahn, CEBS, CMS

Learning Objectives

After completing this chapter, the reader should be able to

- discuss the history and trends of employee benefits management;
- explain the rationale and tax implications of offering benefits in addition
  to compensation and why benefits are critical to the recruitment and
  retention of healthcare staff;
- describe a variety of benefits that may be offered with employment, and
  relate the management implications of offering each;
- relate the knowledge of employee benefits to selected human resources
  management issues and systems development; and
- make suggestions for the design and communication of benefit plans.

Introduction

Benefits are a competitive lever in recruiting and hiring employees. Employment benefits provide additional compensatory value to individuals and their
families through the provision of leave time, insurance against uncertain
events, and additional targeted services. The success of any healthcare organization requires a concerted investment in human capital for many reasons.
Demand for experienced healthcare providers has never been greater, while
competition for clinical staff, including physicians, has intensified. Nonclinical staff are in great demand as well. The labor shortage is compounded by
the fact that capacity at most medical, nursing, and allied health schools does
not meet demand; therefore, fewer students can attend. Replacement costs
and turnover costs far exceed the cost of investing wisely in human capital.

In most healthcare organizations, labor costs are the single largest line
item in the operating budget. An increase in labor cost often has a correlation to
the cost of employer-sponsored benefits; in fact, many fringe benefits are based
on a percentage of employees' salaries. Thus, the cost of fringe benefits can be a

significant line item in any operating budget. Depending on the actual benefits offered and their respective design structures, the average cost of fringe benefits in many healthcare systems can range from 20 percent to 35 percent of salary. The U.S. Chamber of Commerce (2006) projects that, across all industries, employee benefits account for almost 40 percent of total compensation.

Research by the University HealthSystem Consortium (2005; Bragg and Vermoch 2003) indicates that attracting and retaining clinical workforce is one of the top three concerns cited by chief executive officers (CEOs) who participated in the study. Further, another survey of CEOs ranked the retention of the clinical workforce as a top financial concern (ACHE 2005). The significant workforce shortages are exacerbated by the rate of growth in healthcare jobs and the aging workforce. While financial worries are pressing concerns for CEOs, staffing and quality are also at the top of the list (Evans 2006). As such, offering a comprehensive fringe benefits structure is an increasingly important recruitment and retention tool. The introduction of the Internet has made researching potential employers virtually effortless. Candidates, as well as incumbent employees, can access detailed information about employers and are often very well versed in the fringe benefits offered by various companies.

The pressure to offer a benefits package that is competitive in the marketplace is significant in healthcare. This is illustrated in part by the weight that is placed on compensation and benefits packages by organizations that are recognized as "employers of choice." Research by Ahlrichs (2002) indicates that benefits are an important factor to consider in an applicant's decision to accept employment. In addition, offering a good benefits package is part of a health system's acknowledgment of its Magnet status; one of the 14 "forces of magnetism" is Force 4 (ANCC 2007):

> Personnel Policies and Programs: Salaries and benefits are competitive. Creative and flexible staffing models that support a safe and healthy work environment are used. Personnel policies are created with direct care nurse involvement. Significant opportunities for professional growth exist in administrative and clinical tracks. Personnel policies and programs support professional nursing practice, work/life balance, and the delivery of quality care.

Because of the importance of benefits to the entire employee compensation package, many tasks involved in the design, communication, and monitoring of benefit plans are the responsibility of human resources personnel. Knowledge of one's organization, the market in which it competes, and the needs of the workforce is crucial in making decisions of what benefits should be offered. Beyond benefits that are mandated, what other benefits should be offered to employees? To what extent should benefits be offered to different classifications of employees?

This chapter presents an overview of the most common benefits related to employment compensation, describes a variety of benefits that may be offered as well as their tax implications, explains the role of government in benefits management, and discusses key issues in the design and management of benefit plans.

Brief Historical Background

Retirement benefit programs in the United States can be traced back to the Plymouth Colony settlers military retirement program of 1636 (EBRI 2007). Beyond retirement plans, health coverage benefit programs across industries are a development of the late nineteenth and early twentieth century in the United States. In the late 1800s, industries began to employ physicians as a result of the increasing potential for worker injury in a country that was undergoing industrialization. The railroad, mining, and lumber industries offered more extensive medical services, which were necessary because workers were helping in the expansion into areas in the West where care was not available. Companies retained a doctor and made mandatory deductions from workers' salaries to cover the cost of the medical services or the salary of the physician (Starr 1982). The rise in industrialization also led to the creation of disability insurance in the late 1800s. Although coverage was not tied to employment at that time, individuals could purchase coverage that served as assurance that they would still have income in the event of a disability.

Coverage of workers in the railroad, mining, and lumber industries was the stimulus for Justin Ford Kimball to create Baylor University's hospital prepayment plan in 1929; this plan was the precursor to the creation of Blue Cross. The initial arrangement was simple and direct between the university hospital and teachers in the Dallas area (Cunningham and Cunningham 1997). This prepayment plan (which allowed up to 21 days of care in the hospital for 50 cents per month) was different from any type of conventional insurance. Prepayments were made directly to the hospital that was providing the care with no third-party involvement.

The Great Depression, beginning in 1929, shed light on the financial problems faced by the aged, ill, and disabled populations. These concerns led to the passage of the Social Security Act in 1934 and the federal government's involvement in providing retirement income protection. By mandating salary withholding in 1935 as a contribution to the trust fund for Social Security, precedent was set and other benefits coverage began to expand. Social Security provided some retirement benefits and included coverage of categorical programs but not medical coverage for the elderly or poor. Amendments to the Social Security Act in 1956 and 1964 added income protection for the disabled along with health insurance for the elderly and disabled under Medicare (EBRI 2007).

The wage freeze during World War II allowed companies to offer benefits in lieu of wage increases. Employers benefited with federal exemption of defined benefits from the companies' tax liability. Subsequent legislation that permitted tax preferential treatments gave incentives to employers to offer more private, voluntary benefits. Note that a countervailing force against increasing the number and variety of benefits is the inability of companies to subsidize offerings—more simply, providing benefits is becoming less affordable.

Federal and state governments regulate and carefully monitor the tax treatment and administration of benefits. Since the 1950s, a proliferation of legislation has been observed that establishes guidelines to protect individuals and employers in administering employment-related benefits and that monitors public and private benefit plans. Table 12.1 lists federal legislation that affects benefits administration. Employers have the responsibility to ensure that they are in compliance with all of the rules and regulations governing the benefits of their employees. The following section illustrates the regulatory compliance expected of employers using three examples of the most far-reaching legislation.

TABLE 12.1   Legislation that Affects Employee Benefits Administration

Legislation (Acronym)	Major Accomplishment	Legal Citation and Web Address
Uniformed Services Employment and Reemployment Rights Act (USERRA)	Provides continuous employment and benefits for soldiers who are deployed while employed	38 U.S.C. § 4301 www.osc.gov/userra.htm
Economic Growth and Tax Relief Reconciliation Act of 2001 (EGTRRA)	Provides greater flexibility for participants who transfer defined contribution balances at termination of employment and consistencies in deferral amounts, eligibility, and so on among various defined contribution plans	Public Law 107-16, June 7, 2001 www.irs.gov/pub/irs-utl/ egtrra_law.pdf
Health Insurance Portability and Accountability Act of 1996 (HIPAA)	Provides for the elimination of waiting periods when participants move between group health plans; also provides regulations for privacy/security of health-related information within a company that has access to such information and regulations for how an employer may use, store, and transmit such protected information	Public Law 104-191 http://aspe.hhs.gov/ admnsimp/pl104191.htm

TABLE 12.1 Continued

Legislation (Acronym)	Major Accomplishment	Legal Citation and Web Address
Medicare Prescription Drug Improvement and Modernization Act of 2003 (MMA)	Introduced Medicare Part D, prescription drug coverage, and Medicare Advantage products; allows greater choice of coverage as private insurance companies can provide coverage through PPO*, fee-for-service, medical savings accounts, and other special needs plans directly to the Medicare population	Public Law 108-173 www.cms.hhs.gov/ MMAUpdate/downloads/ PL108-173summary.pdf
Government Accounting Standards Board (GASB) No. 43 and No. 45	Rules that require government employers to book the accrued cost of future retiree benefits as a current liability; similar to FASB 106 provisions for publicly traded companies; beginning in 2007 on a phased-in basis	www.gasb.org/project_pages/ opeb_summary.pdf
Pension Protection Act of 2006 (PPA)	Provides additional protection against employers that underfund defined benefit retirement plans by giving additional premiums, closing loopholes, raising caps on minimum amounts that employers must contribute, and requiring measurement of funding levels; also provides additional enhancements in the defined contribution plans; allows for easier implementation of automatic enrollment in deferred savings plans, ensuring participants have greater access to their financial investments and to professional advice	Public Law 109-280 www.dol.gov/ebsa/pdf/ ppa2006.pdf

*PPO: preferred provider organization

Major Federal Legislation

Three major federal laws that affect benefit coverage and administration are the Employee Retirement Income Security Act of 1974 (ERISA), the Consolidated Omnibus Budget Reconciliation Act of 1986 (COBRA), and the Health Insurance Portability and Accountability Act of 1996 (HIPAA). Each of these acts has specific implications for benefits management. ERISA is a federal law administered by the U.S. Department of Labor to establish minimum standards by which many pension and health plans in private industry are governed. Most nongovernmental companies in the United States are covered by ERISA, whereas state or federal agencies are not. The types of protection mandated by ERISA are primarily administrative in nature. For example, employers must maintain plan documents in accordance with applicable federal laws and ensure that definitions for plan eligibility are not discriminatory. ERISA also includes expectations for the fiduciary aspects of administration, requiring plan administrators to appropriately manage and control the assets of the plan, to develop a process by which plan participants can obtain benefits or benefits information, and to inform participants of the right to sue for the company's breach of fiduciary responsibility. The organization must also file annual tax returns after an external audit of the plan has been conducted.

Over the years, ERISA has been amended so that health plans have greater protections. For example, COBRA provides qualifying employees and their families the right to continue to participate in employer-sponsored health coverage for a limited time after certain qualifying changes in family status, such as the loss of a job. Often, buying individual medical insurance directly is much more expensive for an employee, but COBRA helps employees and their spouses and dependents by guaranteeing them continued access to the employer's healthcare plan at the current group rate. The employee pays the full healthcare premium, which is often a less expensive option than buying an individual policy. COBRA covers any group health plan sponsored by an employer with 20 or more employees on more than 50 percent of typical business days in the previous calendar year. In addition, COBRA requires companies to provide timely notification to all covered beneficiaries in the event that a qualified family status change would make those individuals eligible for COBRA. Hefty penalties can be assessed for failure to adhere to these timely notification guidelines.

In 1996, HIPAA was enacted to protect employees and their families who have preexisting medical conditions or who could suffer health-coverage discrimination because of health-related factors. For example, under HIPAA, an individual who changes employment may have no waiting period for preexisting illness if there is less than a 63-day break in healthcare coverage from the prior employer. In addition, the confidentiality of protected health information (PHI) is specifically outlined in HIPAA. For example, details of employees' medical conditions, enrollment forms, medical claims data, or other specific health information must be filed separately from the employees' personnel files to prevent unauthorized or inappropriate access to PHI. Also, HIPAA protects the type of information that can be used in making decisions about coverage or premiums. In short, HIPAA is intended to balance access to claims information or other medical information with the need for an employer to make revenue-driven decisions. Thus, the employers' need to access claims information to make decisions about the coverage it will offer must respect individual privacy requirements. For example, employers cannot make coverage decisions that would have an adverse impact on individuals, such as eliminating coverage for a specific diagnosis because a number of employees have that diagnosis.

In many healthcare organizations, enforcing HIPAA is the responsibility of a compliance officer. Computerized medical records are also protected by HIPAA, as is the disclosure of medical information by staff. HIPAA *does not protect against accidental disclosure,* but it sets up standards that make such an incident less likely and establishes penalties if information is released without following the standards. For example, discussing an interesting case in the lobby of the medical center may be considered a HIPAA violation if PHI is released. The provisions of HIPAA were expanded with inclusion in the Newborns' and Mothers' Health Protection Act, the Mental Health Parity Act, and the Women's Health and Cancer Rights Act.

Audits of compliance can be conducted, and failure to follow the provisions of ERISA, COBRA, or HIPAA can subject the employer to serious financial penalties.

Overview of Employment Benefits

Given the competitive nature of healthcare, administrative staff must understand the full range of benefits that the employer provides, because many, if not most, employees may not realize the richness of their organization's benefits package. For example, a registered nurse may choose to seek employment at another medical center for a modest gain in hourly rate and not realize that the benefits offered by the new employer are not as robust as those given by the current employer. In this example, the healthcare organization will have to recruit and orient a new registered nurse, when in fact the resignation may have been prevented if the individual fully understood the value of the employers' benefits packages.

When educating staff about the value of the benefits package, the organization must stress the concept of total compensation. *Total compensation* is the value of the employee's base salary plus the value of the benefits package. An employer may help articulate this fact in several ways, including the following:

- Add a section on pay advices that notes the value of the employer-paid portion of health insurance.
- Provide benefits calculation tools on the company website or intranet.
- Produce customized benefits statements during the annual open enrollment process.

Communication of the worth of these benefits is essential if an employer intends them to play a part in recruitment and retention.

Following is a description of employee benefits that are mandated by law and those that are voluntary. The tax implications of each benefit are also discussed in this section; some voluntary benefits are entirely taxable, some are tax exempt, and others are tax deferred.

Mandatory Benefits

Social Security and Medicare Part A

The Federal Insurance Contributions Act (FICA) authorizes a payroll tax that funds Social Security, disability, and Medicare Part A. FICA requires Social Security payroll taxes to be collected from the employee and matched by the employer. The 2008 FICA employee contribution is 6.2 percent of wages, up to a taxable wage base of $102,000. The Medicare rate is 1.45 percent of wages, with no wage limit (Social Security Online 2007). Employers must match each of these amounts and send the total withheld and matched amounts to the federal government. Once the taxable wage total is made, only the Medicare Part A deduction with the employer match is sent. The taxable wage base is determined annually by the Internal Revenue Service (IRS) and is subject to change.

Unemployment Compensation

Unemployment compensation is a mandatory assessment of the employer and varies by state. The intention of unemployment compensation is to protect employees who have lost their jobs under certain circumstances, such as being laid off. Voluntary separation and termination for cause that is well documented is typically not covered. The premium amount for unemployment insurance is calculated based on the types of positions in the organization as well as the experience of the company with reductions in force. For example, an organization with a professional staff would likely pay more than one with a sales force, because the amount of salary to supplement for a professional is likely to be higher in the event of a layoff.

Workers' Compensation

Legislation for Workers' Compensation was passed to protect an employer from possible litigation for workplace injuries and to provide wages and benefits, including medical expenses, to employees who are injured on the job. Each state has different rules governing its Workers' Compensation program. Most states mandate that employers have insurance coverage, although some states provide their own Workers' Compensation funds to which employers can contribute. Many organizations choose to self-insure Workers' Compensation to save costs, and this can be very successful if managed well. Workers' Compensation is monitored and enforced by the Occupational Safety and Health Administration (U.S. Department of Labor 2007a). In a healthcare setting, workplace injuries that may initiate a Workers' Compensation claim result from injuries incurred from such events as lifting patients, needlesticks, and exposures to disease.

Voluntary Benefits

Most benefits that employers provide are voluntarily offered and, as such, differentiate one employer from another. Administration of some voluntary benefits may need to follow established rules and guidelines or reporting requirements, and if so, the employer is responsible for ensuring compliance. Following are the most common voluntary benefits offered by an employer.

Vacation leave is fully taxable when taken. Employers establish vacation eligibility according to employee category—salaried or hourly. Length of service usually determines the amount of vacation days that can be accrued and carried over from year to year. Employers must account for accrued vacation liability.

Leave Benefits

    Sick leave allows employees to get paid during time off as a result of illness, injury, or medical appointments. As with vacation leave, employers establish sick and illness leave policies according to category of employee.

    Family and medical leave is covered by the Family and Medical Leave Act (FMLA), which applies to employers that have more than 50 employees. Under FMLA, employers must offer up to 12 weeks of unpaid leave per year for maternity or other medical needs to eligible employees (U.S. Department of Labor 2007b). An employee can take advantage of this benefit if he or she has worked at least one year or has put in 1,250 hours of service in the 12 months before the needed leave. Individual employers may choose to pay for this leave, but that is left to their discretion. Reasons given for an FMLA leave include the birth or adoption of a child, taking care of a family member with a serious illness, or an employee's own ailment. Family leave can be taken on an intermittent basis, and employers need to track the unpaid leave given that the 12-month period in which it can be taken can be based on a fixed (e.g., calendar or fiscal year) or on a rolling basis (e.g., 12 months since the first day of leave). The employer covered by the FMLA must stipulate the basis or standards for this benefit. For example, the employer may request a medical certificate if the employee requests the leave for a medical purpose.

Benefits designed to provide protections and services related to health, dental, vision, life insurance, and disability are typically categorized under health and welfare benefits.

Health and Welfare Benefits

    Employer-sponsored *health insurance* is one of the most expensive items in the budget for employers as a result of escalating costs of healthcare. Although health insurance remains a voluntary benefit, employers, particularly larger organizations, are expected to offer this benefit. Employers that provide health insurance can deduct their expenditures from pretax earnings. Usually, employees are offered a choice of private health insurance plans, including the traditional service benefit coverage and managed care options,

TABLE 12.2   Types of Health Insurance Plans

Type	What Is Covered?	Advantages	Disadvantages
Full Service	First-dollar coverage provided on all medical and hospital services up to a predetermined maximum	Members receive coverage for extensive medical and preventive care, both inpatient and outpatient	• Expensive for employer because of high claims costs • Complexity involved as the plans may pay physician claims and hospital claims differently
Comprehensive	Cost sharing of medical expenses at a predetermined percentage of claims (coinsurance), after an up-front deductible, up to a predetermined maximum where the plan pays 100 percent of claims above the out-of-pocket maximum	Introduced cost sharing with the member as well as other cost-control features, such as second surgical opinion, preadmission review, and full coverage for diagnostic tests	• All cost-control incentives are written on the front of the claim • Provides no incentive to reduce overutilization and use of high-cost providers
Preferred Provider Organization (PPO)	Claims incurred at providers that participate in the insurance carriers' PPO network are paid at a higher level than claims incurred at nonparticipating providers	Claims costs are reduced because of negotiated discounts with the insurance carriers when members use a participating provider	• Potentially substantial cost differential if care is sought at a nonparticipating medical provider • Members must first determine if their provider is participating in the network
Health Maintenance Organization (HMO)	• Only claims incurred at providers that participate in the insurance carriers' HMO network are covered • All specialty care that is directed through the member's gatekeeper or primary care physicians with referrals to the appropriate provider	Primary care physicians are paid by the insurance company to be gatekeepers; this keeps costs down as gatekeepers can manage the care received from a specialist and ensures that the specialists are part of the participating network	• More limited network size, making it more difficult for members to find participating physicians • All care must be directed through the gatekeeper, creating additional visits or time necessary to provide access to specialists

TABLE 12.2   Continued

Type	What Is Covered?	Advantages	Disadvantages
High-Deductible Health Plan (HDHP)	Medical care for the member is not paid until a high deductible is met, typically greater than $2,000; after this deductible is met, claims are paid at a predetermined cost-sharing percentage	• Members are encouraged to understand the costs of medical care as they must meet a high deductible before the employer plan will pay for claims • Usually, preventive care is excluded from the deductible, thus encouraging wellness • Usually provided as part of a consumer-driven health plan and supplemented with health reimbursement accounts or health savings accounts	• Members must pay high-deductible amount out of their own pocket before coverage can begin; members may not have budgeted for these amounts • Providers must get billed amounts from patients instead of insurers • More risk for nonpayment

and this offer extends to employee dependents (spouse, children) as well. Table 12.2 presents various types of health insurance plans, and Table 12.3 lists additional health and welfare benefits.

Some employers opt to self-insure, negotiating with a private health insurance company to administer benefits to employers through an administrative services contract. Self-insured employers may extend coverage not only to dependents but also to domestic partners. Today, domestic partners are not universally considered as dependents. However, several states and companies have provisions that are inclusive of domestic partners.

Self-insured healthcare is attractive for many healthcare organizations because it typically allows greater flexibility in plan design. For example, the plan can be designed to encourage staff to use the employer's providers and facilities by providing financial incentives such as lower copays and out-of-pocket expenses. Such a design can positively affect the cost of administering the health plan because the revenue generated may pay for the cost of paying claims. Self-insured organizations are not obligated to offer state-mandated health benefits. Other large employers are more likely to self-insure if they

TABLE 12.3   Other Health and Welfare Benefits

Benefit	What Is It?	Who Pays?	Who Determines Amount?	Types of Plans
Dental	Covers a percentage of dental care up to an annual maximum	Employer and employee; generally a greater percentage of the cost is borne by the employee	Employer may choose to offer multiple plans; employees elect the plan or the employer provides a single plan	Dental indemnity; dental PPO**; dental HMO*; direct dental
Prescription Drug Coverage	Covers some amount of the cost of prescription medications	May be included in health insurance or as a separate rider to the health insurance policy	Employer may choose to offer multiple plans; employees elect the plan or the employer provides a single plan	Two-tier coverage; three-tier coverage; four-tier coverage; coverage after deductible
Vision	Covers a predetermined amount of expenses for exams, frames, lenses, contacts, among others, during a specified period (annually or biannually)	May be included in health insurance or provided as a voluntary supplemental coverage	Employer may choose to offer multiple plans; employees elect the plan or the employer provides a single plan	Vision PPO; Vision HMO
Stop-loss Coverage	Protects against catastrophic claim amounts either on a single claimant or the total claims expense	Employer pays for protection against unpredicted catastrophic claims	Employer	Specific aggregate
Life	Provides a death benefit for the covered person payable to a predesignated beneficiary	Employer provides a basic level of life insurance; employees may elect to purchase supplemental coverage on themselves, spouse, and/or children	Employer chooses the level of the basic coverage; employees may elect varying levels of supplemental coverage	Group term life; group universal life; group variable life; group variable universal life

TABLE 12.3 Continued

Benefit	What Is It?	Who Pays?	Who Determines Amount?	Types of Plans
Disability	Provides a level of income payable to the employee after a predetermined period out of work as a result of illness, injury, or disease	Employer provides a basic level of coverage; employees may choose to purchase supplemental coverage	Employer chooses the level of the basic coverage; employees may elect varying levels of supplemental coverage	Short-term disability; basic long-term disability, supplemental long-term disability
Flexible Spending Account	Allows employees to deduct a fixed, pretax amount from their paycheck over the plan year either for medical (including dental, vision, and prescription) expenses not covered by insurance or for dependent care expenses for a child under 13 or an adult who requires care because of age or mental handicap	Employee elects the specific payroll amount; employer has the ability to provide a matching dollar amount	Employee determines the amount based on his or her expected expenses in the respective category for the next plan year; must be elected each year, and any monies remaining after the plan year are forfeited back to the employer	Medical care; dependent care
Health Savings Account	A tax-advantaged medical savings account available to taxpayers in the United States who are enrolled in a high-deductible health plan	Employee or employer can make contributions to this plan; contributions can be either through pretax payroll deduction or directly to the financial institution and then claimed as a deduction to gross income on taxes	Amounts deposited within the plan year must not exceed the statutory limit set by the IRS; amounts remaining in the account at the end of the tax year may be rolled forward to next year; amounts are portable when employees leave employment	Health plan only

(Continued)

TABLE 12.3 Continued

Benefit	What Is It?	Who Pays?	Who Determines Amount?	Types of Plans
Health Reimbursement Account	An employer-funded account that reimburses an employee for medical expenses	Must be funded by employer only	Employer provides funding for the account based on its own criteria—no plan requirements; funds may be used to pay health insurance premiums and funds may not be rolled to the next plan year; portability upon termination is possible with constructive receipt issues	Health plan only

*HMO: health maintenance organization; **PPO: preferred provider organization

have a large claims experience and have the funding mechanisms to be able to do so. For healthcare organizations, health benefits coverage presents a unique challenge. While healthcare workers tend to use more health services than employees in other industries, because of their medical knowledge and their proximity to services, the cost of providing care to them is affected by the contracts that third parties, such as managed care companies and insurance companies, have negotiated to pay healthcare providers and facilities.

Note that under the Mental Health Parity Act, mental illness is considered a medical condition and thus requires employers to provide the same level of coverage for mental illness as they would for a physical condition. To contain costs for mental health, an employer can elect to carve out mental health and use a special behavioral health company to focus on mental health needs. Because behavioral health companies are a niche provider, they can provide economies of scale that may not be possible with a larger health insurer. An Employee Assistance Program (EAP) is also effective in controlling mental health costs if such a program is used as a "gatekeeper" to access mental-health-related services. EAPs typically offer a finite number of counseling and therapy sessions with professionals in the field, and all dealings with this group are totally confidential. Some employers provide the option of having a manager make a mandatory referral to the EAP to address concerns about an employee's mental health. Regardless of how employees access EAPs, use of the services in these programs is typically more cost effective than use of a psychiatrist under a healthcare benefit.

Wellness and fitness programs also fall under the health and welfare benefits. The adage "prevention is the best medicine" can be used by employers as a strategy to manage healthcare costs and to increase employee productivity. More and more workplace initiatives are focusing on wellness and fitness, especially in healthcare organizations. Because this trend is relatively new, only limited longitudinal data exist to prove the return on investment of such an offering. However, recent anecdotal articles describe how employer-sponsored wellness and fitness programs can contribute to a healthier and more productive workforce (Bridgeford 2007; Gresham 2007; Smolkin 2007).

Wellness programs may be easier to implement in healthcare than in other industries for several reasons. First, many healthcare organizations require pre-employment health assessments based on the physical requirements of a position. Second, healthcare organizations typically have numerous content experts and other resources on site. Third, healthcare workers are typically more sophisticated consumers of wellness and preventive programs. Despite these reasons, many healthcare employees do not take advantage of services such as free flu shots. The low percentage of healthcare workers who get a flu shot has caused organizations such as the Joint Commission and the Centers for Disease Control and Prevention to bring the matter to the forefront for healthcare administrators. Indeed, one of the Joint Commission's 2007 goals for infection control requires hospitals and health systems to identify the reasons that healthcare staff do not get flu shots and then to use this information to come up with strategies that will increase participation.

There is renewed interest in providing incentives to employees to improve their health and reduce risky behaviors. Many healthcare organizations and insurance companies ask employees to complete personal health assessments to determine current and future risks based on family medical history. Others provide special payments to staff who have normal blood pressure, do not smoke, or have a healthy bodyweight index rating. Regardless of the method used to increase staff participation in wellness activities, the future clearly will bring increased focus on prevention and fitness for duty among healthcare workers. This emphasis will stem the escalating costs of healthcare, encourage better management of chronic diseases, reduce injuries, and increase productivity.

Dental insurance is sometimes offered to employees and their dependents as an addition to health insurance, although many employees expect this coverage. The cost associated with dental insurance is rising as much as the cost of health insurance. An option for a self-insured healthcare organization that is affiliated with a dental school is to contract directly with the school to provide dental care.

Vision coverage is typically an add-on to the health insurance benefit. Vision plans can be basic, which will include coverage for an annual eye exam and contact lenses or glasses. A vision network frequently provides better coverage at a more affordable price. A trend in recent years is the availability of hearing insurance for baby boomers, who are aging yet remain in the workplace. *Hearing insurance* is an example of a benefit that may be dependent on the changing demographics of the workforce.

Prescription drug benefits may be part of the health insurance coverage. Such coverage is costly both to the organization and to the employee even with the use of a drug formulary. Costs will continue to rise with continued acceptance of bioengineered drugs and other new life-saving treatments. The use of a pharmacy network can control costs if the formulary is carefully constructed to encourage employees to use less costly prescriptions, such as substituting generic drugs for name-brand drugs. The use of pharmacy benefit management companies has helped reduce pharmaceutical costs. These companies perform the normal utilization review function, manage the formulary, and negotiate the costs of drugs with pharmaceutical firms; thus, they can leverage the overall expense of providing the benefit.

Flexible spending accounts (FSAs) allow employees to tax defer, via payroll deduction, an amount that can be used to offset qualified expenses for medical care or dependent care. An FSA may be viewed as a "use it or lose it" benefit because it presents a risk to the program participant who does not accurately calculate the amount of unpaid medical or dependent care expenses that will be incurred in the year ahead. The guidelines for medical and dependent care accounts differ slightly. The IRS allows employers to determine the maximum amount that employees may defer for medical spending purposes. Employers tend to be conservative with setting the maximum because an employee can submit expenses at any time in the plan year and the employer must reimburse the employee regardless of the amount that has been deferred already. For example, an employer could elect to have $5,000 as the maximum annual limit for a health FSA. A participating employee who elected to defer the maximum could present the employer with receipts that totaled to $5,000 in January and then quit in February—long before the maximum has been deducted from the employee's paychecks. Because of this risk, employers should carefully consider their likely exposure when determining the maximum deferral allowed.

The IRS has defined guidelines for what is considered a qualified expense (e.g., many cosmetic procedures are not qualified) and has allowed employers to decide whether or not to allow reimbursements for the cost of over-the-counter products. More and more employers are contracting with companies that provide an FSA "debit card" that can be used for qualified expenses. This method typically allows the employer to offer reimbursement of medical expenses, including for over-the-counter products, without requiring cumbersome paper processing and the determination of a qualifying expense by a benefits staff member. Unlike medical FSAs, where the maximum amount of deferred income is determined by the employer, the maximum for dependent care FSAs is determined by the IRS. Current regulations allow $5,000 per household. Unlike for a medical spending account, the employee can only be reimbursed for expenses up to the amount that has actually been tax-deferred via payroll.

Medical and dependent care FSAs are popular with employers because a lowered taxable wage base means less FICA tax paid by both employer and employee. Further, an FSA's use-it-or-lose-it provision means that the employer can keep the funds that are deferred but are not processed for reimbursement. Employers can charge administrative fees for allowing staff to use FSAs, and this is one way to offset the costs of processing.

Long-term disability (LTD) insurance is considered a welfare benefit because it is designed to provide employees with income in the event they become disabled and cannot work. Because of the nature of healthcare work, healthcare employees have a higher risk of disability than workers in many other industries; thus, providing this benefit may provide a competitive advantage for a healthcare organization. Physicians and nurses specifically ask about LTD coverage when comparing benefit packages between healthcare organizations.

A costly manner of providing LTD insurance is through a specialty-specific plan. This is particularly popular among physicians because the definition of a disability is that the injured person can no longer perform the duties of the specialty that the person was practicing at the time of the injury. Thus, under this definition, a surgeon who can no longer see clearly enough to perform surgery is considered disabled and as such can collect disability pay to supplement other incomes—say, as a general practitioner. While popular with employees, specialty-specific plans are very costly, and few insurers even offer them as an option.

LTD insurance typically becomes active after an employee has been unable to work for 180 days or more; however, this feature of the plan can be decided by the employer, and some have determined that 90 days is the "elimination period." The 90-day period is more beneficial to the employee because the waiting period for eligibility is shorter. Most healthcare organizations will likely agree that LTD insurance, unlike health insurance, is too risky to self-insure because of the risk pool it requires. Healthcare employees are faced with physically demanding work and are often prone to injury as well as accidental exposure to diseases and infections. But by being such a risk, LTD insurance is an attractive provision to include in a comprehensive benefits program for healthcare staff.

LTD insurance is frequently bundled with other plans that cover sickness and disability, such as paid time off, sick time accruals, and short-term disability, giving employees more coverage options in the first 90 to 180 days of disability. An organization can choose to report the amount of premiums paid on behalf of employees for LTD insurance as a taxable fringe benefit. The advantage to the employee is that in the event of disability, the income received is not taxed, and not withholding taxes means that the disability income is closer in amount to the predisability pay.

Short-term disability insurance is an optional benefit for which the employee must pay—either for the entire cost or a significant portion of the premium. This insurance may also be an employer-paid benefit (usually in conjunction with paid-time-off benefits), where the benefits are determined according to employee tenure and salary level. With short-term disability insurance, an employee is covered from the time the illness, condition, or disability starts to the time that the eligibility period for long-term disability has been satisfied. Preexisting conditions may be taken into consideration in the approval process to enroll in this type of insurance. Most plans provide 50 percent to 60 percent of salary to those who receive short-term disability.

Long-term care (LTC) insurance usually covers the cost of nursing home, home care, and assisted living. This insurance has become an attractive benefit as baby boomers face decisions about how to care for their parents and plan for their own future. LTC insurance can include a daily allowance for care at a nursing or assisted living facility as well as in-home care. Many plans allow employees to buy inflation protection and extend coverage beyond their employment.

Life insurance is frequently a base benefit offered by employers in all industries. Term group life insurance allows employers to leverage the size of their organization to purchase a more affordable plan. Although all staff who meet eligibility requirements are offered this group insurance, they are no longer covered once they leave the organization. An attractive feature of an employee-sponsored life insurance plan is its portability—that is, an employee's ability to purchase it at the group rate even after he or she resigns. Such portability is offered through a universal life insurance program, which is more expensive for the employer because its benefits extend beyond employment.

Regardless of the type of life insurance offered, the employer must adhere to current IRS regulations that require that the imputed value of policies in excess of $50,000 be calculated and reported to employees as a taxable fringe benefit. The imputed value is actuarially determined; it is not just the cost of the premiums paid by the employer for a policy with a value that is worth more than $50,000. An employer's experience rating as well as actuarial analysis of the demographics of the employee population covered can determine the cost of the plan. The employer decides the amount of the life insurance. Some companies prefer a tiered approach, where the amount is flat and is based on the employee's position level; others base the amount on the employee's salary—for example, the annual salary multiplied by two.

Supplemental life insurance is an optional benefit that many companies allow employees to purchase on behalf of their spouses and children. The ability to buy supplemental insurance at a group rate can be an attractive benefit for some employees. Again, however, portable policies are typically viewed more favorably because the employee can convert an employer-sponsored plan into an individual plan upon termination or resignation from the company. Table 12.4 gives brief definitions of the common types of group life insurance.

Insurance	What Is It?
Term	Covers all benefited employees, provided as a flat amount or multiple of salary from the date of eligibility through the length of employment
Supplemental term	May be purchased by employees to cover themselves, their spouse, and/or their dependent children
Paid up	Life coverage is paid in such a way that all or part of the coverage is fully paid up when the employee retires; as the premium is paid, the amounts of group term coverage are decreased as paid-up amount increases; this type is not commonly used anymore
Permanent	Accrues a cash value over time
Ordinary	Converts to permanent life insurance as the employee contributes to the policy over his or her employment
Variable	Premiums are level over time, but the benefits relate to the value of the assets that are behind the contract at the time the benefits are made payable
Universal	Provides both a term amount of coverage and an accumulating cash value with flexible premium amounts and timing schedules
Variable universal	Provides a guaranteed death benefit with the flexibility of universal premium schedules and the additional investment value of the assets of a variable life insurance policy
Corporate owned	Permanent life insurance purchased for key executives but owned by the organization; at the time of the insured's death, the employer will take the value of what was paid to the policy in premiums and then pay a death benefit to the executive's beneficiaries
Split dollar	Varying forms of permanent life insurance that may be purchased on key executives or company owners; these two parties split both the premium payments and/or the death benefit

TABLE 12.4

Types of Group Life Insurance Plans

Retirement Plans   A retirement plan is often a fundamental cornerstone of a comprehensive benefits plan. The type of plan offered and the amount that the employer contributes to a retirement account can be a valuable recruitment tool. Further, careful plan design can create incentives that will assist retention strategies. Many organizations provide a base contribution to such plans and offer a vehicle for employees to save for their own retirement. The two main types of retirement plans are *defined contribution* and *defined benefit*. Table 12.5 enumerates the differences between these two types and also presents a hybrid of the two.

The IRS further categorizes a retirement plan as either a qualified retirement plan or a nonqualified retirement plan. A *qualified retirement plan* has strict eligibility and vesting requirements and strict taxable limits. For example, at least 70 percent of employees who are not highly compensated must be eligible to participate in a qualified plan. To that end, plans that are covered by ERISA must undergo periodic nondiscrimination testing to ensure that this requirement is met. Qualified retirement plans receive more tax benefits, and typically the employee and employer are not taxed until the time a distribution is made. Most qualified plans allow employees to withdraw monies for "hardships" such as loss of home, college education for children, or excessive medical bills. The employee is taxed for a hardship withdrawal and is charged a penalty for early (before retirement age) withdrawal. *Nonqualified retirement plans* are typically designed to meet the needs of key executives and are not subject to as many government regulations. This condition allows nonqualified plans to exceed some of the limits of qualified plans. Because nonqualified plans do not come with as many restrictions, they are perceived as carrying a risk of forfeiture as creditors may attach to the plan assets.

With *defined contribution plans,* the employer contributes an amount to an employee's individual retirement account. The employer determines the rate of this contribution and has discretion over the methodology to calculate this rate. Contribution amounts can vary and may be based on such factors as salary, years of service, or even a combination of age and years of service. Using age and years of service as a basis for contribution can help attract mid-career employees, because the employer can contribute more to their accounts than to the plans of newer and younger staff for whom retirement may not be as important at this stage in their lives.

In addition, the employer can choose the vendor companies and may approve and restrict investment options for employees within these choices. Employees then determine which vendor to use and the allocation of investments they desire (e.g., maximum risk, low risk). The amount that an employee receives upon retirement is dependent on the value that the employee initially established, continually managed, and grew over the years. The IRS determines the limits on the maximum allowable employer contributions, and these limits are adjusted annually.

TABLE 12.5 Categories of Retirement Plans

Retirement Plan	What Is It?	Types	Advantages	Disadvantages
Defined benefit	Provides a retirement benefit payable to the employee upon attainment of age and years of service, based on a percentage of salary during working years; usually payable monthly for the lifetime of retiree and/or spouse	Final average salary; career average salary; dollars times years of service	• Benefits based on years on the job, encouraging long-term service • Benefits based on salary, usually at the highest level	• Not as portable • Cannot borrow against the plan • Assets not directly allocated to the participant until retirement • Employer must fund account based on future amounts payable • Payable to retiree in either qualified joint and survivor annuity or a life annuity
Defined contribution	Employer provides a contribution to an account based on the employee's current salary/ earnings, and employee can draw on the account after retirement with reduced tax liability	Profit sharing (401k, 401a); employee stock option plans; money purchase plans; tax-deferred savings	• Employee generally allowed to direct the investments • Assets are allocated to employee such that balance is available at any time • At end of employment, assets are transferable to other accounts • Can be paid out in lump sum or in installments over a period of time	• Final balance in account is based on the performance of the market and the selected investments • No guaranteed benefits
Hybrid	Plans that have aspects of both defined benefits and defined contribution	Cash balance; floor offset; pension equity	Balance in account is available to employee	• Complex and not easily understood • Although the account "balance" is available, it may not be in real dollars but may be an actuarially estimated value

Defined benefit plans are group plans, not individual accounts. The contribution amount the employer must make to such a plan is actuarially determined based on the number of participants and their ages, salaries, and projected retirement dates. In theory, the funds contributed to a defined benefits plan should be sufficient to fund all retirees each year. Upon retirement, the actual monetary benefit that the employee receives is determined formulaically and is based on the employee's years of service and salary preceding retirement. Many state-sponsored retirement plans are defined benefit plans. Other benefits of employment may continue with the payment of a cash benefit.

Tax-deferred plans are savings plans that allow staff to contribute to their own retirement. Deferred compensation results in a reduced tax liability for both the employer and the employee, thus making them popular aspects of retirement plan design. Many organizations encourage employees to participate in tax-deferred plans by contributing a "match" to their retirement account.

Recent media coverage has touted the advantage of Roth 401K, Roth 403B, and other nonqualified salary deferral options. Participation by employees and/or employers in nonqualified plans should include research into their potential impacts. The total amount that can be deferred is determined by the IRS and varies annually. Further, the IRS determines the maximum allowable contributions and maximum salary (i.e., $230,000 in 2008) on which not-for-profit companies can contribute (IRS 2008). If an employer offers multiple options, it must consider the total of all contributions. Limits are set based on aggregation of all plans offered and the actual amount of contribution by plan.

Other Voluntary Benefits

Other voluntary benefits may include programs that are offered through the employer that require participating employees to pay for the premiums. These can include benefits such as auto, home, or pet insurance; cancer or other specific disease coverage; supplemental hospitalization and disability payments; will preparation; and concierge services. Many healthcare organizations also offer staff uniform allowances, extensive educational and professional growth opportunities, and tuition reimbursement. Further, with a healthcare workforce that is predominantly female, organizations should consider on-site child care, a benefit offer that can make a health system more competitive from a recruitment and retention standpoint. Assistance with adult day care is another optional benefit that employers are considering.

Perquisites are benefits that may be offered to executives. Such "perks" may include car allowances, cell phones, pagers, personal digital assistants (e.g., a Blackberry), club memberships, and equipment for the home office. Other executive-level benefits may include cash bonuses and awards, stock options, and severance packages for full or early termination of a contract. Many of these benefits are taxable, and organizations should review their tax implications carefully.

Designing a Benefits Plan

Many factors must be considered when designing a benefits structure that meets the needs of the organization, including generational differences, demographics, and organizational budget.

As mentioned earlier, in the current U.S. work environment, more employees from different generations are working side by side than ever before. With such a mixture of employees, employers must be aware of various generational differences when designing a benefits package. For example, baby boomers may be interested in retirement plans and life insurance, whereas Generation Xers may value paid time off and frequent bonuses. An organization can learn these differences or preferences by using methods such as analyzing market data and garnering employee input through opinion surveys or suggestion boxes.

The demographics of the employee population can be a key determinant in benefits package design. For example, because the registered nurse (RN) workforce is predominantly female, the employer can find out the ages of these nurses. By analyzing the age, the employer can then determine whether programs such as prenatal care or annual mammograms drive healthcare costs and, if so, can explore more cost-effective ways to deliver these services to its RN workforce.

Benefits designers should be knowledgeable of the budget that has been allocated for the benefits program so that they can plan accordingly or find possible funding sources. Again, a well-rounded and comprehensive benefits program can help to attract and retain employees in a competitive market, so it must be well designed and cost effective.

An employee is most typically aware of and concerned about the insurance premiums he or she has to pay out-of-pocket and the annual increases in such a deduction. Many employers pass the cost increases to employees by raising the amount deducted from employees for health insurance coverage. This cost-shifting can cause controversy if the employees are paying more than the employer or if the rate of salary raises does not absorb the cost of the benefit increases. Cost-containment strategies could range from raising out-of-pocket expenses for those who do not use the healthcare organization's facilities and providers to hiking up copayments and deductibles. Another effective cost-control strategy is to provide employees an incentive to waive coverage if they can show proof of coverage through their spouse or if they can arrange for retiree health coverage from a former employer. As discussed earlier, employers often outsource certain benefits programs such as pharmacy or mental health coverage. The option to outsource all benefits administration may be another cost-saving option. However, note that with this option the employer may lose the ability to customize the benefits package for its employees and encounter employee dissatisfaction if the customer service provided by the benefits administrator is less than ideal.

Another cost-control strategy is to use cafeteria plans or Section 125 plans, named after the section in the Internal Revenue Services Code that authorizes this method. These plans are popular with employers and employees alike. Employees can elect to pay through payroll deductions for certain qualifying costs on a pretax basis. Examples of qualifying costs include but are not limited to insurance premiums, certain medical expenses not covered by the employer, and expenses associated with dependent care. Also, employees can reduce their overall tax liability and thus increase their take-home pay. The advantage of a cafeteria plan for employers is that the employer match to FICA taxes is reduced and thus can save them large amounts of money. In addition, some states reduce the employer's liability for Workers' Compensation.

In designing a benefits program, employers may choose to self-insure certain benefits rather than fully insure with a third party. *Self-insurance* means that the employer takes the risk to appropriately budget, underwrite, and administer a customized benefit rather than contract for a standard plan. A self-insured plan typically allows the employer greater flexibility in plan design. Self-insured health and dental plans can be structured to provide employees with incentives to seek care for themselves and their families at the facilities of the healthcare organization. If an organization chooses to self-insure, contracting with a third party for stop-loss insurance is a wise move. *Stop-loss insurance* mitigates the risk to the employer in the event that there are large claims in a given plan year. For example, if the employer purchases $200,000 of stop-loss insurance, then that amount is the most that the employer will pay for a given claim; all costs beyond this stop-loss amount is then absorbed by the insurance vendor. Another form of stop-loss insurance is aggregate stop loss, which covers the claims cost that exceed a certain percentage of the underwriter's projected claims costs for the plan year. This is typically priced at 125 percent or 150 percent of the projected claims. An aggregate stop-loss insurance protects an employer not only from a catastrophic claim for a single participant but also from circumstances that result in multiple large claims that accumulate in excess of the aggregate stop-loss level. These tactics help employers hedge against unanticipated large claims and can significantly reduce the amount of actual claims costs as well as administrative fees associated with a self-insured plan.

Managerial Implications

Given the complexities, legalities, and fiduciary requirements associated with all of the benefits described in this chapter, assigning experienced and qualified benefits professionals to the task of designing (or assisting in) a benefits program is advisable. In particular, individuals who are certified employee benefits specialists should be used as they are extremely valuable to this process. Experienced benefits professionals are familiar with the requirements for accounting, audits, tax filing, and other implications of benefits administration.

Further, it is helpful to have the benefits staff collaborate with the budget staff so that accurate projections of changes in plan designs or premiums can be reflected in the organizational budget.

Communication is also key to the administration of a successful benefits plan. Plan administrators should use every opportunity to keep employees abreast of benefits offered. For example, employers should provide employees with regular information and updates about their total compensation, including the value of employer-sponsored benefits and salaries. During open enrollment periods, the employer must circulate detailed information because this is an opportune time to explain the benefits structure. Also, employers should always include a disclaimer that employer-sponsored benefits are subject to change so that staff understand the possibility that some benefits may be eliminated or reduced in the future, based on economic or other operational exigencies. See Table 12.6 for a listing of resources related to employee benefits.

TABLE 12.6 Resources for Additional Information on Employee Benefits

Who?	Where?	What?
U.S. Department of Labor	www.dol.gov/ebsa	Guidance and recent changes in labor laws and regulations as they pertain to employer-sponsored pensions, health plans, and other employee benefits
Internal Revenue Service		
Forms and publications	www.irs.gov/formspubs/index.html	Quick access to all published forms and publications of the IRS; includes searchable database by topic or publication number
Frequently asked questions	www.irs.gov/faqs/index.html	General questions and answers regarding tax regulations; includes searchable database by category or keyword
Federal Register	www.gpoaccess.gov/fr/index.html	Official daily publication for rules, proposed rules, and notices of federal agencies and organizations as well as executive orders and other presidential documents; includes an extensive search capability

(Continued)

TABLE 12.6 Continued

Who?	Where?	What?
Pension Benefit Guaranty Corporation	www.pbgc.gov	Federal corporation created by the Employee Retirement Income Security Act of 1974, which protects the pensions of nearly 44 million U.S. workers and retirees in 30,330 private, single-employer, and multi-employer defined benefit pension plans
Centers for Medicare & Medicaid Services	www.cms.hhs.gov	Access to research, guidance, statistics, resources, and tools related to Medicare, Medicaid, and SCHIP* programs sponsored by the federal government
International Foundation of Employee Benefit Plans	www.ifebp.org	A nonprofit organization dedicated to being a leading objective and independent global source of employee benefits, compensation, and financial literacy education and information in the United States and Canada
Benefitnews	www.benefitnews.com	Comprehensive, high-quality news on the benefits industry; also publishes a weekly magazine called *The Employee Benefit News*
Benefits Link	benefitslink.com/index.html	Portal to news, analysis, opinions, and government documents about employee benefit plans

*SCHIP: State Children's Health Insurance Program

Summary

In the competitive healthcare arena, employers are challenged to offer as comprehensive a benefits package as possible that will attract and retain healthcare workers at all stages of their careers. Employers are further challenged to provide these benefits in a cost-effective manner with careful consideration to designing a structure that will meet the needs of their employees. Attention must be paid to the complex federal guidelines that govern many benefits programs so that compliance standards and fiduciary responsibility are met.

Discussion Questions

1. Describe the concept of total compensation. Why is it important?
2. How did the Social Security Act change the way retirement benefits were viewed?
3. In designing a benefits plan, what are the most important considerations for an employer?
4. Some industries are cutting back on benefits because of globalization and global competitiveness. Will globalization affect benefits offered in healthcare organizations, or is the benefits structure in healthcare insulated from these global pressures?
5. Employers are finding it more difficult to support health insurance coverage as a benefit as it has become more costly than the tax savings for offering it. Is employer-based health insurance on its way out, and if so, is it more or less practical to maintain it as a benefit in a healthcare organization?

Experiential Exercise

The purpose of this exercise is to give readers an opportunity to analyze the benefits provided by a healthcare organization. Visit the human resources department of a local hospital, and answer the following questions:

1. How many total employees are in the department, and how many are assigned to handle benefits administration? How many of the staff are certified employee benefits specialists?
2. How are benefits communicated to employees at this hospital?
3. What benefits are offered to full-time, part-time, and hourly employees?
4. Do physicians receive the same benefits as other employees?
5. What perquisites are offered to executives?
6. Are there any benefits that the organization is considering but are not currently being offered? If yes, what are they and how were they identified? If no, what benefits may be added if the organization can afford to do so?

Begin this exercise by visiting the website (or the human resources web page) of the organization to see how much benefits information is posted online. After visiting the department, write a summary of what was found. In writing up the summary, make an assessment of how comprehensive the benefits package is for employees and how well it is communicated.

References

Ahlrichs, N. S. 2002. *Competing for Talent: Key Recruitment and Retention Strategies for Becoming an Employer of Choice.* Mountain View, CA: Davies-Black Publishing.

American College of Healthcare Executives (ACHE). 2005. "Top Issues Confronting Hospital CEOs: 2005." [Online information; retrieved 3/08.] www.ache.org/PUBS/Releases/123005_Hospital_CEO. pdf.

American Nurses Credentialing Center (ANCC). 2007. "Magnet Recognition Program." [Online information; retrieved 3/08.] www.nursecredentialing.org/magnet/forces.htm.

Bragg, D., and K. Vermoch. 2003. *Workplace of Choice Benchmarking Project Report.* Oakbrook, IL: University HealthSystem Consortium.

Bridgeford, L. 2007. "Snack Attack: Bringing Healthful Snacks to the Workplace." *Employee Benefits News,* April.

Cunningham, R., III, and R. M. Cunningham, Jr. 1997. *The Blues: A History of the Blue Cross and Blue Shield System.* DeKalb, IL: Northern Illinois University Press.

Employee Benefit Research Institute (EBRI). 2007. *EBRI Databook on Employee Benefits,* Online Edition. [Online information; retrieved 3/08.] www.ebri.org.

Evans, M. 2006. "What Really Matters Most." *Modern Healthcare* 36 (2): 8–9, 16.

Gresham, L. 2007. "Manufacturer Adopts Tangerine-Wellness Incentive-based Program to Cut Health Care Costs by 10%." *Employee Benefits News,* April.

Internal Revenue Service (IRS). 2008. "IRS Announces Plan Limitations for 2008." [Online information; retrieved 3/08.] www.irs.gov/newsroom/article/0,,id=174873,00.html.

Smolkin, S. 2007. "Wellness Without Borders: Manufacturer Implements Wellness Programs for Its US, Canadian Staff." *Employee Benefits News,* May.

Social Security Online. 2007. [Online information; retrieved 3/08.] www.socialsecurity.gov/OACT/COLA/cbb.html#Series.

Starr, P. 1982. *The Social Transformation of American Medicine.* New York: Basic Books, Inc.

University HealthSystem Consortium. 2005. *Member Satisfaction Survey, 2004–2005.* Oakbrook, IL: University HealthSystem Consortium.

U.S. Chamber of Commerce. 2006. *Employee Benefits Study.* Washington, DC: U.S. Chamber of Commerce.

U.S. Department of Labor. 2007a. "Benefits: Workers Compensation Programs." [Online information; retrieved 3/08.] www.dol.gov/compliance/topics/benefits-comp.htm.

———. 2007b. "Compliance Assistance: Family and Medical Leave Act." [Online information; retrieved 3/08.] www.dol.gov/esa/whd/fmla/.

HEALTH SAFETY AND PREPAREDNESS

William Gentry

Learning Objectives

After completing this chapter, the reader should be able to

- identify the resources required to develop and maintain a safe and prepared workplace,
- understand the key roles and steps in developing a safe workplace,
- discuss internal and external effects of disasters on the workplace, and
- define how a workplace can recover from an unsafe or a disaster event.

Introduction

In 2006, general medical and surgical hospitals reported more injuries and illnesses than any other organization—more than 264,300 cases (Bureau of Labor Statistics 2007). That is the bad news. The good news is that since 2005 the number and incidence rate of injuries for hospitals have decreased by 3 percent and 5 percent, respectively. Even though *workplace injuries* have been trending down since 2003 and workplace safety awareness, technology improvements, and management commitment have all increased, *disaster-related injuries* and facility damage have risen. The reason is that man-made and natural disasters have been growing in scale, number, and impact. Population density has also been noted in and around high-hazard zones, and the number of healthcare institutions that serve these populations has risen.

    Healthcare institutions are not held to the same standard of safety and preparedness as are other businesses. Rightly or wrongly, the public perceives that healthcare institutions should not only be injury-free and mistake-free but also disaster resistant. This expectation challenges safety and preparedness work within a healthcare environment, because every consequence of adverse events cannot be anticipated. Nevertheless, steps can be taken to decrease the negative impact of a workplace event. Two key steps discussed in this chapter are *hazard analysis* and *proper planning*. Neither is normally budgeted for, and both are labor intensive. So why should we expend the money and energy on these steps? The answer is fundamental: This investment pays big dividends in lives saved, injuries prevented, and costs avoided.

Hazard Analysis for a Healthy and Safe Workplace

A healthy workplace tends to be a safe workplace where fewer employee days are lost, less employment turnover is experienced, and the workplace attitude is more positive. Employees also reward management's investment in a healthy workplace with increased output. Employee health can be influenced by the institution's willingness to provide a suitable healthy and safe workplace, a positive cultural and social environment, and programs that promote healthy lifestyle practices (see Table 13.1)

Having a healthy work environment is a necessary, but not a sufficient, condition for a safe and prepared workplace. Healthcare workers face multiple hazards on the job, including contamination threats, back injuries, allergies, patient demands, violence, and stress. Workplace safety is the responsibility of everyone: Employees should be safety conscious, and every manager should promote and reward safety practices. Efforts must be consistent from management to employees, full time and part time. In other words, a safe workplace is a true team effort that requires time, effort, and commitment.

One way that healthcare institutions can make their facilities safer is to complete a job hazard analysis recommended by the Occupational Safety and Health Administration (OSHA 2002). OSHA is a federal agency that focuses solely on workplace safety and preparedness. Its mission is to help industries prevent workplace injuries and illnesses and comply with the Occupational Safety and Health Act.

A job hazard analysis consists of identifying workplace hazards and then prioritizing the hazardous jobs (see Figure 13.1).

After identifying hazardous jobs and conditions, institutions should develop a step-by-step workplace safety program. Many resources for program development for biological, chemical, physical, and stress-related hazards are available through OSHA, the Centers for Disease Control and Prevention, and the National Institute for Occupational Safety and Health (2007).

In general, healthcare institutions that have successful safety programs do the following:

- Screen prospective employees for prior safety issues; driving records; and, if allowed, drug use.
- Maintain work areas that are clean, free of clutter, and not littered with non-work-related materials.

Health and Safety Factors	Institutional Programs	**TABLE 13.1**
Noise level	On-site medical services	Environmental Workplace Factors and Institutional Programs to Mitigate Them
Work design	Return-to-work initiatives	
Air quality	Daily/weekly/monthly e-mail tips	
Safe lifting	Health and safety fairs	
Ergonomics	Medical surveillance programs	
Employee violence	Disability case management	
Toxic substances	Smoke-free workplace	
Physical demands	Self-defense classes	
Work pace		
Safety guidelines		

Cultural and Social Factors

Balance between work and family	Clear and accurate job descriptions
Employee satisfaction	Time management
Staff involvement in decision making	Management training
Workplace equity	Overtime limit
Flex time	Motivational speakers
Positive supervisor communication and feedback	Breaks outside in natural light
Staff morale	
Peer communication	
Employee recognition	
Employee training and development	
Social atmosphere	

Lifestyle Practices Factors

Smoking cessation	Health and safety fairs
Hygiene	Relaxation training
Healthy weight	Substance abuse programs
Stress management	Active living challenges
Healthy eating	Healthy cooking programs
Coping with shift work	Anger management
Physical activities	
Healthy pregnancy	
Women's health issues	
Alcohol and drug use	

SOURCE: Grey Bruce Health Unit (2007)

- Manage safety by having managers walk around to directly observe workplace practices and to listen to employee concerns about and ideas for safety.
- Expect employees to work safely, instead of constantly trying to catch and punish them for minor infractions.

FIGURE 13.1

Job Hazard
Analysis

Identifying Workplace Hazards

- What can go wrong?
- What are the consequences?
- How could the hazard arise?
- What are contributing factors?
- How likely is it that the hazard will occur?

Priorities for a Job Hazard Analysis

- Jobs with the highest rates of injury or illness
- Jobs with the potential to cause severe or disabling injuries or illness, even if there is no history of previous accidents
- Jobs in which one simple human error could lead to a severe accident or injury
- Jobs that are new to your operation or have undergone changes in processes and procedures
- Jobs that are complex enough to require written instructions

SOURCE: Occupational Safety and Health Administration (2002)

- Provide incentives for workplace safety training certifications, and require managers to attend safety classes with employees.
- Incorporate a safety message, update, or success story into all staff meetings, engendering a proactive safety environment that is openly monitored and discussed by all employees.

Leadership must not only educate the entire workforce on the organization's safety program but must also lead by example, adhering consistently to all safety goals and procedures. Leaders of all levels should view safety as an investment in the workplace that will reduce employee time loss, minimize insurance claims, and increase productivity and morale.

Preparedness for Workplace Disasters

For a healthcare institution, a disaster is any unplanned event that can cause deaths or significant injuries to employees, patients, or the community. It can also be any event that shuts down a facility, disrupts operations, causes physical or environmental damage, or threatens the facility's financial standing or public image (Federal Emergency Management Agency 1993). Disasters can affect the healthcare workplace in two ways: (1) a disaster that affects the facility itself, and (2) a disaster that affects the availability of workers but does not affect the facility. A healthcare organization must be prepared for each of these scenarios.

Healthcare workers do not live within an insular system, and they may be directly and personally affected when a disaster strikes. Adequate staff contingency planning should take this fact into account. Also, workers and their families may be among the victims. For example, after the 2004 tsunami in Indonesia, the provincial health department of the Banda Aceh region reported that only 80 of its 400 workers were accounted for and that approximately 150 of its physicians were missing (Krajewski, Sztajnkrycer, and Báez 2005). In other words, in the aftermath of a disaster, the healthcare facility may remain intact, but its staff may be substantially depleted.

A *planning safety team* may be the best in assessing disaster preparedness in healthcare organizations. However, for a preparedness initiative, funding and staffing are usually inadequate or a luxury for many, except larger institutions. According to the Federal Emergency Management Agency (1993), a planning safety team approach may do the following:

- Encourage awareness and employee investment in the process.
- Increase the amount of time and energy that participants are willing to give.
- Enhance the visibility and stature of the planning process.
- Provide a broad perspective on the issues.

The planning safety team should plan for two distinct types of disasters: (1) a disaster that occurs within the facility that causes a disruption to normal operations, and (2) a disaster that occurs in the community that results in mass casualty events and thus a surge in demand over normal operations. For disasters that are contained in the facility, plans should focus on getting the facility back up and running as safely and expeditiously as possible—action that is often referred to as *business continuity planning*. The key to this planning is to provide a framework of steps that bring the institution back up to service whether or not it is physically intact or is relocated to an alternate site. The main goal of business continuity planning is to provide temporary infrastructure, information technology functions, customer service, and staffing if access to the original office is not possible. For disasters that occur in the community, plans should focus on providing optimum resources and services to the victims while still maintaining current services—action that is referred to as *surge capability*.

Creating an event list with the assistance of the local emergency management office helps guide preparedness planning. Here is an example of a detailed disaster event list:

- Drought/water shortage
- Earthquake
- Fire
- Flood
- Hazardous material spill
- Heat

- Hurricane
- Ice/snow
- Pandemic
- Severe weather
- Staffing shortage
- Terrorism
- Tornado
- Transportation accident
- Utility outage
- Workplace violence

After creating a potential disaster list, managers can then plan how to continue core operations for each type of event on the list. The plan should address the following functions (Federal Emergency Management Agency 1993):

- Administration and logistics
- Communications
- Community outreach
- Direction and control
- Life safety
- Property protection
- Recovery and restoration

These functions are the foundation for the emergency procedures that the facility will follow to protect personnel and equipment and to resume operations. Once developed, the disaster operations plan should be reviewed by the local emergency management office and the institution's legal authority and then approved by the board or chief executive officer. The plan should also be exercised, reviewed annually, and evaluated after actual implementation and then updated by the planning safety team.

Healthcare institutions are not fortresses that are built to stand against all disasters. That myth was dispelled after Hurricane Katrina hit the Gulf Coast, leaving facilities damaged, flooded, and powerless and in some cases while patients and other evacuees were still in the building. Hospitals are not designated as shelters, but public perception is different, forcing facilities to be the best-prepared and best-designed system in the community in the event of a catastrophe. Shelter or not, the public will come, and hospitals need current and comprehensive plans to meet this expectation.

A significant part of organizational preparedness is training all staff on the contents and procedures of the plan. A preparedness program should address individual preparedness as well, emphasizing the point that disaster planning should begin at home. An individual preparedness plan should include a three-day, self-sustaining family kit that includes food, supplies, medicines, and necessary equipment such as a portable radio. Such a plan should also incorporate the needs of specific family members, such as children, elders, and disabled or ill family, as well as pets.

Safety and Preparedness Requirements

Healthcare institutions have a moral and civic duty to promote safety and to work toward disaster resiliency. The public believes that, even in the face of disasters, hospitals will always remain open, their employees will always make it to work, and all services (even scheduled appointments) will always be available. In addition to its moral and civic responsibilities, an institution has to meet regulatory and credentialing requirements that address workplace safety and disaster preparedness. Each healthcare profession has developed workplace safety programs and instituted some disaster initiatives to meet compliance requirements, and OSHA and the Joint Commission have also established compliance regulations most relevant to healthcare organizations.

OSHA's (2002) healthcare safety standards are a recognized subset of the regulations that address general issues in healthcare operations and delivery. OSHA's standards address the following areas:

- Hazard communication
- Bloodborne pathogens
- Ionizing radiation
- Exit routes
- Electrical
- Emergency action plan
- Fire safety
- Medical and first aid
- Personal protective equipment
- Ergonomics, workplace violence, and other workplace issues

In addition to establishing these subset standards, OSHA recognizes that specific healthcare entities require close guidance, including hospitals, laboratories, medical and dental offices, and nursing homes and personal care facilities. OSHA compliance is a daunting task at first glance. However, OSHA has made the process easier by creating step-by-step guidelines on how to recognize compliance requirements, how to build a compliance program, and how to work through compliance inspections. Some states also have an OSHA-approved program—a program that is subject to state occupational safety and health regulations, which may include more stringent or supplemental rules than those required by the federal agency. Also, these state programs provide compliance assistance services.

Even though most of OSHA's site visits or reviews are performed after a reported incident, the agency is becoming more proactive. OSHA works with healthcare institutions in developing a compliance program, conducts site visits (making recommendations only), and provides a wealth of tools in the form of documents and its website. While compliance enforcement is still its key mission, OSHA also provides noncompliance-related visits and assistance because it realizes that being proactive about safety will reduce the number of enforcement issues yearly.

The other organization that provides healthcare-safety-related guidance is the Joint Commission, formerly known as the Joint Commission on Accreditation of Healthcare Organizations or JCAHO. An independent, not-for-profit organization, the Joint Commission (2007) evaluates and accredits more than 15,000 U.S.-based healthcare organizations and programs, including hospitals (general, psychiatric, children, rehabilitation), nursing homes, behavioral and mental facilities and services, and hospices, to name a few. As the predominant healthcare accreditation body in the nation, the Joint Commission's certification process is comprehensive and requires compliance with standards in various functional areas such as patient rights, patient treatment, and infection control. Such standards identify performance expectations for activities that affect the safety and quality of the workplace and patient care. Accreditation is maintained through site visits, documentation, and personnel and patient interviews. The Joint Commission has introduced a host of new changes to its system, and the most significant of these are additions to the emergency management standards and the expansion of the survey role of life-safety specialists, who will conduct site visits at large facilities for two days. Also, the Joint Commission is focusing more on hospitals with fewer than 200 beds.

Note the difference between these two organizations: The Joint Commission provides a professional accreditation, while OSHA manages federal workplace safety requirements.

Measuring Workplace Safety and Preparedness

Measurement of a workplace safety and preparedness program is necessary to document not only concerns but successes as well. Managers need confirmation that safety practices are in place, comply with the law at a minimum, and operate effectively. Measurement should include count reports, trending data, observations, and practical application reviews (e.g., demonstrations, drills). Health and safety performance measurement should seek to answer questions such as the following (Health and Safety Executive 2001):

- Where is the institution now relative to its overall health and safety aims and objectives?
- Where is the institution now in controlling hazards and risks?
- How does the institution compare with others?
- Is the institution getting better or worse over time?

- Is the institutional management of health and safety effective (i.e., are we doing the right things)?
- Is the institutional management of health and safety reliable (i.e., are we doing things right consistently)?
- Is the institutional management of health and safety proportionate to the hazards and risks?
- Is the institutional management of health and safety efficient?
- Is an effective health and safety management system in place across all parts of the organization and being deployed?
- Is the institutional culture supportive of health and safety, particularly in the face of competing demands?

Review of a healthcare institution's safety environment should be conducted quarterly; results should then be developed into an annual safety report. The planning safety team should collect measurement data to construct updated plans, guides, and procedures. Institutions must recognize that no single reliable measure of health and safety performance exists. What is required is a variable approach that provides information on a range of health and safety activities. For example, simply tracking employee illness, injury, and work loss will not provide the overall measurement of a workplace safety program.

Moreover, measuring workplace preparedness is just as important as measuring safety. Preparedness efforts may be measured in drills, exercises, and discussions. Drills and exercises can serve a dual purpose: for measurement and for team building. In addition, measurement considerations should include the use of outside evaluators who can provide an unbiased after-action report. Evaluations and the after-action report should be used by management and the planning safety team to recognize strengths and weaknesses in the institution's preparedness plan.

Summary

A healthy, safe, and prepared workplace is not a naturally occurring phenomenon. It requires both financial and time investment. Healthcare employees are becoming more selective about their working environments as well as their jobs. Workplace safety has required parameters that are monitored at the state and federal levels. Safety requirements, guides, and suggestions are available through federal and state OSHA programs (OSHA 2005).

A healthy and prepared workplace offers many benefits, including fewer employee-days lost, more productivity, and quicker return to normal functionality after a disaster or an emergency event. Health, safety, and preparedness programs begin at the senior management level, are employee driven, and are measured annually. Management's best sources for feedback about the effectiveness of the institution's health, safety, and preparedness efforts are the employees who do the actual day-to-day work. Open communication about these initiatives throughout the institution encourages the creation of comprehensive plans, reveals weaknesses within the system, and results in employee buy-in that in turn strengthens the organizational well-being. Research shows that increasing the stature of workplace health, safety, and preparedness usually produces the following effects (Grey Bruce Health Unit 2007):

- Improvement in workplace morale
- Enhancement of retention and recruitment strategies
- Decrease in benefits costs (e.g., for injury, illness, prescriptions)
- Growth in productivity
- Reduction of absenteeism rates
- Positive impact on the bottom line
- Boost of the corporate image

Healthcare institutions cannot afford to not invest in workplace health, safety, and preparedness. Commitment to, plans for, and reviews of such a program should be ongoing but are especially needed after a major event that causes injuries, fatalities, infrastructure loss, or staffing depletion. Without such an initiative, institutional losses and costs will be higher than the costs of establishing the program.

Discussion Questions

1. What is the public's perception of healthcare institutions as being in a perpetual state of disaster preparedness? How does this view differ from the number of injuries and illnesses reported in hospitals in 2006 (see Bureau of Labor Statistics 2007)?

2. What are the three factors that influence the workplace health and wellness of employees?

3. In addition to workplace preparedness, what other types of preparedness efforts can be promoted at healthcare institutions?

Experiential Exercise

1. The surrounding community of Hospital A has just experienced a debilitating ice storm, with loss of power expected for the next five to seven days. Employees at Hospital A are showing up for work, but they are not alone: Some single parents have brought their children and some have carried along their pets. Still others have come in or have stayed after their shift to have

a warm place to be. How could Hospital A accommodate these groups? If the hospital does not accommodate them, how will it handle or make up for the resulting staff shortage? What steps can Hospital A take in the future to plan for this type of expectation? Look for "win-win" solutions to this challenge.

2. Many of the maintenance staff (who are mostly male) at Hospital B are experiencing back injuries that have caused a shortage of technicians on any given shift. Hospital B recently began staff cutbacks, scheduling no male aids who are trained to assist with patient transfers. What correlations are there between the back injuries and staff cutbacks? What steps can Hospital B take to resolve both issues?

3. Hospital C has made the decision to create a facility emergency plan. Management is considering three options to pursue this decision: (1) have the hospital's safety officer write the plan, (2) form a planning committee to develop the plan, or (3) bring in an experienced contractor to create the plan. Discuss the pros and cons of each option.

4. Hospital D has added a new process to its operations. The hospital has an excellent health and safety record, but its safety officer has just retired. Three weeks after the new process is implemented, employees began complaining of stiff joints, headaches, and tiredness. The timing of such complaints is coinciding with the active flu season. How does Hospital D differentiate between the two possible causes of the symptoms? Is the hospital obligated to pay medical costs associated with any testing? What questions should management ask, and how would management measure the results of its analysis?

References

Bureau of Labor Statistics. 2007. *Workplace Injuries and Illnesses in 2006.* Washington, DC: Government Printing Office.

Federal Emergency Management Agency. 1993. *Emergency Management Guide for Business and Industries.* No. FEMA 141. Washington, DC: Government Printing Office.

Grey Bruce Health Unit. 2007. *A Healthy Workplace Program.* [Online information; retrieved 3/08.] www.publichealthgreybruce.on.ca/WorkplaceWellness/3-Benefits.htm.

Health and Safety Executive. 2001. *A Guide to Measuring Health and Safety Performance.* Suffolk, UK: Health and Safety Executive.

Joint Commission. 2007. *Facts About the Joint Commission.* [Online information; retrieved 3/08.] www.jointcommission.org/AboutUs/joint_commission_facts.htm.

Krajewski, M. J., M. Sztajnkrycer, and A. A. Báez. 2005. "Hospital Disaster Preparedness in the United States: New Issues, New Challenges." *Internet Journal of Rescue and Disaster Medicine* 4 (2). [Online information; retrieved 3/08.] www.ispub.comostia/index.php?xmlFilePath=journals/ijrdm/front.xml.

National Institute for Occupational Safety and Health. 2007. *NIOSH Safety and Health Topic: Health Care Workers.* [Online information; retrieved 3/08.] www.cdc.gov. libproxy.lib.unc.edu/niosh/topics/healthcare/.

Occupational Safety and Health Administration (OSHA). 2002. *Job Hazard Analysis.* No. OSHA 3071. Washington, DC: Government Printing Office.

———. 2005. *Healthcare Facilities Possible Hazards and Solutions: General Solutions.* [Online information; retrieved 3/08.] www.osha.gov.libproxy.lib.unc.edu/SLTC/ healthcarefacilities/recognition.html.

MANAGING WITH ORGANIZED LABOR

Donna Malvey, PhD

Learning Objectives

After completing this chapter, the reader should be able to

- address the relationship of organized labor and management in healthcare,
- distinguish the different phases of the labor relations process,
- describe the evolving role of unions in the healthcare workforce,
- examine legislative and judicial rulings that affect management of organized labor in healthcare settings,
- review emerging healthcare labor trends, and
- consider the potential impact of the Internet on the labor–management relationship.

Introduction

The *labor relations process* occurs when management (as the representative for the employer) and the union (as the exclusive bargaining representative for the employees) jointly determine and administer the rules of the workplace. A *union* is an organization formed by employees for the purpose of acting as a single unit when dealing with management about workplace issues, and hence the term organized labor. Unions are not present in every organization because employees must authorize a union to represent them. Unions typically are viewed as threats by management because they interfere with management's ability to make and implement decisions. Once a union is present, management may no longer unilaterally make decisions about the terms and conditions of work. Instead, management must negotiate these decisions with the union. Similarly, employees may no longer communicate directly with management about work issues but instead must go through the union. Thus, the union functions as a middleman, which is relatively expensive to maintain for both parties. Employees pay union dues, and management incurs additional costs for such things as contract negotiations and any increases in salaries and benefits negotiated by the union (Freeman and Medoff 1984).

In healthcare, because labor costs generally account for 70 percent to 80 percent of expenditures, controlling labor costs is critically important. Thus, even if a union negotiates a minor wage or benefit increase, it will result in a significant increase in total costs. Subsequently, management has a strong incentive to keep unions out of the organization (Scott and Seers 1996). However, given the trends of unionization in healthcare, managers are increasingly forced to work with unions. This chapter examines the phenomenon of healthcare unionization and provides direction for managing with organized labor. In addition, it discusses the possible behaviors and strategies that comprise the labor–management relationship; explains the generic labor relations process of organizing, negotiating, and administering contracts; explores developments in organizing a relatively unorganized healthcare workforce; considers the impact of labor laws, amendments, and rulings on human resources (HR) strategies and goals; and considers the potential impact of the Internet on the labor–management relationship.

Managing with organized labor involves the application and maintenance of a positive labor relations program within the organization. A productive and positive labor–management relationship can only be accomplished through integration with other HR functions. For example, employees expect management to provide environments that are clean and safe from workplace hazards and health-related concerns, such as AIDS and hepatitis B. If management allows the environment to deteriorate, union organizers will focus on these issues (Becker and Rowe 1989; Fennell 1987). In addition, the labor relations process occurs across all levels of the organization and involves all levels of management. Upper-level management will develop objectives and strategies regarding wage rates and staffing ratios while mid-level managers and first-line supervisors will implement these objectives.

Developing strategies and goals to implement a positive labor relations program in healthcare requires an understanding of the generic labor relations process of organizing, negotiating, and administering contracts with a union as well as specific knowledge of emerging healthcare labor trends. A productive and positive labor–management relationship involves compromise by both parties because of the adversarial nature of the relationship. Just because a union has won the right to represent employees does not mean that management has to accept all of its terms. All parties—management, unions, and employees—have a vested interest in the success and survival of the organization; yet they also have opposing or conflicting interests. For example, unions will look toward improving the benefits package for employees, while management, faced with budget cutbacks and declining reimbursements, will have concerns about containing costs. Thus, the challenge for management is working with the union to reconcile differences in a fair and consistent manner.

As Figure 14.1 suggests, the labor–management relationship reflects a continuum of possible behaviors and strategies, ranging from the most

Positive	Neutral	Negative
• Management and union have joint collaboration on the rules of the workplace	• Management and union have a fairly neutral relationship	• Management and union have a mostly adversarial and unstable relationship
• Management and union have a positive relationship, with both parties focusing on the success and survival of the organization	• Management–union relationship is neither oppositional nor supportive	• Contract administration is predominantly oppositional and self-serving
• Management and union proactively respond to external threats	• Management and union focus on maintaining status quo	• Management and union tend to be reactive to external threats

FIGURE 14.1

Ranges of the Labor–Management Relationship in Healthcare

positive or collaborative (in which management and the union share common goals oriented toward the organization's success) to the most negative or oppositional and self-serving. Even if the relationship is neutral and both parties cooperate to maintain the status quo, a variety of factors can cause the relationship to shift in either direction. For instance, restructuring, such as a merger, may create uncertainty for both the union and management and, as a result, may reposition their relationship along the continuum. However, the direction in which the relationship moves will depend largely on the knowledge and understanding of the labor relations process on both sides of the issue.

Overview of Unionization

Union membership has been declining steadily for decades. In the 1950s to 1970s, union membership represented 25 percent to 30 percent of the U.S. workforce. During the 1980s and 1990s, organized labor's influence and bargaining power declined and weakened as the nature of U.S. industries shifted from factories and traditional union strongholds to service and technologies (Fottler et al. 1999). This trend appears to have continued, as evidenced by the fact that organized labor has been unable to make any net gains in membership despite downward pressure on wages, increasing healthcare insurance costs, and outsourcing of service and manufacturing jobs overseas (*Christian Science Monitor* 2004).

Union membership rate has steadily decreased from 20.1 percent in 1983, the first year for which comparable union data are available, to 12 percent in 2006. In 2006, the total number of employees belonging to a union was approximately 15.4 million. Unions appear to be more successful in organizing workers in the public sector than in the private sector and in healthcare rather than in other industries. The union rate for government or public-sector workers has held steady at approximately 36.2 percent since 1983, while the rate for private-industry workers has fallen to 7.4 percent or about half over the same time period. Within the public sector, however, local government workers had the highest union membership rate—41.9 percent. This group reflects several heavily unionized occupations such as teachers, firefighters, and police officers (Bureau of Labor Statistics 2000a, 2000b, 2004, 2006a, 2006b; Scott and Lowery 1994).

The healthcare workforce comprises an estimated 13.1 million workers and represents one of the largest pools of unorganized workers in the United States and a prime target for union organizers. Of the 4.3 million healthcare workers currently employed in hospitals, only 471,000 belong to a union. In addition, just 246,000 of the 5.4 million workers employed in other healthcare sectors, such as nursing homes and clinics, are unionized (Bureau of Labor Statistics 2000b, 2004, 2006a). Furthermore, unions in other healthcare sectors have consistently won a greater percentage of their elections than in the hospital segment or even in other industries (Scott and Seers 1996). Fifteen of the 30 fastest growing occupations are health related, and registered nurses and nursing aides, orderlies, and attendants are projected to experience greater growth during this decade than other health occupations (Hecker 2004). Even though labor surveys indicate that the demand for unions exists, healthcare unions have not yet realized significant membership increases (*Christian Science Monitor* 2004; Kearney 2003). Nevertheless, some labor experts believe that healthcare unions represent one of the few areas in which organized labor has been showing some energy. Healthcare unions are reported to have invested heavily in membership recruitment and helping members gain influence (Evans 2006).

The Labor Relations Process

In an attempt to protect workers' rights to unionize, the U.S. Congress passed the National Labor Relations Act (NLRA) in 1935, which serves as the legal framework for the labor relations process. Although the NLRA has been amended over the years, it remains the only legislation that governs federal labor relations. The law contains significant provisions intended to protect workers' rights to form and join unions and to engage in collective bargaining. The law also defines unfair labor practices, which restrict both unions and employers from interfering with the labor relations process. The NLRA delegates to the National Labor Relations Board (NLRB) the responsibility for overseeing implementation of the NLRA and for investigating and remedying unfair labor practices. NLRB rulemaking occurs on a case-by-case basis.

Key participants in the labor relations process include (1) management officials, who serve as surrogates for the owners or employers of the organization; (2) union officials, who are usually elected by members; (3) the government, which participates through executive, legislative, and judicial branches occurring at federal, state, and local levels; and (4) third-party neutrals such as arbitrators. The process also involves three phases that are equally essential: the recognition phase, the negotiation phase, and the administration phase.

Recognition Phase

During this phase, unions attempt to organize employees and gain representation through either voluntary recognition of the union or a representation election, which certifies that the union has the authority to act on behalf of employees in negotiating a collective bargaining agreement. In rare cases, the NLRB may direct an employer to recognize and bargain with the union if evidence exists that a fair and impartial election would be impossible. During the past two decades, management strategies and tactics have become more aggressive during the recognition phase as management has endeavored to keep unions from becoming the employees' representative. For example, management may institute unfair labor practices such as filing for bankruptcy, illegally firing union supporters, and relocation. Although unions may file grievances with the NLRB over these practices and the use of any illegal or union-busting tactics, legal resolution usually occurs years after the fact and long after union elections have been held. Thus, both unions and management understand that the battle lines are drawn in the recognition phase, and both sides will be fervently engaged in shoring up support.

The desire to unionize is believed to result from three issues: wages, benefits, and employee perceptions about the workplace. Because ascertaining the desires of employees is difficult, management must rely on signals or indicators in the workplace. Table 14.1 summarizes some of the behaviors that may indicate organizing activities or the potential for organizing employees. For example, high turnover of approximately 40 percent characterizes health-care institutions such as hospitals (Swoboda 1999). However, when employees are leaving their jobs for a local competitor, management must investigate the underlying reasons for turnover. Even simple issues, such as an increase in requests for information on policies and procedures, can indicate problems and should not be discounted.

	Increase/	
TABLE 14.1 Warning Indicators for Healthcare Organizations		
Item	*Increase/ Decrease*	*Comment*
Turnover— especially to competitors	Increase	Turnover in healthcare organizations typically is much higher than in organizations in other industries because of enhanced mobility from licensing and standardization; however, if employees are moving to competing organizations in the local area, such movement may indicate dissatisfaction rather than career opportunities
Employee- generated incidents	Increase	Staff members are fighting among themselves; theft or damage to organization's property; insubordination related to routine requests by supervisors
Grievances	Increase	More grievances are being filed with the HR office compared with informal settlements of supervisors and employees
Communication	Decrease	Staff members are reluctant to provide feedback and generally become quiet when management enters the room; suggestion boxes are empty and employees are less willing to avail themselves of the "open door" system or other mechanisms to air dissatisfaction/problems
HR office informational requests	Increase	Employees are interested in policies, procedures, and other matters related to the terms and conditions of employment, and they want this information in writing; verbal responses no longer satisfy them
Off-site meetings	Increase	Employees appear to be congregating more at off-site premises
Grapevine activity	Increase	Rumors increase in number and intensity
Absenteeism and/ or tardiness	Increase	Employees are engaging in union- organizing activities prior to and during work hours

During the recognition phase, the union solicits signed authorization cards that designate the union to act as the employees' collective bargaining representative. When at least 30 percent of employees in the bargaining unit have signed their cards, the union requests the employer to voluntarily recognize the union. Voluntary recognition is rarely granted by employers, however, and occurs less than 2 percent of the time in healthcare organizations. When employers refuse voluntary recognition of the union, the union is then eligible to petition the NLRB for a representation election. In response to the petition, the NLRB verifies the authenticity of the signatures collected by the union, determines the appropriate bargaining unit, and sets a date for a secret-ballot election. Healthcare workers represent a significant number of all workers participating in NLRB elections. In 2005, about 16 percent of the 2,674 NLRB elections held involved healthcare workers, and these workers were more likely to vote for a union compared with all other industries (NLRB 2005).

In recent years, unions have supported legislative efforts that would amend existing labor laws to eliminate secret-ballot elections. Such efforts are perceived to be part of organized labor's strategy to target the union election process itself. Under existing labor law, the period leading up to the election can take several months to a year, during which employers are permitted to contest eligibility of workers to vote in a unit. Subsequent hearings and appeals can further extend the process. Even though it is illegal for employers to intimidate workers during this period, unions allege such tactics. Unions also claim that by the time the election is actually held, workers are too afraid to vote for the union as their representative (Kaira 2005). Although legislative attempts to eliminate secret-ballot elections have been unsuccessful, they reflect the continuing determination of unions to revise the organizing process in their favor.

Bargaining Unit

The NLRB determines which employees are eligible to be in a bargaining unit and thereby eligible to vote in the election. Currently, the NLRB permits a total of eight bargaining units in healthcare settings. The implications of this number and some historical perspective are provided later in this chapter; that section summarizes legislative and judicial rulings. Although the NLRB has modified its criteria over the years, it has not changed its outlook on managerial or supervisory employees, who are ineligible for membership in a bargaining unit. Under a provision of the NLRA (29USCS 152 [11]), an employee is a "supervisor" if the employee has the authority, in the interest of the employer, to engage in specific activities, including responsible direction of other employees, where exercise of such authority requires the use of independent judgment. In a landmark 2006 ruling, the NLRB clarified and set forth guidelines for determining whether an individual is a supervisor under the NLRA. The NLRB ruled that "charge" nurses were supervisors, thereby making them and certain other nurses like them ineligible for bargaining unit representation.

This ruling represents an opportunity to reclassify many nurses as management and thereby potentially decreases the union's ability to recruit new members.

Generally, the union election is scheduled to occur on workplace premises during work hours. The union is permitted to conduct a pre-election campaign in accordance with solicitation rules that are proscribed for both unions and management. For example, patient care areas such as treatment rooms, waiting areas used by patients, and elevators and stairs used in transporting patients are off limits; but kitchens, supply rooms, business areas, and employee lounges are permissible locations. During the campaign, management may not make threats or announce reprisals regarding the outcome of the election, such as telling nurses that layoffs will result if the union is elected or pay raises will be given if the union loses. Management also may not directly ask employees about their attitudes or voting intentions or those of other employees. Management is allowed, however, to conduct captive-audience speeches, which are meetings during work time to inform employees about the changes that certifying a union will mean for the organization and to persuade employees to give management another chance.

To win the election and be certified by the NLRB as representing the bargaining unit, the union must achieve a simple majority or 50 percent plus 1 of those voting. Consequently, if voter turnout is low, the decision to be unionized will be decided by less than a majority of employees eligible to vote. When the union wins the election, it assumes the duties of the exclusive bargaining agent for all employees in the unit even if those employees choose not to join the union and pay membership dues. Similarly, any negotiated agreements will cover all employees in the bargaining unit. If the union loses, however, it can continue to maintain contact with employees and provide certain representational services such as informing them of their rights. The union may lose the right to represent employees in the bargaining unit through a decertification election.

Negotiation Phase

After winning the election, the union will begin to negotiate a contract on behalf of the employees in the bargaining unit. Federal labor laws encourage collective bargaining on the theory that employees and their employers are best able to reach agreement on issues such as wages, hours, and conditions of employment through negotiating their differences. The process of negotiating this contract is referred to as collective bargaining. The NLRA (Section 8 [d], 1935) defines collective bargaining as follows:

> . . . the performance of the mutual obligation of the employer and the representative of the employees to meet at reasonable times and confer in good faith with respect to wages, hours and terms and conditions of employment or the negotiation

of an agreement, or any question arising there under, and the execution of a written contract incorporating any agreement reached requested by either party to agree to a proposal or require the making of a concession.

The NLRA requires an employer to recognize and bargain in good faith with a certified union, but it does not force the employer to agree with the union or make any concessions. The key to satisfying the duty to bargain in good faith is approaching the bargaining table with an open mind and negotiating with the intention of reaching final agreement (LLR 3115: 7888).

Issues for bargaining have evolved over a period of years as the result of NLRB and court decisions. Those issues are categorized as illegal, mandatory, or voluntary (permissive). Illegal subjects, such as age-discrimination employment clauses, may not be considered for bargaining. Mandatory bargaining issues are related to wages, hours, and other conditions of employment; Figure 14.2 provides a partial list of these issues. Mandatory subjects must be bargained if they are introduced for negotiation. Voluntary, or permissive bargaining, issues carry no similar restriction. Examples of voluntary issues include strike insurance and benefits for retired employees.

Prior to bargaining, management will formulate ranges for each issue, which is similar to an opening offer, followed by a series of benchmarks that represent expected levels of settlement. Of course, management must calculate a resistance point beyond which it will cease negotiations. Fisher and Ury (1981) have developed a principled method of negotiation based on the merits or principles of the issues. The following four basic points are involved:

1. *People*. Separate the people from the problem.
2. *Interests*. Focus on interests, not the positions that people hold.
3. *Options*. Generate a variety of alternative possibilities.
4. *Criteria*. Insist that solutions be evaluated using objective standards.

According to this method, management will formulate a best alternative to a negotiated agreement for each issue. In this manner, negotiators evaluate whether the type of agreement that can be reached is better than no agreement at all. By considering mutual options for gain, the negotiator offers a more flexible approach toward bargaining and increases the likelihood of achieving creative solutions.

Collective bargaining is both a laborious and a time-consuming endeavor. Bargaining requires not only listening to others but attempting to understand the motivational force behind the dialogue. Successful negotiators make every effort to understand fully what truly underlies bargaining positions and why they are so fiercely held. Also, negotiators are receptive to any signals that are being communicated, including nonverbal communication

FIGURE 14.2
Mandatory
Bargaining
Issues

- Wages
- Arbitration
- Duration of agreement
- Reinstatement of economic strikers
- Work rules
- Lunch periods
- Bonus payments
- Promotions
- Transfers
- Plant reopening
- Bargaining over "bar list"
- Arrangement for negotiation
- Plant closedown and relocation
- Overtime pay
- Company houses
- Union-imposed production ceiling
- No-strike clause
- Workloads
- Cancellation of security upon relocation of plant
- Employer's insistence on clause, giving arbitrator right to enforce award
- Severance pay
- Safety
- Checkoff
- Hours
- Holidays (paid)
- Grievance procedure
- Change of payment (hourly to salary)

- Merit wage increase
- Pension plan
- Price of company meals
- Seniority
- Plant closing
- Employee physical examination
- Truck rentals
- Change in insurance carrier/benefits
- Profit-sharing plan
- Agency shop
- Subcontracting
- Most-favored-nation clause
- Piece rates
- Change of employee status to independent contractor
- Discounts on company's products
- Clause providing for supervisors' keeping seniority in unit
- Nondiscriminatory hiring hall
- Prohibition against supervisors doing unit work
- Partial plant closing
- Discharge
- Vacations (paid)
- Layoff plan
- Union security and checkoff

- Work schedule
- Retirement age
- Group insurance (health, life, and accident)
- Layoffs
- Job-posting procedures
- Union security
- Musician price list
- Change in operations resulting in reclassifying workers from incentive to straight time, cut workforce, or installation of cost-saving machine
- Motor carrier union agreement
- Sick leave
- Discriminatory racial policies
- Work assignments and transfers
- Stock-purchase plan
- Management rights clause
- Shift differentials
- Procedures for income tax withholding
- Plant rules
- Superseniority for union stewards
- Hunting on employer forest preserve where previously granted

NOTE: This is a list of major items for bargaining; the list does not include subcategories.

such as body language (Fisher and Ury 1981). Bargaining, as depicted in Figure 14.3, can be conceptualized as a continuum of bargaining behaviors and strategies. At one end of the continuum is *concessionary bargaining*, in which the employer asks the union to eliminate, limit, or reduce wages and other commitments in response to financial constraints. This type of bargaining is likely to occur when the organization is in financial jeopardy and is struggling to survive. At the opposite end is *integrative bargaining*, which seeks win-win situations and solutions that creatively respond to both parties' needs. This type of bargaining requires the trust and cooperation of both parties. In the center is *distributive bargaining*, which is a win-lose type in which each party gives up something to gain something else. This type of bargaining is likely when negotiations are contentious and full of conflict.

Even when both parties negotiate in good faith and fulfill the covenants of the NLRA, an agreement still may not be reached at times. When this happens, parties are said to have reached an impasse. To resolve an impasse, a variety of techniques may be implemented. These techniques involve third parties and include mediation, in which a mediator evaluates the dispute and issues nonbinding recommendations. If either party rejects the mediator's recommendations, arbitration is an alternative. Arbitrators, similar to mediators, are neutral third parties, but their decisions are legally binding. For example, arbitrators may recommend that either party's position be accepted as a final offer, or they can attempt to split the differences between the two parties' positions.

If these techniques fail to resolve the impasse, employers or the union can initiate work stoppages that may take the form of lockouts or strikes. A lockout occurs when the employer shuts down operations either during or prior to a dispute. A strike, on the other hand, is employee initiated. Lockouts or strikes can occur during negotiations and also during the life of the contract. Special provisions for these work stoppages in healthcare settings are discussed in the section below on the history of judicial and legislative rulings.

In addition, no-strike and no-lockout clauses can be negotiated in the agreement. No-strike clauses essentially prohibit strikes, either unconditionally or with conditions. An unconditional no-strike clause means that the union and its members will not engage in either a strike or work slow-down

---

Integrative Bargaining (win–win)		Distributive Bargaining (win some–lose some)		Concessionary Bargaining (winner takes all)

FIGURE 14.3
Collective Bargaining Continuum

while the contract is in effect. A conditional no-strike clause bans strikes and slow-downs except in certain situations and under specific conditions, which are delineated in detail in the agreement. Comparable clauses for lockouts exist for employers.

Administration Phase

When an agreement between the union and the employer is reached, it must be recorded in writing and executed in good faith, which means that the terms and conditions of the agreement must be applied and enforced. This agreement will include disciplinary, grievance, and arbitration procedures, many of which have been discussed in other chapters. The collective bargaining agreement imposes limitations on the disciplinary actions that management may take. The right to discharge, suspend, or discipline is clearly enunciated in contractual clauses and in the adoption of rules and procedures that may or may not be incorporated in the agreement.

Management may discipline up through discharge only for sufficient and appropriate reasons and must base all procedures on due process. The union's role in the process is to defend employees and to determine the propriety of management action. The burden of proof rests with management to prove that whatever action was taken was proper and consistent with progressive discipline. If the grievance proceeds to arbitration, arbitrators will usually support management if they find evidence of progressive discipline and evidence that employees were fully aware of the standards against which their behavior was to be measured. These standards include very basic rules and regulations that outline offenses that will subject employees to disciplinary action and the extent of such action.

The heart of administering the collective bargaining agreement is the *grievance procedure*. This procedure is a useful and productive management tool that allows implementation and interpretation of the contract. A grievance must be well defined and restricted to violations of the terms and conditions of the agreement. However, other conditions may give rise to a grievance, including violations of the law or company rules, a change in working conditions or past company practices, or violations of health and safety standards.

The grievance process usually contains a series of steps. The first step always involves the presentation of the grievance by the employee (or representative) to the immediate, first-line supervisor. If the grievance is not resolved at this step, broader action is taken. Because most grievances involve an action by the immediate supervisor, the second step necessarily must occur outside the department and at a higher level; thus, the second step will involve the employee (or representative) and a department head or other administrator. Prior to this meeting the grievance will be written out, dated, and signed by the employee and the union representative. The written grievance will document the events as the employee perceived them, cite the appropriate contract provisions that allegedly had been violated, and indicate the desired resolution or settlement prospects. If the grievance is unresolved at this point, a third step becomes necessary that involves an in-house review by top management. A grievance that remains unresolved at the conclusion of the third step may go to arbitration if provided for in the contract and if the union is in agreement.

Most collective bargaining agreements restrict the arbitrator's decision to application and interpretation of the agreement and make the decision final and binding on both parties. Most agreements also specify methods for selecting arbitrators. If the union agrees to arbitration, it must notify management, and an arbitrator is jointly selected. In evaluating the grievance, arbitrators focus on a variety of criteria, including the actual nature of the offense, the past record of the grieving employee, warnings, knowledge of rules, past practices, and discriminatory treatment. Thus, a large number of factors interact, making arbitration a complex process.

An arbitration hearing permits each side an opportunity to present its case. Similar to a court hearing, witnesses, cross-examinations, transcripts, and legal counsel may be used. As with a court hearing, the nature of arbitration is adversarial. Thus, cases may be lost because of poor preparation and presentation. Generally, the courts will enforce an arbitrator's decision unless it is shown to be unreasonable, unsound, or capricious relative to the issues under consideration. Also, if an arbitrator has exceeded his or her authority or issued an order that violates existing state or federal law, the decision may be vacated. Consistent and fair adjudication of grievances is the hallmark of a sound labor–management relationship.

In healthcare settings, the strike is the most severe form of a labor–management dispute. A critical part of planning for negotiations is an honest assessment of strike potential. This involves identifying strike issues that are likely to be critical for all parties. Although estimating the impact of possible strikes, including economic pressures from lost wages and revenues, is essential, the key to a successful strike from the perspective of the union is to impose enough pressure on management to expedite movement toward a compromise. Pressure may be psychological as well as economic. In healthcare settings, the real losers in a strike are the patients and their families. During a strike, patients may be denied services or forced to postpone treatment, be relocated to another institution, or even be discharged prematurely.

Management must be aware of critical factors that affect its ability and willingness to withstand a strike. When attempting to estimate the impact of these factors, managers will evaluate several key indicators, including revenue losses, timing of the strike, and availability of replacements for striking workers. However, management must also contemplate factors that affect the union, such as the question of whether striking employees will be entitled to strike benefits, especially health benefits. If so, for how long? Both parties must also consider the impact of outside assistance to avoid or settle a strike.

A Review of Legislative and Judicial Rulings

Table 14.2 summarizes important legislative and judicial rulings and their impact on healthcare settings. As the table indicates, in recent years significant rulings have centered primarily on organizing issues, mostly involving physicians and nurses and their eligibility for inclusion in bargaining units. In 2004, the focus appeared to shift to financial issues such as changes to the Fair Labor Standards Act, which exempted most nurses from overtime pay. Unions were also affected by changes to the Labor Management and Disclosure Act. Stricter reporting requirements were required that aimed at increased transparency and accountability for how unions spend dues money (*Harvard Law Review* 2004). In 2006, much attention was directed toward organizing issues, specifically the determination of who is a supervisor; a supervisor, after all, is excluded from the bargaining unit.

As management structures have grown increasingly flat and less hierarchical, many jobs have assumed expanded duties that include a managerial component. Accordingly, determining who is a supervisor has become challenging, especially with regard to health professionals who operate with some autonomy (Von Bergen 2006). Of particular significance for healthcare are two decisions that concern supervisory status. First, there is the U.S. Supreme Court decision in the case of the NLRB v. Kentucky River Community Care, Inc. The Supreme Court criticized the NLRB's lack of clarity in its interpretation of the term *independent judgment* to determine supervisory status. Subsequently, the NLRB addressed its definition of supervisory status. In a landmark case, Oakwood Healthcare, Inc., 348 NRB No. 37 (September 29, 2006), the NLRB ruled that permanent charge nurses employed by acute care hospital Oakwood Heritage Hospital in Taylor, Michigan, exercised supervisory authority in assigning employees within the meaning of Section 2 (11) of the NLRA. In this ruling, the NLRB reexamined and clarified its interpretations of the terms "independent judgment," "assign," and "responsibility to direct." At issue was whether nurses at Oakwood assigned and directed other nurses using their own judgment rather than following written instructions or orders from a supervisor. The NLRB held that charge nurses who usually assign work and monitor care during a shift were supervisors and hence excluded from the bargaining unit. Nurses who handled such responsibilities on a part-time basis were not considered to be supervisors and therefore would remain eligible for union membership (Evans 2006; *PR Newswire* 2006).

TABLE 14.2
Summary of
Important
Legislative
and Judicial
Rulings

Year	Legislation/Judicial Ruling	Impact on Healthcare Organizations
1947	Taft-Hartley amendments to NLRA	Exempted not-for-profit hospitals from NLRA coverage, including collective bargaining
1962	Executive Order #10988	Permitted federally supported hospitals to bargain collectively
1974	Healthcare amendments to NLRA	Extended NLRA coverage to private, not-for-profit hospitals and healthcare institutions; special provisions for strikes, pickets, and impasses
1976	NLRB ruling: Cedars-Sinai Medical Center, Los Angeles	Ruled that medical residents, interns, and fellows (house staff) are students and excluded from collective bargaining
1989/ 1991	NLRB ruling/Supreme Court affirmation on multiple bargaining units: PL 93-360	Expanded the number of bargaining units in acute care hospitals from three to eight
1999	NLRB Ruling: Boston Medical Center	Reversed Cedars-Sinai Medical Center decision and ruled that house staff are employees, not students, and can therefore be included in collective bargaining
2001	Supreme Court decision regarding nurse supervisors: NLRB v. Kentucky River Community Care, Inc.	Court ruled that registered nurses who use independent judgment in directing employees are supervisors. Expected impact: limiting unions' ability to organize nurses
2003	U.S. Department of Labor adopted a rule that increases union financial reporting requirements (19 C.F.R. pts 403 and 408) to provide for transparency of union financial structures and accountability of how unions spend their dues	
2004	U.S. Department of Labor issued new rules that make most nurses ineligible for overtime pay under Part 541 of the Fair Labor Standards Act	
2006	NLRB ruling: Oakwood Heritage Hospital, Taylor, Michigan	NLRB addressed supervisory status in response to the Supreme Court's decision in the Kentucky River case; issued guidelines for determining whether an individual is a supervisor under the NLRA; and reclassified certain nurses (i.e., charge nurses) as management and thus are ineligible to join unions

Expected impact: Reduce potential for union recruitment, and it could permit employers to challenge existing contracts and remove nurses from bargaining units |

The impact of this ruling could be consequential for union membership because the ruling substantially limits the ability of unions to recruit nurses. Also, it can make organizing a union in a hospital or other healthcare facility more difficult because of fewer eligible workers. Healthcare employers can challenge union elections and attempt to decertify nurses who are no longer protected by the collective bargaining agreements (Harrell 2006). However, employers may also face union challenges and may be called upon to demonstrate that supervisory assignments were consistent with the NLRB guidelines. Because the answer to "who is a charge nurse?" varies from hospital to hospital, gray areas are left to be settled. These gray areas are what unions will ultimately challenge (Evans 2006; Alexander 2006). In addition, unions will likely fight for contract provisions to keep supervisory nurses in the union.

The Taft-Hartley Act (Taft-Hartley) amended the NLRA in 1947. The primary intent of these amendments was to strike a balance in the NLRA, because most of its protections and rights applied to workers and employers needed a means for redress. Taft-Hartley also gave states federal permission to enact right-to-work laws, which essentially prohibit employees from being forced to join unions as a condition of employment. Currently, 21 states, mostly in the South and West, have enacted such laws. Unions oppose right-to-work laws in part because under the NLRA, unions are responsible for representing all employees in the bargaining unit, even those members who choose not to join the union and consequently pay no union dues. (Nonunion members of the bargaining unit are often referred to as "free riders" because they acquire all of the benefits of union membership without any cost. Meanwhile, proponents of right-to-work laws maintain that no one should be forced to join a private organization, especially if that organization is using dues money to support causes that contravene an individual's moral or religious beliefs.)

Although the NLRA, as it was initially enacted in 1935, did not exempt healthcare employees explicitly, court interpretations tended to exclude healthcare workers from its regulations, until later amendments asserted jurisdiction over a variety of healthcare institutions. Taft-Hartley had a significant impact on healthcare workers because Section 2 (2) specifically excluded from the definition of "employer" those private, not-for-profit hospitals and healthcare institutions. However, the NLRB asserted jurisdiction over proprietary hospitals and nursing homes, and the 1974 Health Care Amendments, Public Law 93-360, brought the private, not-for-profit healthcare industry within the jurisdiction of federal labor law.

Approximately 2 million additional healthcare workers became eligible for representation with the 1974 Health Care Amendments (Stickler 1990). These amendments afforded stringent protections regarding work stoppages to safeguard patient care. Table 14.3 summarizes the provisions for strikes and pickets as well as impasse requirements. In drafting the 1974 amendments, the congressional committee specifically included a ten-day strike and picket notice provision, a requirement that had not been applied to other industries. The committee did so to ensure that healthcare institutions would have sufficient advance notice of a strike. Furthermore, the committee report of the amendments held that a union is in violation if it has a strike at a facility more

1974 Healthcare Amendments to the Taft-Hartley Act	General NLRA Provisions	
30-day "reasonable" time to picket following which a representation petition must be filed by the union with NLRB	Similar requirement	**TABLE 14.3** Comparison of Provisions for Strike or Picket Notification and Impasse Requirements
90-day notice for modifying an existing collective bargaining agreement	60-day requirement	
60-day notice to FMCS* of impending expiration of existing collective bargaining agreement	30-day requirement	
Following FMCS notification, contract must remain in effect for 60 days without any strikes or lockouts	30-day requirement	
30-day notice of a dispute must be given to FMCS and appropriate state agency during initial negotiations	No similar requirement	
The director of FMCS is authorized to appoint a board of inquiry in the event of a threatened or actual work stoppage	No similar authority	
10-day written notice to employer and FMCS of strikes or pickets required of healthcare unions [Note: this notice cannot occur before either (1) the end of the 90-day notice to modify the existing contract or (2) the 30-day notice in the case of an impasse during negotiations of the new contract.]	No similar requirement	
A new Section 19 provides for an alternate, a contribution to designated 501(c)(3) charities, for the payment of union dues for persons with religious convictions against making such payments	No similar requirement	

* Federal Mediation and Conciliation Service

than 72 hours after the designated notice time, unless the parties agreed to a new time or the union issued a new ten-day notice. In addition, if the union does not begin the strike or other job action at the time designated in the initial ten-day notice, it must provide the healthcare facility with at least 12 hours' notice before the actual beginning of the action. Thus, the 12-hour "warning" must fall completely within the 72-hour notice period. Repeatedly serving ten-day notices on the employer also constitutes evidence of a refusal to bargain in good faith and is a violation of the NLRA.

The reprisals for violating the ten-day notice are substantial. For example, workers engaged in work stoppage in violation of the strike notice lose their status as employees and are subsequently unprotected by the NLRA provisions. Exceptions to the requirements for unions to provide notices are provided as well. If the employer has committed a flagrant or serious, unfair labor practice, then notices are not required. In addition, the employer may not use the ten-day notice period to essentially undermine the bargaining relationship that otherwise exists. For example, the facility can receive supplies, but it is not free to stockpile supplies for an unduly extended period. Similarly, the facility cannot bring in large numbers of personnel from other facilities for the purpose of replacing striking workers (Metzger, Ferentino, and Kruger 1984).

In 1989, an NLRB ruling established eight units for the purpose of collective bargaining in acute care hospitals: (1) physicians, (2) nurses, (3) all other professionals, (4) technical employees, (5) business office clerical employees, (6) skilled maintenance employees, (7) guards, and (8) all other nonprofessionals. Figure 14.4 provides more detail on the various occupations that fall within the eight designated categories. As with all bargaining unit determinations, supervisors are excluded from unit membership. The American Hospital Association (1991) strongly opposed the ruling and appealed to the U.S. Supreme Court, protesting that eight units would lead to a proliferation of bargaining units in the hospital, further fragmenting healthcare collective bargaining; increasing bargaining costs; making implementation of hospitalwide policies more difficult; and ultimately inflating the cost of healthcare and rendering the bargaining process more complicated, lengthy, and subject to legal appeals and challenges. The Supreme Court disagreed, affirming the NLRB's ruling in 1991. Although little empirical evidence specifically evaluates the impact of the eight-unit ruling (Hirsch and Schumacher 1998), election activity and the union win rate within these eight units have increased. Table 14.4 presents election information for the period 1995 through 1999.

Finally, despite lobbying campaigns, unions have failed consistently in their attempts to eliminate secret-ballot NLRB elections. As discussed earlier, unions prefer to revise the organizing process in their favor by calling

1. Physicians
2. Nurses:
   - registered nurses
   - graduate nurses
   - non-nursing department nurses
   - nurse anesthetists
   - nurse instructors
   - nurse practitioners
3. All professionals, except for registered nurses and physicians:
   - audiologists
   - chemists
   - counselors
   - dietitians
   - educational programmers
   - educators
   - medical artists
   - nuclear physicists
   - pharmacists
   - social workers
   - technologists
   - therapists
   - utilization review coordinators
4. Technical employees:
   - infant-care technicians
   - laboratory technicians
   - licensed practical nurses
   - operating room technicians
   - orthopedic technicians
   - physical therapy assistants
   - psychiatric technicians
   - respiratory therapy technicians
   - surgical assistants
   - x-ray technicians
5. Business office clerical employees
6. Skilled maintenance employees
7. Guards
8. All other nonprofessional employees

FIGURE 14.4

Eight Categories of Workers Specified in NLRB Bargaining Rules

for a card-check method instead of an election. An example of such an effort is the Employee Free Choice legislation, including Senator Ted Kennedy's Employee Free Choice Act of 2007 (Senate Bill 1041). This act sought to amend labor laws to eliminate elections for certification. Although the union has not yet achieved legislative success, it is likely to continue to push for change.

TABLE 14.4
Summary of
Election
Activity in
Health Services
Elections,
1995–1999

Year	Total Elections	Union Wins
1995	291	156
1996	370	205
1997	407	258
1998	486	290
1999	517	333

SOURCE: Industrial Distribution of Representation Elections Held in Cases Closed, FY 1995–1999. Annual Reports of the NLRB.

Developments in Organizing Healthcare Workers

Unions

The union landscape shifted dramatically in 2005, when the SEIU (Service Employees International Union) ended its relationship with the AFL-CIO (American Federation of Labor and Congress of Industrial Organizations) because of a failure to pursue aggressive strategies to recruit new members. The SEIU subsequently aligned itself with the Change to Win federation, joining six other former AFL-CIO affiliates that similarly chose to sever ties. The SEIU action was consequential as it reduced the AFL-CIO membership of 13 million by about a third. In 2007, the SEIU, which reportedly represents 1.9 million members, announced the formation of a separate national healthcare union—SEIU Healthcare—that focuses exclusively on healthcare workers. The SEIU has been visible in its support of efforts to expand nurse–patient ratios and efforts to organize physicians. In addition to its focus on hospital, nursing, and long-term care workers, SEIU Healthcare will target employees in ambulatory surgery centers, laboratories, clinics, and other healthcare areas (Siderius 2005; SEIU 2007). To date, the local unions of SEIU Healthcare have been visibly active in recruitment and bargaining. Recently, SEIU Healthcare successfully negotiated one of the largest labor contracts with HCA, a private-sector hospital chain. The contract covers six facilities and 4,000 workers across HCA hospitals in Florida and includes a wage increase (Dorschner 2007).

The AFL-CIO has also increased its healthcare organizing efforts, creating an alliance of eight of its unions to recruit nurses. This alliance of nursing unions includes United American Nurses (UAN)—the labor arm of the American Nurses Association and one of the largest nurses' unions, with a membership of approximately 104,000 members. In 2007, the California Nurses Association (CNA) also joined the AFL-CIO, bringing along an estimated

71,000 nurses and thus increasing the total number of AFL-CIO's nurse membership to 325,000. The CNA has been aggressive with recruitment efforts and is looking to build membership nationwide. The CNA's organizing arm, the National Nurses Organizing Committee, aims to expand membership nationally, even though its attempt to unionize nurses at Mt. Sinai Hospital in Chicago failed in 2006 (*Modern Healthcare* 2006; Evans 2007a, 2007b).

Physicians

Historically, physicians resisted union organizing for various professional and philosophical reasons. In fact, much of the American Medical Association (AMA) membership generally views unionism as antithetical to professionalism and unions as economic devices that extract benefits for their members at the expense of patient trust and confidence. In addition, organizing physicians presented legal challenges because the majority of physicians are independent contractors and thus are technically ineligible for union membership. Only "employed" physicians, including those employed in academic settings, are authorized to bargain collectively. Physicians who practice as independent contractors are restricted from collective bargaining by the Sherman Antitrust Act of 1890, which prohibits all business combinations that restrain free trade. Therefore, these physicians cannot legally talk with one another about price of service. Subsequently, independent contractors who engage in collective bargaining with entities such as health plans and insurers risk exposure to federal antitrust suits (AAMC 1999; Anthony and Erf 2000; Cohen 1999).

Nonetheless, the growth of "tight" managed care in the 1990s provided a powerful incentive for the rise of the physician union movement in the United States. The vast majority of physician complaints and efforts to unionize derived from corporate interference in medical decision making and coercive practices of managed care organizations (Anawis 2002; Luepke 1999). At its annual meeting in June 1999, the AMA House of Delegates approved a controversial resolution, creating a national "bargaining unit" for physicians. The bargaining unit—Physicians for Responsible Negotiations (PRN)—permitted employed physicians to bargain with health plans and insurers. The resolution was controversial because the AMA, which traditionally opposed physician unions, reversed its position. In so doing, the AMA recognized collective bargaining as an acceptable professional mechanism for interacting with government and other third-party payers. Federal and state legislation also was proposed in support of amending antitrust laws to permit independent physicians to unionize. However, this legislation did not gain widespread support and was subsequently abandoned.

The PRN struggled for survival and recruited few members. In 2002, the AMA reduced its financial support for the PRN, only guaranteeing the union's survival through the year 2003. In March 2004, the AMA, with little press attention, severed its relationship with the PRN. In June 2004, the PRN partnered with SEIU and its two other affiliated doctors' unions—The Doctors Council and the National Doctors Alliance. This affiliation represents the largest collection of unionized physicians in the United States, including approximately 20,000 members made up of salaried and private-practice physicians as well as medical residents and interns (Michels 2004; Romano 2004). Although little evidence exists to explain why the PRN was not well supported by physicians, the loosening of managed care was likely a dominant factor. Increases in consumer choice and open access effectively reduced many of the physician complaints and problems that previously substantiated interest in unionizing. For example, by the late 1990s, specialty physicians were regaining status as revenue and profit generators. Still, physicians also likely recognized the potential for obtaining judicial relief when they filed and won a class-action suit for reimbursement disputes against Aetna (Casalino, Pham, and Bazzoli 2004; Martinez 2003).

House Staff (Medical Residents, Interns, and Fellows) and Medical Students

In 1999, the NLRB ruled that house staff at Boston Medical Center were employees, not students. The impact of this ruling is that house staff in private hospitals are now legally entitled to bargain collectively. This determination was a reversal of a 1976 ruling for Cedars-Sinai Medical Center in Los Angeles in which house staff were classified as students (Yacht 2000). In 2001, medical residents at 525-bed Brookdale University Hospital and Medical Center in New York became the first private-sector hospital physicians in the United States to ratify a collective bargaining agreement since that right was affirmed by the NLRB (*Modern Healthcare* 2001). Opponents of house staff unionization suggest that union activity will create adversarial relationships between house staff and instructors. For example, unions can negotiate resident promotions and fight against disciplinary actions and dismissal of poorly performing house staff (Levenson 1999).

Nurses

Nurses are predominantly employed in hospitals, where they represent the largest service and thus a significant labor cost. Nurses play a key role in patient care, providing care 24 hours a day, 7 days a week. Historically, nurses have struggled with conflict among their obligation to their patients, their profession, and union representation. Approximately 2.5 million registered nurses (RNs) work in the United States and, despite uneven salary levels across the profession and widespread, persistent discontent with working conditions, the majority of these nurses do not belong to a union. Approximately 18 percent of RNs are unionized (Bureau of Labor Statistics 2006b; Leung 1999). In addition, because of a 2006 NLRB landmark ruling concerning supervisory status, many nurses may no longer be eligible for union membership (see Table 14.2).

Unlike physicians, whose workplace problems and needs seem to be addressed without the help of unions, nurses currently have a different experience. As the Interview with a Nurse Activist section (at the end of the chapter) explains, nurse–management relationships are strained. National nurse shortages and pressures on hospitals to trim labor costs have increased nursing workloads and hours and thus the potential for nurses to commit errors during long shifts. In Massachusetts, work hours are a contentious nursing issue and have led to work stoppages and strike threats during contract negotiations (Kowalczyk 2004; Rowland 2006). Research affirms that for nurses to vote in favor of a union, they must believe that joining a union will help them gain greater control over patient care (Clark et al. 2000). Thus, patient care issues appear to be motivating many nurses to unionize (DeMoro 2002; Meier 2000).

Nurse activism remains ongoing and widespread. From informational pickets and protests to threats of strikes, nurses appear prepared to take action to ensure patient safety, adequate staffing, wages, and benefits. For example, in December 2006, nurses filed a class-action antitrust lawsuit against hospitals and health systems in the Detroit area. The suit alleged a collusion among these facilities to fix wages at below-market levels, and it is only one among similar class-action cases filed on behalf of nurses in other states, including Arizona, Illinois, New York, Tennessee, and Texas (Taylor 2006). In May 2007, judges allowed the nurse class-action case in Tennessee to continue despite attempts by the employing hospitals to have the case dismissed. The judge ruled that the nurses had facts that are sufficient to support claims of a conspiracy to depress nurses' wages (Evans 2007c).

The UAN looks to increase support and influence and to bring aggressiveness to organizing and other union activities. Although some state affiliates, such as the CNA, have chosen to align with the AFL-CIO, others such as the Massachusetts Nurses Association (MNA) have opted to go it alone and thus far have been successful. For example, the MNA, which represents 23,000 nurses, used the threat of a strike to negotiate a contract for nurses at Brigham and Women's Hospital; the contract makes nurses at Brigham and Women's Hospital among the highest paid in the state. The MNA also won key contract language that keeps supervisory nurses in the union (Rowland 2006). The move toward increased aggressiveness through union activism derives primarily from problems related to staffing and stress, especially managed care's pressure to reduce hospital lengths of stay. Priority issues for nurses center on patient loads, mandatory overtime, staffing cuts, "floating" to unfamiliar areas, and benefits such as wages and pensions (Meier 2000; Spetz and Given 2003; Rowland 2006).

By joining and becoming active in unions, nurses are exercising their voice and using tools of unionism such as election petitions, contract negotiations, and work stoppages such as sick-outs and strikes. Nurses are capturing the public's attention and using their influence to obtain community support (see Interview with a Nurse Activist section). To date, however, aggression and activism have yielded mixed results. Their efforts to influence patient safety and quality-of-care legislation have been successful at the state level but not at the federal level. For example, California enacted the first law that establishes nurse-to-patient staffing ratios. This law, in effect, requires hospitals to reduce nurse workloads and improve patient safety by guaranteeing minimum nurse-to-patient ratios. It also serves as a framework for mandates in other states and at the federal level (Benko 2004). Similarly, nursing unions have achieved success at the state level with mandatory overtime legislation. State laws that prohibit or limit mandatory overtime have been enacted in five states—Maine, Minnesota, New Jersey, Oregon, and Washington. However, corresponding federal legislation has not been enacted despite heavy union opposition to mandatory overtime. Nursing unions also failed to stop revisions to the Fair Labor Standards Act, which effectively exempts most nurses from overtime pay (see Table 14.2).

The Impact of the Internet

The role of the Internet in union organizing and solicitation campaigns and in collective bargaining and contract administration has received little attention. However, the Internet is expected to be an influential tool, as it has been for many other causes. Union websites offer up-to-date information on union activities and developments and promote membership benefits. Because unions must observe specific rules about visiting work premises to solicit during union recognition campaigns, the Internet offers unprecedented opportunities to communicate with employees without time and place restrictions.

With e-mails, websites, and blogs, unions are equipped with communication channels that can reach prospective members without alerting their employers. Some websites, such as the CNA's, offer sample contracts for nurses to use in bargaining with employers. Similarly, employers have the ability to disseminate information via the Internet. Furthermore, various websites and blogs are dedicated to sharing negative information about unions, such as the number of unfair labor practices filed against unions for coercive or intimidating behavior exhibited toward employees. Enhanced communication also means transparency, and the Internet offers both employers and unions unprecedented insight and information regarding each other's efforts.

For example, when the SEIU began efforts to organize at teaching hospitals in Boston, it sent out a letter to some trustees of Beth Israel Deaconess Medical Center, a teaching hospital, alleging that the hospital had potentially misrepresented its charity care in financial statements (Strom 2008). In response, the chief executive officer (CEO) of Beth Israel Deaconess Medical Center used his widely read blog to accuse the union of unfair tactics, such as attacking the reputation of teaching hospitals, their senior management, and their trustees. The SEIU's response to the CEO's blog was posted on its website and was e-mailed (Cooney 2007). Judging from this example alone, the Internet seems to have enhanced the ability of all parties (employees, employers, and unions) to communicate about the labor-management process. How the Internet will affect the labor–management relationship remains to be seen.

Management Guidelines

Following are key points to remember about labor relations.

1. *Whether a healthcare organization is union or nonunion, it should have a policy on unionism, and this policy should be communicated to current and prospective employees.* A positive labor–management relationship begins with the screening process. All prospective employees should be given information about the institution's position toward unions as well as its goals and strategies of fair and consistent dealings with unions. Employee handbooks and orientation represent other opportunities to communicate management's commitment to provide equitable treatment to all employees concerning wages, benefits, hours, and conditions of employment. Furthermore, management must also communicate that each employee is important and deserves respect and that adequate funds and management time have been designated to maintain effective employee relations (Rutkowski and Rutkowski 1984).

2. *Management not only must have effective policies and procedures for selection of new employees but also must ensure proper fit of personnel with specific jobs.* Job analyses, job descriptions, and job evaluations, as well as fair wage and salary programs, are essential in establishing a fundamental basis for fair representation. Management must not make promises that cannot be fulfilled; at the same time, it should strive to do whatever is possible to improve employee relations. Monitoring employee attitudes through surveys is essential; otherwise, management is dependent on the union for communicating worker problems or change in attitudes.

3. *Management must fulfill its roles and responsibilities to employees by providing necessary training, especially for first-line supervisors who are instrumental in determining how policies are implemented and in serving as liaisons between management and employees.* If supervisors are not properly trained, grievances are less likely to be settled quickly and are more likely to escalate into substantive formal disputes. Training is especially critical in healthcare settings because of constant and rapid changes in technology and workplace safety issues. Management's commitment to training must be consistent with fair and honest

treatment of employees. Similarly, if management fails to establish objective performance policies and does not ensure that they are done routinely, the labor–management relationship is affected. Employees may perceive inequities and unfairness and experience problems of declining morale and productivity because rewards are not matched with performance.

4. *Inconsistent and unfair application of disciplinary policies and procedures can create unnecessary grievance problems.* At a minimum, the principle of just cause should guide the disciplinary process. When employees file grievances, they expect prompt attention to their requests. Delay in responding or ignoring complaints is a clear signal to employees that management does not care about their problems and thus cannot be trusted. Furthermore, management's credibility with employees will then deteriorate, creating an imbalance in the labor–management relationship that leads to employee perception that the union's position is the most honest.

5. *Each phase of the labor-relations process is interrelated and can affect the outcome of other phases.* For example, if the union is able to obtain representation through voluntary recognition, the negotiations for a collective bargaining agreement will likely be less adversarial than a representation election. Similarly, if the negotiations for a collective bargaining agreement are contentious, difficulties may occur in administering the contract. Thus, having a full understanding of each phase and its potential to enhance or impede the overall process of labor relations is essential.

Summary

As this chapter describes, managing with organized labor is challenging. Even though unionism has been declining nationally for decades, the relatively unorganized healthcare workforce has continued to grow and as such has become a serious target for unions. Since 2001, 1.7 million new jobs have been added to the healthcare industry, far surpassing the rest of the labor market. Unlike many other industries, healthcare requires a wide range of personnel, from home health aides to nurses to technicians to physicians (Mandel and Weber 2006). Because union membership and election activity have increased in healthcare settings, managers must devote high-level attention to the application and maintenance of a positive labor-relations program that integrates human resources functions. Unfortunately for healthcare, the rise of claims of unfair labor practices and the increase in threats of strikes, walkouts, and other work stoppages suggest that the labor–management relationship is strained. Thus, it is incumbent on management to create strategies and goals to implement a positive labor-relations program that addresses employee-related challenges. The formation of the SEIU healthcare union, a landmark ruling by the NLRB regarding nursing supervisors, and increased use of the Internet to expand communication channels signal major changes for human resources practices and the labor-relations process.

Discussion Questions

1. Why should management have a policy on unionism? What purpose does such a policy serve?
2. Describe the three phases of the labor-relations process. Why are all phases equally important?
3. What are some of the behaviors that may indicate to managers that organizing activities are occurring?
4. Explain the potential far-reaching impact of the NLRB ruling on nursing supervisors. Will this ruling have a chilling effect on nursing unions?

Experiential Exercises

Case The CEO of a mid-size urban hospital was late one Friday evening, so he took a short cut that caused him to walk by the employee lounge. He walked inside and shook his head. With all the problems of budget cuts and trying to make ends meet, he realized that little money had been available for upkeep of nonpatient areas such as the employee lounge. The carpet was dirty and worn, the coffee mugs were chipped, the wallpaper was torn, and the refrigerator groaned as it cycled on and off. The CEO decided enough was enough. The employees had worked hard and should, at minimum, have an employee lounge that was inviting and pleasant.

He marched back to his office and called the COO to instruct her to create a weekend miracle by calling in the work crews to update and refurbish the employee lounge. He ordered new carpets, new wallpaper, and new appliances, and he wanted it all done by Monday. The CEO told the COO, "I keep telling the employees how much I appreciate their help, especially in these financially tight times, but now I am going to show them. And be sure to replace those old, chipped coffee mugs." Early on Monday morning, the CEO walked by the employee lounge. It looked terrific, and someone had already made coffee. He made a note to himself to tell the COO what a great job she had done.

When he got to his office, he found the union steward sitting on the couch. "I need to have a word with you," the union steward said. He had several words, as it turned out: He said that the CEO had violated the collective bargaining contract and that refurbishing the employee lounge should have been, at minimum, discussed with the union. The union steward spent 20 minutes complaining about violations and procedures. After he left, the CEO called the COO and told her to put the lounge back the way it was, including the chipped coffee mugs. Then the CEO muttered to himself, "That is the last time I try to do anything nice for anyone around here. I have learned my lesson."

Interview with a Nurse Activist

Note: This interview was conducted on May 25, 2004, with the cochair of the nurses' union at a large, urban hospital in the northeast. She has more than 20 years experience as a nurse and definitely considers herself a nurse activist. Although the interview was conducted four years ago, the issues discussed are still relevant today.

Times have changed in nursing. The nurse activist explained that now you cannot trust management, as they will tell nurses anything just to get what they want. In her opinion, even nurses who are promoted to management cannot be trusted. "Management lies," she said. She explained that, at the end of a recent negotiation, management and union representatives did not even shake hands. There has been a loss of respect on both sides. It is ironic that at a time when management and nursing need to work together, a chasm of mistrust separates them. The main issues are not money, but human resources—that is, staffing, mandatory overtime, and workloads. Nurses are working harder and longer shifts; the potential for error increases in such environments. Patient safety and quality of care are at stake. According to the nurse activist, she was eight months pregnant and coming off of an eight-hour shift when she was or-

Case Questions

1. What is the problem in this case?
2. Would you respond in the same way? Why, or why not?
3. What, if anything, can be done at this point?

dered to work an additional four hours. "We are playing a game with patient safety," she said. "Management should be held accountable for what they are doing." As a result, nurses are going to the bargaining table to hold management responsible for the staffing decisions that are threatening patient care.

Nurses are also taking their case to the public. The nurse activist routinely appears on local television and radio shows to gather support for nurses. The community is a key stakeholder. After all, she explained, patients make up the community, and they recall who actually "cared" for them during hospital visits: It was the nurse with the bedpan at 2:00 a.m., or it was the nurse giving comfort to the parents of a sick child. It was not management. With issues of patient safety and medication errors, nurses find it straightforward to get the community on their side in demands for staffing and work hours.

Interestingly enough, Peter Drucker, who invented the field of management study, may agree with this nurse activist. He cited management for not treating nurses as professionals who know their jobs. Although he acknowledged that management is under a lot of financial pressure, Drucker said that instead of telling nurses what to do, management should invite nurses to find solutions to the problems (Petzinger 1999).

Exercise 1 Think of a healthcare facility in your community. Consider its nursing situation. Then, answer the following questions:

1. Are the nurses treated as professionals? Why, or why not?
2. If given the opportunity, do you think these nurses are likely or unlikely to join a labor union in the future? Why, or why not?

Exercise 2 Refer to Table 14.1. Using the indicators listed in the table, conduct an audit of a hospital or a healthcare organization. Determine if the organization has experienced an increase or a decrease in any of the indicators. Then, explain the possible reasons for these increases or decreases.

Exercise 3 Refer to Figure 14.1. Using the figure as a guide, complete the table below by listing specific goals for the union and the organization. Once the table is completed, identify the following:

- Which goals are similar?
- Which goals have the potential for conflict?

Goal Areas	Union Goals	Organization Goals
Survival		
Growth		
Profitability		
Competitiveness		
Recruitment and retention of employees		
Motivation of employees		
Flexibility		
Decision making		
Effective use of human resources		
Communication		

Web Resources

1. For online listings of Private and Public Sector Agreements (Collective Bargaining Agreements) go to www.bls.gov/cba/cbaindex.htm. For example, agreements for Kaiser Permanente facilities can be found under "K" on the Private Sector Agreements web page.
2. At this time, the website for the California Nurses Association contains model RN contracts. The website also provides a listing of salaries and differentials, benefits, working conditions, staffing and professional practices, and performance committees, among other information. Sample contracts are also available for downloading, and these contracts will be updated per current bargaining. Because this is a union website, the information posted here will likely change over time. Visit www.calnurses.org/membership/model-contracts/?print=t.

References

Alexander, A. 2006. "Charge Nurses Can Take Part in Vote to Unionize." *Knight Ridder Tribune Business News.* [Online article; retrieved 9/17/07.] ABI/Inform Global Database, www.proquest.com.

American Hospital Association. 1991. "Legal Memorandum Number 16: Collective Bargaining Units in the Health Care Industry." Chicago: American Hospital Association.

Anawis, M. A. 2002. "The Ethics of Physician Unionization: What Will Happen If Your Doctor Becomes a Teamster?" *De Paul Journal of Health Care Law* 6 (1): 83–110.

Anthony, M. F., and S. Erf. 2000. "Can Physician Unionization Succeed?" *Healthcare Executive* (March/April): 50.

Association of American Medical Colleges (AAMC) Executive Council. 1999. "AAMC Statement on Negotiating Units for Physicians." *AAMC Reporter* 9 (2): 7.

Becker, W. L., and A. M. Rowe. 1989. "Update on Union Organization in Health Care." *Review of Federation of American Health Systems* 22 (5): 11–12, 14–16.

Benko, L. B. 2004. "Workforce Report 2004. Ratio Fight Goes National." *Modern Healthcare* 34 (24): 23, 30.

Bureau of Labor Statistics. 2000a. "Union Membership Edges Up but Share Continues to Fall." [Online news release; retrieved 12/5/01.] http://stats.bls.gov/opub/ted.

———. 2000b. "Unpublished Tabulations from Current Population Surveys, Union Membership Tables, 1999 Annual Averages." Washington, DC: U.S. Government Printing Office.

———. 2004. "Union Members in 2003." [Online news release; retrieved 7/6/04.] www.bls.gov/news.release/union2.nr0.htm.

———. 2006a. "Union Members in 2006." [Online news release; retrieved 08/15/07.] www.bls.gov/news.release/union2.nr0.htm.

———. 2006b. "Current Population Survey (CPS), Table 3, Union Affiliation of Employed Wage and Salary Workers by Occupation and Industry." [Online information; retrieved 10/29/07.] www.bls.gov/news.release/union2.t03.htm.

Casalino, L. P., H. Pham, and G. Bazzoli. 2004. "Growth of Single-Specialty Medical Groups." *Health Affairs* 23 (2): 82–90.

Christian Science Monitor. 2004. "A Worker-Union Disconnect." *Christian Science Monitor* 96 (83).

Clark, D. A., P. F. Clark, D. Day, and D. Shea. 2000. "The Relationship Between Health Care Reform and Nurses' Interest in Union Representation: The Role of Workplace Climate." *Journal of Professional Nursing* 16 (2): 92–96.

Cohen, J. J. 1999. "Unions Are Bad Medicine for Doctors." *Academic Medicine* 74 (8): 905.

Cooney, E. 2007. "Beth Israel Deaconess CEO and Union Lock Horns." [Online information; retrieved 10/8/07.] www.boston.com/news/globe/health_science/articles/2007/08/06/ceo_and_union_lock_horns/.

DeMoro, R. A. 2002. "What California Has Started: Staffing Ratios, Union Activism Are National Solutions to the Nurse Shortage." *Modern Healthcare* 32 (13): 26.

Dorschner, J. 2007. "Union Strikes a Bargain with 6 Hospitals in Chain: Six Hospitals Agree to a Union Contract that Will Increase Wages and May Increase Nurse-Patient Ratios." *Knight Ridder Tribune Business News.* [Online article; retrieved 9/17/07.] ABI/Inform Global Database, www.proquest.com.

Evans, M. 2006. "Nurses Ready to Fight Back." *Modern Health Care* 6 (40): 6–9.

———. 2007a. "California Nurses Association Joins AFL-CIO." [Online article; retrieved 5/22/07] *Modern Healthcare*'s Daily Dose, dailydose@modernhealthcare.com.

———. 2007b. "Chicago Hospital's Nurses Reject California Union." [Online article; retrieved 8/7/07.] *Modern Healthcare*'s Daily Dose, dailydose@modernhealthcare.com.

———. 2007c. "Judge Lets Nurses' Class-Action Case Continue." [Online article; retrieved 5/21/07.] *Modern Healthcare*'s Daily Dose, dailydose@modernhealthcare.com.

Fennell, K. S. 1987. "The Unionization of the Healthcare Industry: General Trends and Emerging Issues." *Journal of Health in Human Resources Administration* 10 (1): 66–81.

Fisher, R., and W. Ury. 1981. "Getting to Yes—Negotiating an Agreement Without Giving In." In *Harvard Negotiation Project,* edited by B. Patton, 21–53. Boston: Houghton Mifflin.

Fottler, M. D., R. A. Johnson, K. J. McGlown, and E. W. Ford. 1999. "Attitudes of Organized Labor Officials Toward Health Care Issues: An Exploratory Survey of Alabama Labor Officials." *Health Care Management Review* 24 (2): 71–82.

Freeman, R. B., and J. L. Medoff. 1984. *What Do Unions Do?* New York: Basic Books.

Harrell, J. 2006. "National Labor Relations Board to Send Labor Up the River." *Long Island Business News Ronkonkoma.* [Online article; retrieved 7/28/06.] ABI/Inform Global Database, www.proquest.com.

Harvard Law Review. 2004. "Labor Law: Department of Labor Increases Union Financial Reporting Requirements." *Harvard Law Review* 117 (5): 1734–40.

Hecker, D. E. 2004. "Occupational Employment Projections to 2012." *Monthly Labor Review* 127 (2): 80–105.

Hirsch, B. T., and E. J. Schumacher. 1998. "Union Wages, Rents and Skills in Health Care Labor Markets." *Journal of Labor Research* 19 (Winter): 125–47.

Kaira, R. 2005. "Labor Paints a Target on Union-Election Law." *Knight Ridder Tribune Business News.* [Online article; retrieved 6/14/05.] ABI/Inform Global Database, www.proquest.com.

Kearney, R. C. 2003. "Patterns of Union Decline and Growth: An Organizational Ecology Perspective." *Journal of Labor Research* 24 (4): 561–78.

Kowalczyk, L. 2004. "University of Pennsylvania Study Links Long Hours, Nurse Errors." *Knight Ridder Tribune Business News* (July 7): 1.

Leung, S. 1999. "More Nurses Join Unions Across State." *Wall Street Journal* (September 15).

Levenson, D. 1999. "Private Hospitals Worry NLRB Ruling Will Spark Intern, Resident Disputes." *AHA News* 35 (47): 1–2.

Luepke, E. 1999. "White Coat, Blue Collar: Physician Unionization and Managed Care." *Annals of Health Law* (8): 275–98.

Mandel, M., and J. Weber. 2006. "What's Really Propping Up the Economy." [Online article; retrieved 1/7/07.] *BusinessWeek* Online, www.businessweek.com/print/magazine/content/06_39/b4002001.htm?chan=gl.

Martinez, B. 2003. "Aetna to Announce Settlement with Physicians." *Wall Street Journal* Eastern Edition 241 (100): A3.

Meier, E. 2000. "Is Unionization the Answer for Nurses and Nursing?" *Nursing Economics* 18 (1): 36–38.

Metzger, N., J. Ferentino, and K. Kruger. 1984. *When Health Care Employees Strike.* Rockville, MD: Aspen.

Michels, T. J. 2004. "Three Doctors' Unions Form Partnership to Unite Resident, Salaried, and Private Practice Physicians." SEIU Press Release. [Online information; retrieved 10/24/07.] www.seiu.org/media/pressreleases.

Modern Healthcare. 2001. "The Labor Picture." Modern Healthcare 31 (May).

———. 2006. "Eight Unions to Team Up on Nurse Organizing Efforts." [Online article; retrieved 2/22/06.] *Modern Healthcare*'s Daily Dose, dailydose[modernhealthcare.com.

National Labor Relations Board (NLRB). 2005. *Annual Report.* Washington, DC: National Labor Relations Board.

Petzinger, T., Jr. 1999. "A Special Report: Industry & Economics—Talking About Tomorrow—Peter Drucker: The 'Arch-Guru of Capitalism' Argues that We Need a New Economic Theory and New Management Model." *Wall Street Journal* Eastern Edition (December 31): R34.

PR Newswire. 2006. "NLRB Issues Lead Case Addressing Supervisory Status in Response to Supreme Court's Decision in Kentucky River." [Online article; retrieved 9/17/07.] ABI/Inform Global Database, www.proquest.com.

Romano, M. 2004. "Labor Union Didn't Work." *Modern Healthcare* 34 (22): 32–34.

Rowland, C. 2006. "Nurses Union Flexing Clout in Contract Talks." *Knight Ridder Tribune Business News.* [Online article; retrieved 9/17/07.] ABI/Inform Global Database, www.proquest.com.

Rutkowski, A. D., and B. L. Rutkowski. 1984. *Labor Relations in Hospitals.* Rockville, MD: Aspen.

Scott, C., and C. M. Lowery. 1994. "Union Election Activity in the Health Care Industry." *Health Care Management Review* 19 (1): 18–27.

Scott, C., and A. Seers. 1996. "Determinants of Union Election Outcomes in the Non-Hospital Health Care Industry." *Journal of Labor Research* 17 (4): 701–15.

SEIU. 2007. "SEIU Plans to Form Healthcare Unit." [Online information; retrieved 8/28/07.] www.fiercehealthcare.com.

Siderius, C. 2005. "Union Official Rallies Nurses at Swedish." *Seattle Times.* [Online information; retrieved 8/28/07.] http://seattletimes.nwsourcecom/cgi-bin.

Spetz, J., and R. Given. 2003. "The Future of the Nurse Shortage: Will Wage Increases Close the Gap?" *Health Affairs* 22 (6): 199–206.

Stickler, K. B. 1990. "Union Organizing Will Be Divisive and Costly." *Hospitals* (July 5): 68–70.

Strom, S. 2008. "Hospital's Accounting Is Under Fire by a Union." *New York Times.* [Online article; retrieved 2/28/08.] www.nytimes.com/2008/02/20/us/20 hosp.html?ref=us.

Swoboda, F. 1999. "A Healthy Sign for Organized Labor; Vote by L. A. Caregivers Called Historic." *Washington Post* (February 27).

Taylor, M. 2006. "Nurses Sue Detroit-Area Hospitals." [Online article; retrieved 12/20/06.] *Modern Healthcare*'s Daily Dose, dailydose@modernhealthcare.com.

Von Bergen, J. M. 2006. "Testing Unions' Clout: Pivotal Cases: For Some Employees, their Union Status Hinges on an NLRB Decision that Will Define the Word Supervisor." *Knight Ridder Tribune Business News*. [Online article; retrieved 9/17/07.] ABI/Inform Global Database, www.proquest.com.

Yacht, A. C. 2000. "Unionization of House Officers: The Experience at One Medical Center." *New England Journal of Medicine* 342 (6): 429–31.

NURSE WORKLOAD, STAFFING, AND MEASUREMENT

Cheryl B. Jones, PhD, RN, and George H. Pink, PhD

Learning Objectives

After completing this chapter, the reader should be able to

- list the factors that affect nurse workload and staffing;
- discuss the influence of nursing shortages on the deployment of nursing staff and on the ability of a healthcare organization to deliver quality patient care;
- compare and contrast the terms nurse workload and nurse staffing;
- recognize the types of licensed and unlicensed nursing personnel employed in patient care delivery, and describe how different types of personnel affect nurse workload and staffing decisions;
- identify three primary reasons for measuring nurse workload;
- explain how an organization's philosophy influences nurse workload and staffing decisions, and be aware of various stakeholder perspectives on staffing and workload issues;
- understand how patient classification systems are used in calculating nurse workload, and discuss the strengths and weaknesses of these systems;
- be familiar with the types of information needed to calculate nursing full-time equivalents and the process for acquiring and using this information; and
- address the impact of nurse workload and staffing on nurse stress and burnout and on the quality of patient care.

Introduction

Nurses are the constant in healthcare organizations. They are on the front-line and at the point of care, 24 hours a day, 7 days a week. They are the most visible faces in these highly complex organizations, where outcomes are critical and where services often are provided under difficult and unpredictable conditions. Nurses provide a critical surveillance function in healthcare organizations, particularly in hospitals, by monitoring care and safeguarding patients; thus, the availability and work of nurses affect quality of care and patient safety (Aiken et al. 2003a). Nurses are a primary determinant of patient satisfaction (Abramowitz, Cote, and Berry 1987; Greeneich 1993; Vahey et al. 2004)—an outcome that takes high priority in a competitive healthcare environment. Clearly, a well-trained, motivated, and appropriately deployed nursing staff have a strong influence on a healthcare organization's ability to provide effective and efficient patient care.

A critical problem for healthcare administrators is deciding how best to deploy nursing staff while considering the quality and costs of care delivered. This challenge is complicated by recurring nursing shortages and by the fierce competition for these professionals. During shortages, healthcare administrators often must take extraordinary steps (such as closing beds or hiring temporary nurses) to ensure that sufficient numbers of nurses are available to care for patients, and these steps are often taken under constrained budgets and without knowing the specific impact on patient outcomes. Managers must be aware of the implications of nurse workload and staffing decisions, particularly during times of nurse shortages, because such decisions may affect staff morale and increase turnover. A basic understanding of nurse workload and staffing issues allows managers to meet day-to-day patient care requirements as well as changing patient care demands, personnel, reimbursement, and regulations.

This chapter provides an overview of nurse staffing, workload, and measurement and the issues that pertain to nurse workload. An understanding of these issues and how to address them is essential for managers who oversee the planning, staffing, budgeting, and evaluation of patient care delivery on units and in departments. Also, in this chapter, the types of nursing professionals are discussed, the terms nurse workload and nurse staffing are defined, the approaches used in different healthcare setting to measure nurse workload are examined, the perspectives of different stakeholders on workload measurement are provided, and nurse staffing metrics are presented along with examples of staffing calculations.

Types of Nursing Personnel

In the United States, licensed and unlicensed nursing personnel differ in terms of education; knowledge, skills, and abilities; and patient care responsibilities. These differences must be taken into account when planning nurse workloads and staffing.

Licensed nursing personnel include those who work under a specific scope of practice set by state and/or national regulatory requirements (Bureau of Labor Statistics 2008). There are two types of licensed nurses: registered nurses (RNs) and licensed practical nurses (LPNs)[1]; the educational, licensure, and practice requirements for one group differ from those of the other. Healthcare organizations require proof of licensure from both types of nurses. Unlicensed nursing personnel, such as nursing assistants, provide support services to licensed nurses and other healthcare professionals. Characteristics of licensed and unlicensed nursing personnel are summarized in Table 15.1.

TABLE 15.1   Description of Licensed and Unlicensed Nursing Staff

	Licensed Nursing Personnel		Unlicensed Nursing Personnel
	RN	**LPN**	**NA***
Educational Preparation	3-year diploma (hospital-based program[a]); 2-year associate degree; 4-year baccalaureate degree[b] Some master's and doctoral programs also exist for entry-level preparation	1–2 years of training at a technical or vocational school	Varies; some healthcare organizations have mandatory training requirements and certification requirements; some states have a registry of those certified
Licensure Required	Issued by states; examination required	Issued by states; examination required	Certification by an accrediting body may or may not be required
Duties	Provide complex nursing care to promote patient health, prevent disease, and help patients cope with illness Observe, assess, and evaluate patient conditions Work with patients, families, and other healthcare professionals to develop and manage patient plans of care May function independently, often work in collaboration with physicians and other healthcare professionals	Provide routine nursing care, which may include taking patient vital signs, administering medications as regulated by the state and/or agency of practice, monitoring patient reactions to routine medications and treatments, assisting with personal hygiene and activities of daily living, collecting patient samples, performing routine lab tests, teaching simple tasks to patients and families, and performing some clerical duties	Provide support services to licensed nurses and other healthcare professionals Provide routine assistive care to patients, such as answering call lights, serving meals, assisting in patient feeding and hygiene care, taking patient vital signs, preparing equipment for patient procedures and treatment, assisting with certain procedures, stocking patient supplies, and performing some clerical duties

(Continued)

TABLE 15.1 Continued

	RN	LPN	NA*
Duties (continued)	May supervise other licensed and unlicensed nursing personnel	In skilled nursing facilities, may evaluate patient needs	In skilled nursing facilities, develop relationships with patients and families
Supervised by	May function independently within scope of practice, or may be supervised by other RNs and in some cases physicians	RN and/or physician, may also supervise other LPNs and/or unlicensed nursing personnel	RN and/or physician, sometimes by LPN

*NA represents nursing aides, nursing assistants, patient care assistants, and orderlies.

a. The number of these programs has been in decline in the last three decades.

b. Advanced practice nurses (i.e., clinical nurse specialist, nurse practitioner, nurse midwife, nurse anesthetist) require a master's or higher-level degree and/or certification in nursing.

SOURCE: Bureau of Labor Statistics (2008)

Healthcare organizations employ a mix of nursing personnel to meet patient care needs. Decisions about the numbers and types of nursing personnel to hire reflect an organization's philosophy about the role and importance of nursing; patient safety and satisfaction; quality of care; and the job satisfaction, perceived value, and safety of nurses and other nursing staff. In short, nurse staffing decisions represent the value that the unit, department, or organization places on nursing practice and on patient care delivery (Van Slyck 1991). This value then is the foundation on which nurse workload and resource allocation decisions are based.

Definitions and Measurement

The terms "nurse workload" and "nurse staffing" are often used interchangeably and inconsistently. For the purposes of this chapter, the following definitions will be used:

- *Nurse workload* means (1) the number of patients or patient days for which nursing care is required on a unit or within a department or organization or (2) the number of patients cared for by an individual nurse (i.e., often referred to as the patient-to-nurse ratio).
- *Nurse staffing* means (1) the number of nurses deployed (also called staffing level) or (2) the process by which the appropriate number and type of nursing personnel are deployed to satisfy nurse workload requirements.

Nurse workload thus refers to a quantity of nursing services, while nurse staffing comprises the planning, budgeting, and costing aspects of providing nursing services.

A review of the literature reveals that researchers define and measure nurse staffing in different ways. These include (1) the number of nursing personnel, by type of nurse; (2) the type of nursing personnel hours (e.g., RN hours) as a percentage of total nursing care hours; (3) the number of personnel (i.e., head count) as a percentage of total nursing staff; (4) the number of FTEs (full-time equivalent) for specific nursing personnel; and (5) the percentage of total nursing FTEs, by type of nurse (e.g., RN FTEs) (Mark, Hughes, and Jones 2004; Seago 2001). As discussed later in this chapter, the relationship between nurse staffing and adverse patient events has been documented in various studies (see, for example, integrative reviews conducted by Kane et al. 2007; Lankshear, Sheldon, and Maynard 2005; and Thungjaroenkul, Cummings, and Embleton 2007). However, comparing the findings from these studies is difficult because of the inconsistencies and variation in the definition and measurement used.

In addition, disagreement abounds in the nursing field about how to best ensure that staffing levels are adequate to meet patient care demands and to keep patients safe. According to the American Nurses Association (ANA 2008), three general approaches have been used to address the appropriateness of nurse staffing levels. The first is a regulatory approach that holds healthcare organizations accountable for establishing and implementing staffing plans based on patient need and other nursing-related criteria, and with input from frontline staff nurses. The second is a legislative approach, whereby specific nurse staffing ratios are mandated by state law. The third is a combination approach that requires organizational nurse staffing plans to be in accordance with specific, legislated nurse staffing ratios.

In 1999, California was the first state to pass nurse staffing legislation for hospitals, setting a minimum nurse-to-patient ratio of 1:6 beginning in 2004, with the ratio declining to 1:5 in 2005. These ratios were established on the assumption that higher nurse staffing levels would lead to improved patient care. However, little or no evidence exists to support the specific ratios selected, and disagreement about whether or not nurse staffing levels should be legislated still exists. Recognizing these arguments, California followed the 1999 staffing legislation with other bills that call for the evaluation of the mandated ratios and the development of staffing plans in hospitals. In 2005, California's governor attempted to halt implementation of the legislated nurse-to-patient ratio of 1:5, but this suspension was later overturned by the courts. Other states have taken similar actions by introducing legislation to mandate the development and implementation of specific nurse staffing plans, minimum staffing ratios, or some combination of both (ANA 2008).

Although nurse staffing legislation influences administrative decision making in some states, these laws do not cover all nursing personnel or patient care situations. In most states, nurse staffing legislation does not exist at all. As a result, administrators still struggle with several important questions:

- What numbers of nursing staff are needed to provide care for patients?
- What types of nursing staff are needed to provide care for patients?
- What mix of nursing staff is needed to provide quality care and ensure patient safety?
- What numbers, types, and mix of nursing staff can the organization afford?
- How does the mix of nursing staff vary by patient care area?

Finkler, Kovner, and Jones (2007) define nurse workload as the volume of work required to deliver nursing care for a patient care unit or department.[2] To facilitate the calculation of nurse workload, unidimensional metrics such as patients or patient days are used. However, in using this approach, the manager should appreciate that these metrics do not capture the complexity of nursing "work," which is multifaceted, requires specialized knowledge and skills, and entails more than the amount of time spent with patients. Unfortunately, we currently lack adequate quantitative tools to capture the complexities of nursing work. This deficiency necessitates that the unit manager take this complexity into account when determining nurse staffing and strive for a "balance of [nursing] job demands with sufficient resources (adequate staffing, time available) to plan and carry out work" (Koehoorn et al. 2002, 6).

Table 15.2 presents four scenarios to illustrate the basic components of average nurse workload. Scenario 1 shows that, given a constant nurse workload (number of patients), a decrease in nurse staffing (the number of nurses) increases the average workload (the number of patients per nurse). Scenario 2 shows that, given a constant nurse staffing, an increase in nurse workload also increases the average workload. Scenario 3 shows that average nurse workload does not change if the number of patients and the number of staff change at the same rate. Scenario 4 shows that the average nurse workload increases if the number of patients increases at a rate faster than the number of staff. These scenarios illustrate the following points: (1) an increase in the average nurse workload may be the result of more patients, fewer nurses, or both and (2) the average nurse workload is not reduced by an increase in nurse staffing if the workload (number of patients) increases at a faster rate. Of course, in the real world, nurse workload is seldom constant and the work of an individual nurse usually fluctuates as patients' numbers and conditions change. Nevertheless, the average nurse workload may be considered a crude measure of the adequacy of nurse staffing.

TABLE 15.2   Basic Components of the Average Nursing Workload

Scenario	Nurse Workload (No. of Patients)	Nurse Staffing (No. of Nurses)	Average Nurse Workload (No. of Patients per Nurse)
1. Constant number of patients, decreasing number of nurses	25	6	4.2
	25	5	5.0
	25	4	6.3
2. Increasing number of patients, constant number of nurses	20	5	4.0
	25	5	5.0
	30	5	6.0
3. Increasing number of patients and nurses with same rate of change	20	4	5.0
	25	5	5.0
	30	6	5.0
4. Increasing number of patients and nurses with different rates of change	20	4	5.0
	25	4.5	5.6
	30	5	6.0

Most healthcare organizations use formal nurse staffing processes to reasonably, fairly, and safely address nurse workload issues. These processes include the use of committees with nursing representatives, such as quality of care and patient safety; the development and implementation of staffing policies and procedures, including standards for the number and skill mix of nursing staff; and the determination of hours-of-care requirements for different types of patients. In addition, nurse staffing issues are usually part of the collective bargaining agreement between employers and nurse unions.

Use of Measures

Nurse workload is measured for three primary reasons: (1) to inform the budgeting process; (2) to meet regulatory and accreditation standards; and (3) to inform the development, implementation, and evaluation of staffing plans. The budgeting process necessitates the calculation of nurse workload to prepare an organization's operating budget and, specifically, to determine nursing personnel requirements and costs (Finkler, Kovner, and Jones 2007). The budgeting process involves decision making about the level and mix of nurse staffing, the workload that nurses will assume, and the allocation of resources. Regulatory requirements and accreditation standards necessitate that healthcare organizations comply with regulations of the Centers for Medicare & Medicaid Services and with the standards of the Joint Commission (2006). For example, in 2002, the Joint Commission instituted a staffing effectiveness requirement for hospital accreditation. Nurse workload systems may be used to gather staffing and outcomes data to document compliance with this requirement.

Nurse staffing plans, on the other hand, are blueprints for meeting specific patient care and regulatory requirements and for deploying nursing personnel efficiently and effectively. Staffing plans also enable managers to develop policies for reasonable work schedules, which promote a positive work environment, and for accommodating operational uncertainties and contingencies.

Nurse workload measures differ across types of healthcare settings. For example, nurse workload can be measured in terms of the number of patients or number of patient days in hospitals, the number of residents or resident days in long-term-care facilities, the number of clinic visits in ambulatory clinics, the number of home visits in home health care services, the number of deliveries in maternity wards, and the number of procedures in day surgery or operating rooms (Finkler, Kovner, and Jones 2007). Measurement systems have been developed to assess nurse workload in these different settings. These systems (usually electronic) capture the variable nature of nursing care requirements across different types of patients and healthcare settings, and they are used to determine the number of nurses required to care for different types of patients (Edwardson and Giovannetti 1994). In short, these systems provide critical information that aids in decision making and in nursing resource allocation (O'Brien et al. 2002).

Perspectives of Stakeholders

Obviously, patients and their families want to be assured that a sufficient number of nurses is available and appropriate patient–nurse ratios are in place so that they can receive individualized care and timely, relevant communications about their condition and treatment (O'Brien et al. 2002). Patients' perceptions are therefore important to healthcare organizations. However, nurse workload measures or systems do not take into account consumers' preferences and desires.

Healthcare administrators, including patient care unit or nursing managers, are concerned about nurse workload measurement for several reasons. First, they are responsible for allocating nursing resources—a decision that ensures patient care needs are met. For example, on a day-to-day basis, nurse managers[3] must modify staffing levels as necessary to meet nurse workload requirements. This may mean using agency or per diem nursing staff to cover for permanent staff who call in sick or are on vacation, to cover ongoing position vacancies that result from turnover or the development of new staffing plans or programs, and/or to respond to unexpected variations in patient care requirements. Second, they have to balance the costs of delivering nursing care with organizational reimbursements. If the nursing staff is too large (i.e., too few patients per nurse), the costs of providing nursing services may be unnecessarily high. On the other hand, if the nursing staff is too small (i.e., too many patients per nurse), costs may be lower in the short run; however, the work under this condition may increase nursing errors, stress, burnout, dissatisfaction, absenteeism, and turnover, which likely will lead to higher costs over the long run. Thus, administrators must ensure that nurse workloads are reasonable and fair, allowing nurses to deliver the level of nursing care needed by patients.

Insurer and payer perspectives have a financial basis as well. In some cases, an increase in charges as a result of nurse workload and staffing can hike up reimbursements. An increase in overall healthcare costs because of workload and staffing also increases the costs of coverage, which are then passed along to consumers. In turn, employers and consumers need to make a decision about whether or not to retain coverage with the insurer, and if so, whether to keep the same level of coverage.

Policymakers view nurse workload in terms of ensuring that nursing resources are sufficient in providing safe, effective care to communities and in meeting changing patient care demands. For example, the aging U.S. population means that, in the future, more nursing resources will be needed to care for the elderly and long-standing nursing shortages in many geographic areas will increase the gap between supply and demand. Policymakers must see to it that government and industry workforce policies recognize changing demographics and support human resources adjustment, such as providing incentives to nurses and other healthcare providers to enter the geriatric care field and educating nurses and other caregivers about long-term care. In addition, policymakers must develop guidelines to ensure that nurse staffing levels are safe and do not place patients at risk of harm or injury.

Nurses view many aspects of workload and staffing in terms of how they are directly affected. These include volume of work; responsibility to their patients, themselves, and their unit; multiple, concurrent, and often competing demands on their time; their feelings of overload and inability to complete work; having to deal with unexpected events or with interruptions; their familiarity with and support of work requirements; the abilities of other caregivers with whom they work; the degree to which the workload spills into their personal lives; their level of emotional and physical exhaustion from work; and their lack of control over workload (Gaudine 2000).

Measurement of Nurse Staffing

Nurse staffing involves determining the numbers and types of nursing personnel employed on a patient care unit in a hospital, long-term-care facility, emergency department, ambulatory clinic, or community health center. Decisions about the numbers and types of nurses employed on a patient care unit are based on (1) the patient population, (2) the nurses' education and skills, and (3) the organization's philosophy about nursing and patient care delivery.

Full-Time Equivalent

The metric for determining the numbers and types of nurses is the full-time equivalent or FTE. Nursing FTE calculations are used to determine unit and departmental staffing needs and are the key input to the budgeting process. An FTE is based on the concept of one individual working full time for a year—or 40 hours a week, 2,080 hours for a 52-week period (Finkler, Kovner, and Jones 2007).[4] FTE calculations include both productive and nonproductive time. Strasen (1987) defines *productive time* as time spent on providing care to patients and *nonproductive time* as time spent not giving care. Nonproductive time includes sick, vacation, holiday, and professional development days as well as other paid time off that is part of the employment benefit. The amount of nonproductive time for different types of personnel is based on organizational policy and may be associated with the individual's length of service to the organization. Although the amount of nonproductive time paid varies by organization, only productive time is used in calculating the amount of nurse workload available to deliver care to patients. For example, if organizational policy indicates that 90 percent of nurses' paid time is considered productive, and 10 percent is vacation, sick time, professional development, and non-patient-care time, then there is $0.90 \times 2,080$ hours paid/FTE = 1,872 productive hours/FTE.

Today, 12-hour shifts and other flexible schedules are commonplace. Under these arrangements, nurses may actually work less or more than 40 hours per week (Strasen 1987). Thus, the number of hours worked must be considered along with the policy regarding paid hours (i.e., productive and nonproductive, or total hours), and the number of productive hours per FTE must be taken into account when calculating unit FTEs (Finkler, Kovner, and Jones 2007). Nurse staffing calculations must take into account the fact that not all nursing personnel work full time. Many nurses work part time, providing managers with some degree of flexibility in staffing a patient care unit. On any particular patient care unit, FTEs may be composed of full-time staff only, part-time staff only, or most likely a mix of full-time and part-time staff. For example, on a patient care unit where full-time nurses work 7 days of 12-hour shifts in a 2-week pay period, the time per position exceeds 1 FTE:

$$12 \text{ hours/day} \times 7 \text{ days} = 84 \text{ hours in 2 weeks/80 hours in 2 weeks}$$
$$= 1.05 \text{ FTE.}$$

Alternatively, if full-time nurses on a patient care unit work 6 days of 12-hour shifts in a 2-week pay period, the time per position is less than 1 FTE:

12 hours/day $\times$ 6 days = 72 hours in 2 weeks/80 hours in 2 weeks
= 0.90 FTE.

Various data are needed to determine nursing FTEs and staffing (Finkler, Kovner, and Jones 2007):

- *Projected patient days.* A patient day is an accounting term that represents the concept of 1 patient that is cared for during a 24-hour period. Projected patient days are an estimate of future workload needs.
- *Nursing care hours (productive time) per patient day.* This is time spent delivering care to patients during a 24-hour period and is generally reported as a monthly average.
- *Staffing mix.* This is the proportion of RNs, LPNs, and unlicensed nursing personnel used to provide care in a 24-hour period.

For illustration purposes, consider this example: A patient care unit that averages 25 patients per day during a 30-day month pays for 6,000 RN hours. Of these 6,000 RN hours, 90 percent are considered productive. What are the paid nursing hours per day and per patient day? How many nursing care hours per patient day are involved? Here are the calculations:

- *Paid nursing hours*

6,000 nursing hours paid per month/30 days in the month =
200 paid nursing hours per day

200 hours of nursing care per day/25 patients per day =
8.0 nursing hours paid per patient per day

- *Nursing care hours*

6,000 nursing hours paid per month $\times$ 90 percent productive =
5,400 nursing care hours per month

5,400 nursing care hours per month/30 days in the month =
180 nursing care hours per day

180 hours of nursing care per day/25 patients per day =
7.2 nursing care hours per patient per day

Patient Classification System

Another important source of workload data is the patient classification or acuity system. Patient classification systems (either a manual, paper-and-pencil tool or an electronic system) categorize individual patient demands and nursing care requirements (Huckabay 1984) based on patient acuity or severity of illness,[5] not on diagnostic category. These systems provide a standard measure of nursing care for classes of patients (generally measured in hours of nursing care required per patient day) and provide a way of matching patient needs with nursing requirements. Commercial patient classification systems include GRASP, Medicus, and Quadramed, and some of these products can be customized by organizations to meet their needs and integrate with other management information systems. Individual organizations also create their own patient classification systems.

The potential for patient classification systems is great because they can be used to project nurse staffing needs, develop unit budgets, establish costs for nursing services, and inform risk management and quality improvement initiatives (DeGroot 1989; Seago 2001; Van Slyck 2000). Unfortunately, patient classification systems are often not used to their potential, are generally distrusted by nurses and administrators as not reliable or valid, and consequently are often not employed in decision making. More specifically, patient classification scores are based on nurses' ratings of patients' characteristics, severity of illness, and required number and complexity of treatment interventions (Van Ruiswyk et al. 1992). Because of the way in which patient scores are obtained, some claim that nurses may actually inflate patient ratings (which is also known as *acuity* or *classification creep*) to increase unit staffing (hence reducing nurse workload) or to prevent staff from being pulled[6] to work on another unit that may be understaffed (Malloch and Conovaloff 1999). On the other hand, some nurses believe that managers are not responsive and do not increase the number of staff when ratings suggest that more nurses are needed. Patient classification systems generally do not take into account the nurses' educational level, years of experience, or knowledge and cannot match the skills of individual nurses with the needs of individual patients. Thus, while these systems may be commonly used to estimate staffing and workload, they do not replace a manager's judgment and staff input for day-to-day or shift-to-shift staffing (Seago 2001).

Historical Data

Other information is needed to inform staffing assessment and measurement. Historical data help to understand variations in patient care on a unit, such as the following:

- *Utilization data*
  - —Average daily census (the average number of patients cared for per day over a defined time period) helps in determining a staffing standard on numbers and mix of nursing personnel by shift.
  - —Occupancy rate (average daily census or average number of patient days divided by the number of beds on the unit) aids in examining the extent to which unit capacity is reached.
  - —Admissions, discharges, and transfers and information on short-stay patients provide insight into patient turnover and work requirements.
  - —Temporal variations in care reveal factors that may affect patient admissions and requirements. For example, the flu season may

increase admissions on certain units, especially on units that provide geriatric care.

- *Payroll data*
  —Productive and nonproductive time paid data assist in determining paid hours per patient day.

- *Human resources data*
  —Staffing vacancies or the number of open positions help in estimating future staffing needs.
  —Nurse turnover rates, or the number of nursing staff who leave over a defined time period, facilitate the estimates of the percentage of productive hours and determine budget adjustments for the time period.
  —Collective agreements account for personnel contract changes.
  —Numbers of new versus experienced nurses aid in identifying productivity differences between new and experienced staff.

Unit and Organizational Knowledge

Efficient nurse staffing hinges on unit and organizational knowledge. First, knowledge of clinical policies is critical. For example, a manager who is staffing an oncology unit must be aware of the unit's clinical policy about patients on certain chemotherapeutic agents, the type of nursing personnel required to observe patients during treatment, the number of patients who typically receive these medications and treatments during a period of time, and the associated risks of the treatment. Second, knowledge of internal organizational changes in care delivery is needed to estimate the effect of changes in programs, procedures, or treatment protocols on staffing requirements. For example, if a new clinical guideline is developed regarding treatment of a particular type of oncology patient, the manager must understand the implications of guideline implementation on the numbers and types of staff required as well as their educational needs.

Third, knowledge of collective agreements is needed to ensure that staffing is in compliance with provisions agreed upon. For example, if staff on the oncology unit can work no more than 60 hours per week and if there are staffing vacancies, the manager will need to develop a plan in accordance with policy that covers shifts when unit needs exceed the supply and availability of existing staff. Fourth, knowledge of the internal and external organizational environment, such as anticipated structural changes or policy developments, is important. For example, if a second oncology unit will be opening to provide care to a specific group of patients, a plan must be in place to transition relevant existing staff to the new unit, cover the original unit, and hire additional staff as needed. Each of these pieces of information should be taken into account when calculating nurse staffing needs. Appendix B (see the end of the chapter) provides a detailed example of FTE and nurse staffing calculations.

Key Issues in Managing Nurse Staffing and Workload

When organizational revenues fall short of expenditures or when healthcare costs rise, labor—a large expense for healthcare organizations—often becomes a target of budget cuts. Organizations have engaged in such strategies as implementing nurse staffing plans that reduce the number of nurses, increase nurse workloads, or increase the number of hours worked by nurses (including overtime). In the long run, these strategies may be counterproductive and may negatively affect a manager's ability to appropriately staff a unit.

Managers should consider several issues as they reconcile budgetary and staffing issues, which are outlined in Figure 15.1 and discussed in greater detail in the following sections. Healthcare administrators, especially first-line patient care unit or nurse managers, should be aware of such issues and the impact of staffing decisions on nurses and nurse perceptions as well as on patients, care delivery, and overall organizational performance.

Workload Stress and Burnout

Workload is one of the most significant predictors of negative health outcomes, stress, decreased job satisfaction, and burnout. Burke (2003) studied the relationship between changing nurse–patient ratios and nurse perceptions of workload, job satisfaction, psychological well-being, and effectiveness of their institutions. According to this study, nurses who are assigned high patient–nurse ratios report heavier workloads, lower job satisfaction, poorer psychological health, and decreased view of hospital effectiveness. This study suggests that when nurses perceive excessive workloads (that is, they feel they have too much work to complete during work hours), they become stressed and burned out, which, in turn, lead to feelings of anger. Nurses in this situation may be more likely to call in sick or leave the organization altogether. High nurse workloads also have been associated with higher 30-day patient mortality and increased levels of nurse burnout and dissatisfaction (Aiken et al. 2002); high levels of nurse burnout and emotional exhaustion have been linked to low levels of patient satisfaction (Vahey et al. 2004).

FIGURE 15.1
Key Issues in
Managing
Nurse Staffing

- Workload stress and staff burnout
- Staff turnover, recruitment, and retention
- Aging of the nursing workforce
- The nature of nursing work
- Union versus nonunion environment
- Nurse–physician relationship
- Workforce diversity
- Balancing quality and costs of care

Healthcare managers must be sensitive to the potential effects of nurse workload stress and burnout. They must design staffing strategies that minimize potential lapses in patient care quality and patient satisfaction. Following are a few simple approaches to address staff concerns about workload and overload (Gaudine 2000; Prescott and Soeken 1996):

- Involve nurses in unit decision making, including the establishment of appropriate workloads.
- Engage nurses in contingency planning on how to deal with sudden changes in patient care needs or conditions and to manage fluctuations in staffing (e.g., call outs, vacations, educational leaves).
- Be aware of changes in clinical practice policies and providers that can affect nurse workload.
- Examine workload and quality data to help make a case for adequate nursing resource allocation.
- Provide adequate and less costly support staff (e.g., clerks) who can assist nursing personnel in carrying out non-nursing tasks and thus relieve nurses to care for patients.
- Develop strategies to give nurses as much control as possible over their workload to reduce their perception of overload. For example, ask nurses for input on the timing of patient admissions, the temporary closing of beds, and approaches to staffing and scheduling.

Staff Turnover, Recruitment, and Retention

Staff retention and turnover become a primary concern for unit managers during times of staff shortages. When staff are in short supply, more job-change opportunities are available within and outside the organization. But if turnover becomes excessive, it may bring about additional turnover, as staff lose their valued friends and colleagues, work teams become disrupted, and staff reflect more on their work environment and wages relative to those provided by competitors in the market (Jones 2004). High levels of turnover can also make recruiting new staff into a work unit difficult, because when there are so many vacancies, working conditions suffer; this information then gets communicated into the market through social and professional networks.

More importantly, however, turnover is costly, with some estimates indicating that the cost per nurse turnover is more than $60,000 (Advisory Board Company 1999) or 1.3 times a departing nurse's salary (Jones 2005). In addition to its quantifiable costs, turnover also presents qualitative costs, such as those that affect quality of care and patient safety as staff leave and enter patient care teams. For example, a nurse who leaves takes with him or her valuable human capital in the form of knowledge, skills, and experiences that are specific to the work unit and the patient populations served by the organization. This loss then affects the work of the entire team until or unless a comparable replacement is hired. While aspects of this human capital loss are quantifiable (e.g., the costs of advertising for a replacement), other elements are harder to put a dollar-figure on—that is, we cannot measure the cost of losing an individual's knowledge, skills, and experiences.

Following are several steps that healthcare administrators can take to deal with staff turnover:

- *Become familiar with organizational systems for tracking nurse turnover.* These systems are often monitored by the human resources department, but line managers typically receive ongoing reports that compare their unit's turnover rate with that of other units and even other organizations.
- *Establish a unit-level database with more detailed nurse turnover information that can be used in managing existing staff, looking for appropriate replacements, and identifying opportunities for growth.* Organizational systems to monitor staff turnover rarely contain fine-grained data, such as the level of expertise that is lost when a particular staff member leaves.
- *Create a process for tracking retention and determining a retention rate.* This is a different process than tracking turnover. Examining retention requires that the manager follow individuals (or cohorts of individuals) over time, beginning at their initial employment date (Waldman and Arora 2004).
- *Establish a mechanism for gathering ongoing feedback about why nurses leave, why they stay, and their perceptions of the work environment.* This will help the manager understand staff concerns, examine trends over time, and identify areas for future improvement.

Aging of the Nursing Workforce

A great deal has been written about the aging of the nursing workforce, highlighting the fact that the current number of younger nurses is insufficient to replace those who will retire over the next 20 years. According to a nationally representative sample of U.S. nurses in a 2004 study, the average age of RNs was 47, with 41 percent older than age 50 and only 8 percent under age 30 (Bureau of Health Professions 2006). These numbers reflect a dramatic shift in the nursing workforce since 1980, when only 25 percent of the workforce were older than 50 years and 25 percent were younger than 30 years. In fact, aging of the nursing workforce has been cited as a reason that the current nursing shortage is different and perhaps more severe than past shortages (Buerhaus, Staiger, and Auerbach 2000, 2004).

For the first time in nursing history, four different generations of nurses are working side-by-side: Gen Yers (or Nexters), born before 1980; Generation Xers, born between 1960 and 1980; baby boomers, born between 1943 and 1960; and veterans, born between 1922 and 1943 (Swearingen and

Lieberman 2004). Members of each generation pose different needs and desires that drive their expectations about work and the workplace. They also have different perspectives on and degree of comfort with technology. Some simply use e-mail or other electronic systems during the process of routine activities, while others tote personal digital assistants and specific pieces of equipment in caring for patients. In turn, these generational differences in needs, desires, and expectations may create conditions that bring out intergenerational conflicts (Greene 2005; Swearingen and Lieberman 2004).

Age and generational issues, combined with changes in healthcare organizations and patient populations, require special attention from the manager. For example, patients today are sicker, have shorter lengths of stay, and require more intensive nursing care than patients in the past. This change in patient needs is the result of many factors, including technological capabilities that enable the delivery of more complex care; an increase in obesity rate, which leads to health problems; and a longer life expectancy, which typically means additional health concerns. These and other factors combine to exert more physical stress and strain on nurses and put them at risk for physical injury.

Creating a positive work environment for nurses requires sensitivity to generational needs. Following are some strategies toward that end (Greene 2005; Swearingen and Lieberman 2004):

- Conduct an ergonomic evaluation of the work environment and address necessary concerns.
- Give adequate support in terms of patient transportation, lifting, and moving.
- Offer adequate training on the multitude of technological devices and equipment used on the unit.
- Provide adequate staffing so that meals and "mental" breaks can be taken from the sometimes relentless bombardment of cognitive and physical demands.
- Put a process in place to stay in touch with generational perceptions and expectations of nurses pertaining to such issues as types of rewards and recognition, job satisfaction, and organizational commitment (Kovner et al. 2006).

The Nature of Nursing Work

Nurses' work has been characterized as complex, fragmented, and unpredictable (Tucker and Spear 2006); ambiguous and dangerous (Philbin 2007); and physically demanding. Potter and colleagues (2004) combined qualitative and human factors methods to examine the work of nursing. They reported that nurses often traverse long and repetitive distances, even when based on a single patient care unit. Nurses' work is also intellectually, emotionally, and psychologically demanding because of its composition and context. For example, the work environment is often chaotic, requiring nurses to perform at an intense cognitive level and to make numerous judgments about patients' conditions, many of which are of an urgent nature and must be made under pressure. Some nursing judgments entail actions that must be taken on behalf of patients, while other judgments involve contacting and interacting with physicians and other care providers to respond to changing patient conditions. According to Potter and colleagues, nurses' work is nonlinear and is plagued with numerous interruptions, which these researchers determined through the use of cognitive mapping. Nurses juggle numerous competing priorities during a shift, and the order of priorities can change quickly as patients' conditions change. In fact, Wolf and colleagues (2006) used human factors engineering and qualitative methods to study the nature of nursing work and reported that nurses often "stack" up to ten or more tasks at one time and experience more than three interruptions per hour. Such practices create conditions that are conducive to mistakes and omissions in care.

Others studies report on the effects of work strains that prevent nurses from recovering from work and gaining sufficient rest. Winwood and Lushington (2006) found that the high-paced work environment exacerbates nurses' psychological strains, which inhibit their ability to sleep and potentially lead to long-term health problems and withdrawal from the workforce. Other studies observed that nurses' work hours (frequently 12-hour shifts or longer) and the subsequent fatigue jeopardize quality of care and patient safety (Dean, Scott, and Rogers 2006; Rogers et al. 2004; Scott et al. 2006).

To address the complexity of nurses' work, managers can engage nurses in a dialogue to gain insights into current processes and systems that support or impede nurses' ability to do their job. This dialogue can be used to identify strategies to reduce the number of interruptions that nurses experience and to give nurses the tools to minimize the cognitive stacking of a great number of tasks and priorities. Many nurses do not get meal or short breaks during their shift or skip breaks to complete their work. Strategies can be developed to ensure that a sufficient number of staff is available to cover breaks and mealtimes so that nurses can get a mental respite and better focus on meeting patient needs.

Union Versus Nonunion Environment

Approximately 19 percent of the U.S. nursing labor market is covered by a union agreement, and 38 percent of hospitals operate under a union contract (Center for American Nurses 2005; Lovell 2006). Nursing unions are not without detractors, who claim that nurses' participation in union activities is unprofessional and associated with decreased job satisfaction and morale (Seago and Ash 2002; Fitzpatrick 2001). However, the following concerns converged in the late 1990s and early 2000s to bring about nurses' renewed interest in unions: declining nurse staffing levels, growing nursing shortage, increasing patient acuity, decreasing patient lengths of stay, proliferation of managed care, decreasing reimbursements, and widespread layoffs (Lovell 2006; Forman and Davis 2002; Schraeder and Friedman 2002; Steltzer 2001). For a detailed discussion of unionization in healthcare, see Chapter 14.

Several interesting observations have been made about unionization of nursing. Lovell (2006) reported that unions increase wages for both union and nonunion nurses in certain geographic markets. Lovell's study indicated that nurses who work in the most unionized states earn roughly 28 percent more than nurses who work in the least unionized states. Similarly, Lovell suggested that the presence of unions increases nurse staffing: Approximately 18 percent more nurses work in the most unionized cities than in the least unionized cities, which in turn improves the quality of care. Another study has found this same correlation. Seago and Ash (2002) examined the relationship between the presence of a union and the outcomes of hospitalized patients with acute myocardial infarction in California. According to that study, patients cared for in unionized hospitals had a 5.7 percent lower mortality rate than patients cared for in nonunion hospitals, after controlling for risk factors. The authors further suggested that the mechanisms through which patient outcomes may be affected include staff stability, staff autonomy, and nurse–physician relationships, all of which improve the work environment and ultimately care delivery.

Unionization is typically viewed as the result of an adversarial relationship or irreconcilable differences between management and staff. Unfortunately, as Forman and Davis (2002, 377) report, nurses have "identified their manager as their greatest source of stress—even greater than heavy patient loads." Managers, whether in a union organization or not, should realize that nurses typically seek out unions when they believe that they do not have a voice in issues that pertain directly to their work and the delivery of patient care (Schraeder and Friedman 2002; Forman and Davis 2002). In fact, many staffing concerns are focused on issues that pertain to communication, such as lack of input into decision making, feeling undervalued, and perceptions of fear and intimidation from organizational leaders (Fitzpatrick 2001).

Managers in unionized hospitals must obviously understand the collective bargaining process and the terms and conditions of the specific agreement at their organization. They also need to develop a strong relationship with the human resources department and consult with its personnel to address staff questions that pertain to the agreement. Managers must also be knowledgeable about dispute resolution and grievance and disciplinary processes, and they must be comfortable with addressing disagreements that may arise between the organization and the union (Forman and Davis 2002). In the worst case, or if disputes cannot be resolved and a strike ensues, managers should have a contingency staffing plan in place.

Time and again, frontline managers have been found to play a critical role in shaping nurse satisfaction and retention. The most important step that frontline managers can take, regardless of whether or not their hospital is under a union agreement, is to maintain open, honest, and consistent dialogue with the nursing staff (Schraeder and Friedman 2002). This simple strategy alone may divert union disagreements, strikes, or union-organizing activities. Managers who do not work in unionized hospitals should be aware of organizing activities in the event that nurses initiate a union campaign within the institution (Forman and Powell 2003). The bottom line is to keep the lines of communication open; to focus on patient care, protecting the safety, security, and well-being of patients and nurses; and to always take the high road by using factual data and acting in a professional manner (Block and Jamerson 2005). Porter-O'Grady (2001) recommends that managers view the union as a partner instead of an adversary and work from the mutual understanding that both sides can achieve positive outcomes and benefits. By doing so, managers and their organizations can take advantage of what nurses actually seek through unionization activities—namely, improving the work environment, nurse staffing levels, and the quality of care received by patients.

Nurse–Physician Relationship

The nurse–physician relationship is a key ingredient in sustaining a healthy work environment but is one of the greatest impediments to an improved workplace. When nurse–physician relationships are collegial, collaborative, and founded on open communications, nurses tend to be more satisfied with their work environment and are more likely to remain in their positions (Jansky 2004; O'Brien-Pallas et al. 2005). When nurse–physician relationships are caustic, over time, nurses become dissatisfied, demoralized, undervalued, and burned out—feelings that may cause them to leave their jobs. In the long run, patient care may suffer.

Because both nurses and physicians work for the good of the patients and to promote quality care, one would expect their relationships would be positive. However, nurse–physician relationships, in general, have been characterized as dysfunctional and in some cases pathologic (Stein 1967). A recent meta-analysis reported a strong and inverse relationship between nurse–physician collaboration and nurse job stress (right behind nurse job satisfaction) (Zangaro and Soeken 2007). Schmalenberg and colleagues (2005) argue that, although both nurses and physicians rate their relationship as important, literature on the topic has appeared primarily in nursing journals. Another study of nurses and physicians reported that both groups acknowledged the presence of disruptive physician behavior in their organization (Rosenstein 2002). However, in a follow-up study conducted in 50 hospitals, nurses were reported to misbehave almost as often as physicians, and respondents believed that poor nurse–physician relationships caused stress, frustration, and burnout and had a negative impact on concentration, communication, collaboration, information transfer, and workplace relationships (Rosenstein and O'Daniel 2005). Nurse–physician relationships also are purported to influence nurses' perceptions of staffing adequacy (O'Brien-Pallas et al. 2005; Laschinger and Leiter 2006), which may be attributed to nurse perception of a work overload when they are frequently involved in negative and emotionally draining interactions with physicians. Poor nurse–physician relationships place an added burden on nurses and physicians, often requiring additional communications, unnecessary follow-up, and perhaps even disciplinary actions for those who may already feel fragmented and stretched thin because of increased patient demands or short staffing. Poor nurse–physician relationships may also be linked to difficulties in recruiting new staff to the unit during times of shortage. For example, if nurse–physician relationships on a particular unit are known to be poor, other units likely know about it; as this information spreads, potential new hires may be deterred from working on the unit.

Despite the hardships that a poor relationship creates for the individuals involved, the bigger concern is that it affects the quality of patient care. Rosenstein and O'Daniel (2005) report that nurses and physicians perceived that negative relationships potentially affect patient care and outcomes, resulting in adverse events, medical errors, compromised patient safety, increased patient mortality, and lowered patient satisfaction. Other studies have found a link between good relationships and high patient satisfaction, minimized patient mortalities, fewer ICU readmissions, decreased length of stay, lowered costs, and perception of higher quality of care (O'Brien-Pallas et al. 2005; Schmalenberg et al. 2005).

Following are important recommendations for managers to improve nurse–physician relationships on their unit or in their organization:

- Conduct training workshops on interdisciplinary collaboration, communication, and coordination (O'Brien-Pallas et al. 2005).
- Hold joint, interdisciplinary staff meetings, rounds, and/or case reviews (O'Brien-Pallas et al. 2005; Schmalenberg et al. 2005).
- Articulate expectations clearly regarding nurse–physician relationships (Matthews and Lankshear 2003; Schmalenberg et al. 2005).
- Facilitate the development of joint critical pathways and protocols (Schmalenberg et al. 2005).
- Keep patient care as the shared, superseding goal (Schmalenberg et al. 2005).
- Develop and articulate clear processes for conflict resolution (Schmalenberg et al. 2005).
- Manage conflicts constructively when they occur (Schmalenberg et al. 2005).

- Role-model positive interactions with physicians and the medical director (Schmalenberg et al. 2005).
- Foster nurse competence through educational offerings (Schmalenberg et al. 2005).
- Create a positive culture that puts patients first, empowers nurses and builds their confidence, values teamwork and collegiality, builds trust, and respects each individual (Schmalenberg et al. 2005).

Walking rounds by the manager will also provide opportunities to observe nurse–physician interactions and to address concerns that may affect the work environment. Above all, managers play a fundamental role in fostering positive nurse–physician relationships, which in turn affects patients and potentially future unit staffing.

Workforce Diversity

One of many recommendations for addressing the nursing shortage has been to increase diversity in the nursing workforce (AACN 2001; Joint Commission 2002). In fact, the "Nursing's Agenda for the Future"—a document compiled by 19 U.S. nursing organizations, with input from more than 60 public and private organizations—lists diversity as one of its ten strategic goals for 2010 (Nursing's Agenda for the Future Steering Committee 2002). The Joint Commission (2002, 24) also recommends diversifying the nursing workforce as a recommendation for addressing the nursing shortage "to broaden the base of potential workers and to improve patient safety and health care quality for patients of all origins and backgrounds."

Nursing always has been and still is predominantly composed of white females. Currently only about 5.8 percent of the nursing workforce is made up of males (Bureau of Health Professions 2006). While this number represents a 14.5 percent increase in male nurses since 2000 (and a 273 percent increase since the baseline National Sample Survey of Registered Nurses conducted in 1980), males still represent a very small percentage of the nursing workforce overall. Additionally, approximately 11 percent of the nursing workforce is made up of nonwhite Latino, which is a decline from the 12.4 percent reported in 2000 (Bureau of Health Professions 2006).[7] Like the percentage of males in nursing, however, nurses of diverse racial and ethnic backgrounds still represent a very small proportion of the overall nursing workforce. This does not mirror the composition of the U.S. population at large.

Literature on the effects of workforce diversity on nurse staffing is largely absent. However, growing evidence suggests that individuals prefer to receive care from healthcare professionals who share their racial background and that healthcare professionals are more sensitive to the values and beliefs of patients from their own racial background (Coffman, Rosenoff, and Grumbach 2001;

Institute of Medicine 2004). Although the composition of the nursing work-force is changing, progress in achieving diversity in the last 20 years has been slow when compared to changes in the U.S. population. These changes may be partly the result of problems in the nursing work environment, slowly rising nursing wages, and other issues associated with the nursing shortage. However, they may also reflect the opportunities available to individuals from diverse backgrounds, their cultural beliefs, and even the slow progress in achieving cultural competence in the healthcare workplace. However, much is unknown, and this is an area ripe for research.

Several documents offer recommendations for healthcare leaders and managers toward building a more diverse workplace (Institute of Medicine 2004; Nursing's Agenda for the Future Steering Committee 2002):

- Create diversity and cultural competence through educational programs and standards.
- Provide opportunities for individuals of diverse racial and ethnic backgrounds to receive mentoring and guidance from leaders of similar and different backgrounds.
- Recognize the value of diversity on the patient care team, and promote diversity through hiring practices.
- Engage staff in developing a unit-based diversity plan.
- Seek information from nurses of diverse backgrounds to target recruitment and retention programs to diverse populations.
- Involve staff in recruitment and hiring decisions.
- Create leadership career paths for nurses from diverse backgrounds.

Balancing Quality and Costs of Care

Healthcare organizations are feeling increasing pressure to improve the quality of care while at the same time operating under a constrained financial environment. Also, during times when organizational revenues fall short of expenditures and/or healthcare costs rise, labor often becomes the target of budget cuts. This cost-cutting measure puts pressure on nurses because they are typically the largest group of professionals in the organization. Nurse staffing often comes under scrutiny in cases when the organization is considering whether the number of nurses can be reduced or whether the nurse workload and work hours can be increased.

Nurse staffing has received a great deal of attention in the last decade because of society's increasing concerns about patient safety and the high-profile reports that document the relationship between low nurse-staffing levels and adverse patient events (Aiken et al. 2002, 2003b; Kovner and Gergen 1998; Kovner et al. 2002; Mark, Harless, and Berman 2007; Mark et al. 2004; McGillis Hall et al. 2003; McGillis Hall, Doran, and Pink 2004; Needleman et al. 2002, 2006). For example, Aiken and colleagues (2003b) document that higher patient-to-nurse ratios are associated with a higher risk of mortal-ity and failure to rescue among surgical patients. Specifically, the risk of death is 14 percent higher in hospitals where workloads or ratios are six or more pa-tients per one nurse, and this risk is 31 percent higher in hospitals with work-loads of eight or more patients per one nurse, relative to hospitals where nurse workloads are four or fewer patients per one nurse. This study also documents a relationship between nurses' educational level and patient mortality, citing that hospitals that employ higher numbers of nurses with a baccalaureate (or higher) degree have lower patient mortality rates than hospitals that employ fewer nurses with a baccalaureate (or higher) degree.

Pay-for-performance (P4P) programs, which strive to compensate healthcare providers based on achieving certain patient outcomes, are becom-ing commonplace in the U.S healthcare system. For example, the Centers for Medicare & Medicaid Services (CMS) oversees Medicare's P4P program. The Hospital Quality Alliance program rewards hospitals on achieving a certain threshold on a set of ten quality indicators (e.g., care for myocardial infarc-tion) (CMS 2005). Hospitals that submit data on these ten indicators receive full, DRG-based (diagnosis-related groups) payment. Premier Hospital Qual-ity Demonstration reimburses hospitals based on 34 quality measures in five broad categories (acute myocardial infarction, congestive heart failure, coro-nary artery bypass graft, pneumonia, and hip and knee replacement); hospi-tals that score in the top 10 percent receive an added bonus of 2 percent, and hospitals that score in the second 10 percent receive a 1 percent bonus. Con-flicting evidence exists regarding the effectiveness of P4P, but given that pri-vate groups, such as the Leapfrog Group, are also reimbursing providers based on a P4P system, this payment scheme will likely become the standard for re-imbursing hospitals in the future.

Evidence that suggests that the lowest cost mix of nursing staff may not be the best option to improve quality of care and patient outcomes is grow-ing. In fact, Needleman and colleagues (2006) provide what they call an "un-equivocal" business case for nurse staffing. Using existing data, they con-ducted three different nurse staffing simulations to determine associated costs: (1) increasing the proportion of RN nursing care hours per day to the 75th percentile for hospitals below that level; (2) increasing the number of nursing care hours per day to the 75th percentile for both RNs and LPNs, again for hospitals below that percentile; and (3) using a combination of the first two options. The results of these simulations indicate that increasing nurse staffing under the first option provided the greatest return on invest-ment. That is, increasing RN hours only without increasing the total hours of licensed nursing staff was associated with a net reduction in costs.

Given that a richer RN staff has been documented to improve quality and to save money, changing nurse staffing to optimize patient outcomes may well be one of the best solutions for a unit or hospital to consider when examining ways to improve quality scores and in turn increase reimbursements. As Litvak and colleagues (2005) suggest, if one considers all of the patient safety measures currently being implemented, none of them can substitute for adequate nurse staffing. To ensure adequate staffing, managers can take several steps:

1. Managers should stay up-to-date on current research to be familiar with evidence that can help build their case for justifying changes or modifications in nurse staffing.
2. Managers should work with financial staff to develop and put in place a process for evaluating staffing costs relative to patient outcomes and quality. This kind of evaluation can be used to determine returns on investments made in modifying staffing levels and to develop a business case for modifying nurse staffing levels. It will also help managers understand how variations in staffing may affect patient and organizational outcomes.
3. Managers must involve staff in any attempts to address quality of care or cost concerns through modifications in nurse staffing. By involving staff in decisions regarding a change in the numbers and/or types of unit-based staff, the manager will gain insights from front-line caregivers regarding how potential staff changes may affect patient care and staff. The net result likely will be an improved overall staffing strategy for the unit.

Future Directions and Challenges

Measuring nurse workload and staffing and acting on the results are issues that have occupied healthcare administrators and researchers for decades. As Edwardson and Giovannetti (1994) suggest, many thought that patient classification systems would identify the right numbers of staff to provide care for certain patients. However, these systems have proven to be problematic, especially in terms of their reliability and validity, leaving managers faced with the need to establish nurse workloads and calculate nurse staffing needs for their units. Also, many healthcare organizations still lack the ability to free nurses from non-nursing tasks (e.g., retrieving medications from the pharmacy) that further increase nurse workloads but do not require specific nursing knowledge to carry out (Moody 2004).

Moody (2004) advocates a nurse workload approach that is grounded in human capital theory. This approach uses a nursing productivity index that takes into account nurses' knowledge, skills, and abilities (i.e., human capital) and the needs of patients for whom they provide care. This type of workload model is based on Peter Drucker's (1994) *knowledge worker* concept that values nurses based on their thought processes and judgments, and this system, although difficult to quantify, more adequately reflects the complex nature of nursing work. Moody proposes that this model captures data on patient intensity, nurse staffing, infection and error rates, organizational resources (financial and human), patient outcomes, patient ability to provide self-care, and provider outcomes. In addition, Moody advocates for the costs of nursing turnover to be included in the workload model (because nurse turnover reflects a human capital loss that should be considered in valuing nurses and their work) and for determining replacement costs for nurses who leave (Jones 2005). Details of this valuation are not provided, but the concept of valuing nursing work based on knowledge, skills, and abilities is intuitively appealing.

Various nurse staffing studies have documented the important relationship between nurse staffing and patient care outcomes, yet further research is needed to explain this relationship. For example, conceptually cogent and consistent measures of nurse staffing can facilitate the comparison of findings across studies and the identification of specific patient outcomes that are sensitive to changes in nurse staffing for different patient populations. Furthermore, much of the nurse staffing research is generally atheoretical. Thus, theory-driven research in this area is direly needed to help explain the how and why behind the relationship between nurse staffing and patient outcomes (Mark, Hughes, and Jones 2004).

Nurse workload systems are needed that take into account short-term staffing contingencies and variability in patient demand, improve the deployment of nursing personnel, and facilitate the development of long-term staffing plans. Moreover, information systems that link nursing workloads and patient outcomes are needed to improve the quality of patient care. Litvak and colleagues (2005) address the challenges that managers face in managing uncertainty and unnecessary variability in patient demands, which stresses staffing plans, adds strain to nurse workloads, and may compromise patient safety. Litvak and colleagues suggest that variability in hospital workload can be attributed to natural or uncontrollable variability that is largely patient and disease driven (such as patient admissions through the emergency department) and to controllable variability that is largely imposed by providers (such as scheduling elective surgeries and hospital discharges). These types of variability translate into necessary and unnecessary resources and dollars spent on healthcare. The latter type of variability, according to Litvak and colleagues, can be minimized to even out demand peaks and valleys, for it is during the valleys that most organizational resources are wasted. For example, in the past, hospitals have staffed nurses based on the number of beds, regardless of whether the beds were occupied. This system worked well when patient demand was high and nurses were in sufficient supply, but it wasted nursing resources when demand was low. During the 1990s, hospitals cut the numbers of nurses and staffed based on low and average demand, but this often resulted in understaffing that in turn caused stress for nurses and quality concerns for patients.

Litvak and colleagues and Pickard and Warner (2007) call for demand-based staffing. Litvak and colleagues suggest that organizations must understand and manage their sources of controllable variability and must recognize that predicting when patients will come to the emergency department is as possible as predicting elective procedures. Queuing theory and other operations management techniques can be used to understand and manage variability, smooth the extremes of demand, and reduce stress on the system. By eliminating or minimizing the controllable variability (e.g., appropriate use of block scheduling for physicians' operating room time, more coordinated discharge planning), the organization can then better staff for the uncontrollable or patient-driven demand.

Pickard and Warner (2007) present a demand management model to support staffing that is based on patient outcomes, measured in real time, and that is used to project future short-term patient demand (i.e., days). These requirements are embedded in a decision-support system that uses electronically captured data. This approach forecasts demand for controllable and uncontrollable variability by incorporating progress patterns for different types of patients; scheduled and predicted unscheduled admissions (based on staff input and historical data); and staffing information to help identify demand by unit, by day, and by hour and shift, which can be used in turn in making short-term staffing projections. Staffing is continuously updated based on patient outcomes and progress.

Although electronic systems such as the demand management system described earlier will become commonplace in the future, there is no substitute for the critical judgments of managers, who possess unique knowledge of nurse workload measurement, the work of nurses, clinical care processes, and the patients whom nurses serve. Healthcare administrators can contribute unique insights into nurse staffing to proactively plan and ensure that (1) nurses are involved in decisions that affect unit operations and nurse workloads, (2) adequate nursing resources are available to provide patient care, and (3) adequate support services are in place to support nurses and relieve them of performing nonessential tasks (Burke 2003).

Summary

Nurses are key members of the healthcare team. Understanding how best to deploy nurses while balancing quality and costs is an important ongoing function for healthcare administrators that may be especially challenging during periods of nursing shortage, when adequate numbers and types of nurses needed to ensure the delivery of safe, high-quality care may be in short supply. This chapter provides an overview of important tools and techniques that calculate nurse workload, and it presents examples to illustrate these calculations. Use of these tools and techniques aids in the routine planning of patient care delivery, development of unit and organizational budgets, and the equitable distribution of nursing staff. More importantly, however, use of these practices will foster the creation of an environment that increases nurse job satisfaction and well-being and that decreases the stress and burnout often associated with high workloads and inadequate staffing. Over the long run, sensitivity to nurse workload and staffing issues will contribute to the delivery of high-quality patient care, the formation of high-performing patient care teams, and improvements in overall organizational performance.

Discussion Questions

1. What are the various elements that compose nurse workload?
2. How is nurse workload related to nurse staffing?
3. What critical data are necessary to assemble before calculating nurse staffing needs?
4. How is organizational philosophy reflected in the measurement of nurse workload?
5. What other workforce issues may affect nurse staffing? How and why do these issues relate to nurse staffing and workload?

Experiential Exercises

Exercise 1   Jack Needleman and colleagues examine different nurse staffing arrangements in their 2006 *Health Affairs* article entitled "Nurse Staffing in Hospitals: Is There a Business Case for Quality?" (see the Reference list for a complete citation of the article). In this study, the authors used nurse staffing and patient discharge data from 799 U.S. hospitals to simulate three different nurse staffing approaches and to determine which of these options produced the greatest cost savings. Read this article, and then answer the following questions.

Exercise 1 Questions

1. Assume that you are the manager of a 30-bed general medical-surgical unit at a 200-bed community hospital. How can you use the findings from this article to help make staffing decisions on your unit?

2. What other important data sources will you examine before making a decision to increase or decrease the nurse-to-patient ratio?
3. Now consider that you are the chief executive officer at a large academic health hospital in an urban setting. Over the next two years, the nurse staffing ratio on the general medical-surgical units in your facility is projected to decrease from 1 nurse per 6 patients to 1 nurse per 4 patients. How will you estimate the costs and savings of such a change? Be sure to consider the organization's philosophy of care in your evaluation plan.

Exercise 2   The Joint Commission's staffing effectiveness standard defines staffing effectiveness as "the number, competency, and skill mix of staff in relation to the provision of needed care and treatment" (see www.jointcommission.org/NR/rdonlyres/979B4315-F409-476B-810C-22F0F0CB3BD5/0/hap_cah_sii_hr130.pd). Most healthcare organizations must meet this requirement to receive Joint Commission accreditation, and that accreditation is paramount to the ability of hospitals to operate and receive reimbursement.

Exercise 2 Questions

Visit two patient care units at a local hospital, and talk to the manager in each one. Ask the following questions of each manager:

1. How has your unit implemented the Joint Commission's staffing effectiveness standards?
2. How have unit operations changed as a result of this implementation?
3. How has this implementation affected the quality of care delivered to patients on your unit?
4. How has the nursing staff on your unit responded to this implementation?

   Following the interview, compare and contrast the two approaches followed by each manager for meeting the required staffing effectiveness standards. Is one approach better than the other? How can you use the experiences of these two unit managers to inform your own nurse workload and staffing decisions in the future?

Exercise 3 Susan Moore is the nurse manager in charge of a 25-bed medical unit at St. Eligius Hospital. She is currently preparing the nurse staffing plan for the next fiscal year. Hospital management has provided all nurse managers with a list of assumptions for staff planning, most of which are to use last year's numbers as first estimates for next year. Susan has assembled the following data for last year:

- The percentage of productive nursing hours was 83 percent.
- Fifty-two percent of nursing staff worked days, and 48 percent worked nights.
- The nursing staff was made up of 74 percent RNs, 16 percent LPNs, and 10 percent NAs.
- At St. Eligius Hospital, 1.0 FTE = 2,080 hours.

   From the hospital's patient classification system, Susan also assembled the following information for last year:

Patient Classification Level	Historical Patient Days	Historical Average Care Hours per Patient Day	Historical Total Unit Workload
1	1,000	4	4,000
2	2,000	6	12,000
3	3,000	10	30,000
4	2,000	14	28,000
5	1,000	18	18,000
Total	9,000		92,000

However, Susan is an experienced manager and is aware of several changes that will affect the nursing unit in the next year. More specifically, Dr. Smith, a senior physician who accounted for a large proportion of the unit's admissions, has just retired. In recent years, Dr. Smith has limited his practice to simpler medical cases, referring more complex cases to specialists who do not admit to the medical unit.

Dr. Jones just started at the hospital; she was recruited to replace Dr. Smith. Dr. Jones is a recent graduate who intends to care for many of the complex patients whom Dr. Smith previously referred to other specialists. Although the hospital projects that the unit's patient days will not differ from historical patient days, Susan is projecting a change in the mix of patients because of the arrival of Dr. Jones: 500 Level-1 patient days, 1,500 Level-2 days, 3,000 Level-3 days, 2,500 Level-4 days, and 1,500 Level-5 days.

Susan also knows that Dr. Jones plans to do more complex treatments during the day, which will (1) increase the nursing staff who work days to 57 percent and reduce the staff who work nights to 43 percent and (2) increase the nursing staff who are RNs to 78 percent, who are LPNs to 14 percent, and who are NAs to 8 percent.

Exercise 3 Questions

1. Based on Susan's projection of patient days, what is the projected total unit workload by patient classification level? What differences do you notice between the projected and the historic total unit workload?
2. Calculate the historical number of FTEs by staff type and by shift. Based on Susan's projection of patient days, calculate the projected number of FTEs by staff type and shift. What differences do you notice between the projected and historic FTEs?

Notes

1. LPNs are known as licensed vocational nurses (LVNs) in California and Texas (Bureau of Labor Statistics 2008).
2. For budgeting purposes, the patient care unit or department represents a cost center or entity for which nursing workload is determined.
3. Nurse managers oversee the day-to-day operations of patient care units. Other healthcare administrators may serve in this capacity as well. However, nurse managers commonly fill this role because they understand clinical care processes, the implications of nursing practice, and the scope of practice for different types of nursing personnel at the point of care delivery.
4. In a two-week pay period, 1 FTE equals 80 hours.
5. Patient needs and care requirements vary, even within the same disease category or classification.
6. The practice of pulling nurses from their regularly assigned unit to work on another understaffed unit is often referred to as *floating*.
7. This decline may be a function of data-collection procedures, study methodology, and nurse responses rather than an actual decline in the number and percentage of nonwhite, Hispanic nurses. However, we cannot know the exact explanation for this decline.

References

Abramowitz, S., A. A. Cote, and E. Berry. 1987. "Analyzing Patient Satisfaction: A Multianalytic Approach." *Quality Review Bulletin* 13 (4): 122–30.

Advisory Board Company. 1999. "A Misplaced Focus: Reexamining the Recruiting/Retention Trade-Off." *Nursing Watch* 11: 1–14.

Aiken, L. H., S. P. Clarke, D. M. Sloane, J. Sochalski, and J. H. Silber. 2002. "Hospital Nurse Staffing and Patient Mortality, Nurse Burnout, and Job Dissatisfaction." *JAMA* 288 (16): 1987–93.

Aiken, L. H., S. P. Clarke, J. H. Silber, and D. M. Sloane. 2003a. "Hospital Nurse Staffing, Education, and Patient Mortality." *LDI Issue Brief* 9 (2): 1–4.

Aiken, L. H., S. P. Clarke, R. B. Cheung, D. M. Sloane, and J. H. Silber. 2003b. "Educational Levels of Hospital Nurses and Surgical Patient Mortality." *JAMA* 290 (12): 1617–23.

American Association of Colleges of Nursing (AACN). 2001. "Effective Strategies for Increasing Diversity in Nursing Programs." [Online article; retrieved 3/8/08.] www.aacn.nche.edu/Publications/issues/dec01.htm.

American Nurses Association (ANA). 2008. "Nurse Staffing Plans and Ratios." [Online article; retrieved 7/17/07] http://nursingworld.org/MainMenuCategories/ANAPoliticalPower/State/StateLegislativeAgenda/StaffingPlansandRatios_1.aspx.

Block, V. J., and P. A. Jamerson. 2005. "Running a Successful Campaign Against Unionization." *Journal of Nursing Administration* 35 (1): 29–34.

Buerhaus, P., D. Staiger, and D. Auerbach. 2000. "Implications of an Aging Registered Nurse Workforce." *JAMA* 283 (22): 2948–54.

———. 2004. "New Signs of a Strengthening U.S. Nurse Labor Market?" *Health Affairs* Web Exclusive (W4): 526–33.

Bureau of Health Professions, U.S. Department of Health and Human Services. 2006. *The Registered Nurse Population, Findings from the National Sample Survey of Registered Nurses, March 2004.* Health Resources and Services Administration. [Online report; retrieved 7/19/07.] ftp://ftp.hrsa.gov/bhpr/workforce/0306rnss.pdf.

Bureau of Labor Statistics, U.S. Department of Labor. 2008. *Occupational Outlook Handbook, 2008–09 Edition.* [Online information; retrieved 3/4/08.] www.bls.gov/oco/.

Burke, R. J. 2003. "Hospital Restructuring, Workload, and Nursing Staff Satisfaction and Work Experiences." *The Health Care Manager* 22 (2): 99–107.

Center for American Nurses. 2005. "Workplace of the Future: Spotlight on the Mature Nursing Workforce." [Online proceedings; retrieved 7/25/07.] http://nursingworld. org/center/ebook/download/maturemonograph.pdf.

Centers for Medicare & Medicaid Services (CMS). 2005. *Medicare Pay for Performance (P4P) Initiatives.* [Online document; retrieved 7/30/07.] www.cms.hhs.gov/apps/media/ press/release.asp?Counter=1343.

Coffman, J. M., E. Rosenoff, and K. Grumbach. 2001. "Racial/Ethnic Disparities in Nursing." *Health Affairs* 20 (3): 263–72.

Dean, G. E., L. D. Scott, and A. E. Rogers. 2006. "Infants at Risk: When Nurse Fatigue Jeopardizes Quality Care." *Advances in Neonatal Care* 6 (3): 120–26.

DeGroot, H. A. 1989. "Patient Classification System Evaluation: Part 2, System Selection and Implementation." *Journal of Nursing Administration* 19 (7): 24–30.

Drucker, P. F. 1994. "The Age of Social Transformation." *Atlantic Monthly* 274 (5): 53–80.

Edwardson, S. R., and P. B. Giovannetti. 1994. "Nursing Workload Measurement Systems." In *Annual Review of Nursing Research*, Volume 12, edited by J. J. Fitzpatrick and J. S. Stevenson, 95–123. New York: Springer.

Finkler, S. A., C. T. Kovner, and C. B. Jones. 2007. *Financial Management for Nurse Managers and Executives*, 3rd Edition. Philadelphia, PA: W.B. Saunders Company.

Fitzpatrick, M. A. 2001. "Collective Bargaining, Part 1: A Vulnerability Assessment." *Nursing Management* 32 (2): 41–42.

Forman, H., and G. A. Davis. 2002. "The Rising Tide of Healthcare Labor Unions in Nursing." *Journal of Nursing Administration* 32 (7/8): 376–78.

Forman, H., and T. A. Powell. 2003. "Managing During an Employee Walkout." *Journal of Nursing Administration* 33 (9): 430–33.

Gaudine, A. P. 2000. "What Do Nurses Mean by Workload and Work Overload?" *Canadian Journal of Nursing Leadership* 13 (2): 22–27.

Greene, J. 2005. "What Nurses Want: Different Generations, Different Expectations." Hospitalconnect.com [Online information; retrieved 7/18/07.] www.hhnmag.com/hhnmag_app/hospitalconnect/search/article.jsp?dcrpath=HHNMAG/PubsNewsArticle/data/0503HHN_FEA_CoverStory&domain=HHNMAG.

Greeneich, D. 1993. "The Link Between New and Return Business and Quality Care: Patient Satisfaction." *Advances in Nursing Science* 16 (1): 62–72.

Huckabay, L. M. 1984. *Patient Classification: A Basis for Staffing*. National League for Nursing Publications, #20. New York: NLN.

Institute of Medicine. 2004. *In the Nation's Compelling Interest: Ensuring Diversity in the Health Care Workforce*. Washington, DC: National Academies Press.

Jansky, S. 2004. "The Nurse–Physician Relationship: Is Collaboration the Answer?" *Journal of Practical Nursing* 54: 28–30.

Joint Commission. 2002. "Health Care at the Crossroads: Strategies for Addressing the Evolving Nursing Crisis." [Online information; retrieved 3/08/08.] www.jointcommission.org/NR/rdonlyres/5C138711-ED76-4D6F-909F-B06E0309F36D/0/health_care_at_the_crossroads.pdf.

———. 2006. "Staffing Effectiveness." [Online information; retrieved 3/08/08.] www.jointcommission.org/AccreditationPrograms/Hospitals/Standards/FAQ/Manage+Human+Res/Planning/staff_effectiveness.htm.

Jones, C. B. 2004. "The Costs of Nursing Turnover, Part 1: An Economic Perspective." *Journal of Nursing Administration* 34 (12): 562–70.

———. 2005. "The Costs of Nursing Turnover, Part 2: Application of the Nursing Turnover Cost Calculation Methodology." *Journal of Nursing Administration* 35 (1): 41–49.

Kane, R. L., T. Shamliyan, C. Mueller, S. Duval, and T. Wilt. 2007. *Nursing Staffing and Quality of Patient Care*. Evidence Report/Technology Assessment No. 151 (Prepared by the Minnesota Evidence-based Practice Center under Contract No. 290-02-0009.) AHRQ Publication No. 07-E005. Rockville, MD: Agency for Healthcare Research and Quality.

Koehoorn, M., G. S. Lowe, K. V. Rondeau, G. S. Schellenberg, and T. H. Wagar. 2002. *Creating High-Quality Healthcare Workplaces*. Ottawa, Canada: Canadian Policy Research Networks and Canadian Health Services Research Foundation.

Kovner, C. T., C. Brewer, Y. Wu, Y. Cheng, and M. Suzuki. 2006. "Factors Associated with Work Satisfaction of Registered Nurses." *Journal of Nursing Scholarship* 38 (1): 71–79.

Kovner, C. T., and P. J. Gergen. 1998. "Nurse Staffing Levels and Adverse Events Following Surgery in U.S. Hospitals." *Image: Journal of Nursing Scholarship* 30 (4): 315–21.

Kovner, C. T., C. B. Jones, C. Zahn, P. Gergen, and J. Basu. 2002. "Nurse Staffing and Post Surgical Adverse Events: An Analysis of Administrative Data from a Sample of U.S. Hospitals, 1990–1996." *Health Services Research* 37 (3): 611–29.

Lankshear, A. J., T. A. Sheldon, and A. Maynard. 2005. "Nurse Staffing and Healthcare Outcomes: A Systematic Review of the International Research Evidence." *Advances in Nursing Science* 28 (2): 163–74.

Laschinger, H. K. S., and M. P. Leiter. 2006. "The Impact of Nursing Work Environments on Patient Safety Outcomes: The Mediating Role of Burnout/Engagement." *Journal of Nursing Administration* 36 (5): 259–67.

Litvak, E., P. I. Buerhaus, F. Davidof, M. C. Long, M. L. McManus, and D. M. Berwick. 2005. "Managing Unnecessary Variability in Patient Demand to Reduce Nursing Stress and Improve Patient Safety." *Journal of Quality and Patient Safety* 31 (6): 330–38.

Lovell, V. 2006. *Solving the Nursing Shortage Through Higher Wages.* Institute for Women's Policy Research. [Online report; retrieved 7/26/07.] www.iwpr.org/pdf/C363.pdf.

Malloch, K., and A. Conovaloff. 1999. "Patient Classification Systems, Part 1: The Third Generation." *Journal of Nursing Administration* 29 (7/8): 49–56.

Mark, B. A., D. W. Harless, and W. F. Berman. 2007. "Nurse Staffing and Adverse Events in Hospitalized Children." *Policy, Politics and Nursing Practice* 8 (2): 83–92.

Mark, B. A., D. W. Harless, M. McCue, and Y. Xu. 2004. "A Longitudinal Examination of Hospital Registered Nurse Staffing and Quality of Care." *Health Services Research* 39 (2): 279–300.

Mark, B. A., L. C. Hughes, and C. B. Jones. 2004. "The Role of Theory in Improving Patient Safety and Quality Health Care." *Nursing Outlook* 52 (1): 11–16.

Matthews, S., and S. Lankshear. 2003. "Describing the Essential Elements of a Professional Practice Structure." *Canadian Journal of Nursing Leadership* 16 (2): 63–73.

McGillis Hall, L., D. Doran, G. R. Baker, G. H. Pink, S. Sidani, L. O'Brien-Pallas, and G. J. Donner. 2003. "Nurse Staffing Models as Predictors of Patient Outcomes." *Medical Care* 41 (9): 1096–109.

McGillis Hall, L., D. Doran, and G. H. Pink. 2004. "Nurse Staffing Models, Nursing Hours, and Patient Safety Outcomes." *Journal of Nursing Administration* 34 (1): 41–45.

Moody, R. C. 2004. "Nurse Productivity Measures for the 21st Century." *Health Care Management Review* 29 (2): 98–106.

Needleman, J., P. Buerhaus, S. Mattke, M. Stewart, and K. Zelevinsky. 2002. "Nurse-Staffing Levels and the Quality of Care in Hospitals." *New England Journal of Medicine* 346 (22): 1715–22.

Needleman, J., P. I. Buerhaus, M. Stewart, K. Zelevinsky, and S. Mattke. 2006. "Nurse Staffing in Hospitals: Is There a Business Case for Quality?" *Health Affairs* 25 (1): 204–11.

Nursing's Agenda for the Future Steering Committee. 2002. "Nursing's Agenda for the Future: A Call to the Nation." [Online publication; retrieved 8/19/07.] www.nursingworld.org/MainMenuCategories/HealthcareandPolicyIssues/Reports/AgendafortheFuture.aspx.

O'Brien, A. J., M. Abas, J. Christensen, T. H. Nicholls, T. L. Prou, A. Hekau, and J. Vanderpyl. 2002. *Nursing Workload Measurement in Acute Mental Health Inpatient Units: A Report for the Mental Health Research and Development Strategy.* Auckland, New Zealand: Health Research Council of New Zealand.

O'Brien-Pallas, L., J. Hiroz, A. Cook, and B. Mildon. 2005. *Nurse–Physician Relationships: Solutions & Recommendations for Change.* Comprehensive Report for the Nursing Secretariat and Ministry of Health and Long-Term Care Research Unit, Ontario, Canada. MOHLTC Grant # 06221.

Philbin, S. 2007. "Managing Ambiguity and Danger in an Intensive Therapy Unit: Ritual Practices and Sequestration." *Nursing Inquiry* 14 (1): 51–59.

Pickard, B., and M. Warner. 2007. "Demand Management: A Methodology for Outcomes-Driven Staffing and Patient Flow Management." *Nurse Leader* 4 (2): 30–34.

Porter-O'Grady, T. 2001. "Collective Bargaining, Part 3: The Union as Partner." *Nursing Management* 32 (6): 30–32.

Potter, P., S. Boxerman, L. Wolf, J. Marshall, D. Grayson, J. Sledge, and B. Evanoff. 2004. "Mapping the Nursing Process: A New Approach for Understanding the Work of Nursing." *Journal of Nursing Administration* 34 (2): 101–09.

Prescott, P. A., and K. L. Soeken. 1996. "Measuring Nursing Intensity in Ambulatory Care, Part I: Approaches to and Uses of Patient Classification Systems." *Nursing Economics* 14 (1): 14–21, 33.

Rogers, A. E., W. T. Hwang, L. D. Scott, L. H. Aiken, and D. F. Dinges. 2004. "The Working Hours of Hospital Staff Nurses and Patient Safety." *Health Affairs* 23 (4): 202–12.

Rosenstein, A. H. 2002. "Nurse–Physician Relationships: Impact on Nurse Satisfaction and Retention." *American Journal of Nursing* 102 (6): 26–34.

Rosenstein, A. H., and M. O'Daniel. 2005. "Disruptive Behavior and Clinical Outcomes: Perceptions of Nurses and Physicians." *American Journal of Nursing* 105 (1): 54–64.

Schmalenberg, C., M. Kramer, C. R. King, M. Krugman, C. Lund, D. Poduska, and D. Rapp. 2005. "Excellence Through Evidence Securing Collegial/Collaborative Nurse–Physician Relationships, Part 1." *Journal of Nursing Administration* 35 (10): 450–58.

Schraeder, M., and L. H. Friedman. 2002. "Collective Bargaining in the Nursing Profession: Salient Issues and Recent Developments in Healthcare Reform." *Hospital Topics* 80 (3): 21–24.

Scott, L. D., A. E. Rogers, W. T. Hwang, and Y. Zhang. 2006. "Effects of Critical Care Nurses' Work Hours on Vigilance and Patients' Safety." *American Journal of Critical Care* 15 (1): 30–37.

Seago, J. A. 2001. "Nurse Staffing, Models of Care Delivery, and Interventions." In *Making Health Care Safer: A Critical Analysis of Patient Safety Practices,* edited by K. G. Shojania, B. W. Duncan, K. M. McDonald, and R. M. Wachter. Evidence Report/Technology Assessment: Number 43. AHRQ Publication No. 01-E058. Rockville, MD: Agency for Healthcare Research and Quality.

Seago, J., and M. Ash. 2002. "Registered Nurse Unions and Patient Outcomes." *Journal of Nursing Administration* 32 (3): 143–51.

Stein, L. I. 1967. "The Doctor–Nurse Game." *Archives of General Psychiatry* 16 (6): 699–703.

Steltzer, T. M. 2001. "Collective Bargaining, Part 2: A Wake-Up Call." *Nursing Management* 32 (4): 35–48.

Strasen, L. 1987. *Key Business Skills for Nurse Managers.* Philadelphia, PA: J.B. Lippincott Company.

Swearingen, S., and A. Lieberman. 2004. "Nursing Generations: An Expanded Look at the Emergence of Conflict and its Resolution." *Health Care Manager* 23 (1): 54–64.

Thungjaroenkul, P., G. G. Cummings, and A. Embleton. 2007. "The Impact of Nurse Staffing on Hospital Costs and Patient Length of Stay: A Systematic Review." *Nursing Economics* 25 (5): 255–67.

Tucker, A. L., and S. J. Spear. 2006. "Operational Failures and Interruptions in Hospital Nursing." *Health Services Research* 41 (3 Pt 1): 643–62.

Vahey, D. C., L. H. Aiken, D. M. Sloane, S. P. Clarke, and D. Vargas. 2004. "Nurse Burnout and Patient Satisfaction." *Medical Care* 42 (2 Suppl): 1157–66.

Van Ruiswyk, J., A. Hartz, C. Guse, P. Sigmann, C. Porth, and K. Buck. 1992. "Nursing Assessments: Patient Severity of Illness." *Nursing Management* 23 (9): 44–46, 48.

Van Slyck, A. 1991. "A Systems Approach to the Management of Nursing Services, Part II: Patient Classification System." *Nursing Management* 22 (4): 23–25.

———. 2000. "Patient Classification Systems: Not a Proxy for Nurse 'Busyness'." *Nursing Administration Quarterly* 24 (4): 60–65.

Waldman, J. D., and S. Arora. 2004. "Measuring Retention Rather than Turnover: A Different and Complementary HR Calculus." *Human Resource Planning* 27 (3): 6–9.

Winwood, P. C., and K. Lushington. 2006. "Disentangling the Effects of Psychological and Physical Work Demands on Sleep, Recovery and Maladaptive Chronic Stress Outcomes within a Large Sample of Australian Nurses." *Journal of Advanced Nursing* 56 (6): 679–89.

Wolf, L. D., P. Potter, J. A. Sledge, S. B. Boxerman, D. Grayson, and B. Evanoff. 2006. "Describing Nurses' Work: Combining Quantitative and Qualitative Analysis." *Human Factors* (48) 1: 5–15.

Zangaro, G. A., and K. L. Soeken. 2007. "A Meta-Analysis of Studies of Nurses' Job Satisfaction." *Research in Nursing and Health* 30 (4): 445–58.

APPENDIX B

An Example of FTE and Nurse Staffing Calculations

Consider the annual nurse staffing needs for a busy, 30-bed inpatient pediatric unit at an academic health center. The nurse manager for the unit must determine the total unit workload, or nursing care hours, for the coming year using patient classification system data and patient days projected from historical data. The total workload for this unit is shown in Table 15.3.

The number of FTEs required to staff the unit over a year must be calculated and then distributed across the day shift and the night shift. FTEs must also be further divided according to the types of nurses required for each shift. The nurse manager also knows the following:

- 1.0 FTE = 2,080 hours paid.
- The percentage of productive nursing hours on the unit is 85 percent (an average of 1,768 productive hours/FTE).
- Nursing personnel on this unit are scheduled to work based on a staffing standard of 55 percent for the day shift and 45 percent for the night shift.
- The staff mix is 75 percent RNs, 15 percent LPNs, and 10 percent NAs.

The overall number of FTEs required to staff this unit is determined as follows:

91,300 total hours of care required per year/1,768 productive hours per FTE = 51.6 FTEs for year-round nursing care coverage.

The number of nursing FTEs required to staff day and night shifts for the year (shown in Table 15.4) is calculated as follows:

- Day shift coverage (annual projections)
  - 51.6 FTEs × 55% × 75% RNs = 21.3 RN FTEs
  - 51.6 FTEs × 55% × 15% LPNs = 4.3 LPN FTEs

TABLE 15.3

Total Unit Workload for a 30-Bed Inpatient Unit

Patient Classification Rating	Average Care Hours (ACH) per Patient Day	Projected Patient Days (PD)	Total Unit Workload (ACH × PD)
1	3.5	1,500	5,250
2	5	2,500	12,500
3	9	3,000	27,000
4	13	2,100	27,300
5	17.5	1,100	19,250
Total		10,200	91,300

TABLE 15.4

Full-Time Equivalent Calculations

Staff	Days	Nights	Total
RNs	21.3	17.4	38.7
LPNs	4.3	3.5	7.7
NAs	2.8	2.3	5.2
Total FTEs	28.4	23.2	51.6

APPENDIX B
Continued

−51.6 FTEs × 55% × 10% NAs = 2.8 NA FTEs
−51.6 FTEs × 55% = 28.4 total FTEs

- Night shift coverage (annual projections)
  −51.6 FTEs × 45% × 75% RNs = 17.4 RN FTEs
  −51.6 FTEs × 45% × 15% LPN = 3.5 LPN FTEs
  −51.6 FTEs × 45% × 10% NAs = 2.32 NA FTEs
  −51.6 FTEs × 45% = 23.2 total FTEs

The 51.6 FTEs are scheduled such that nursing and shift requirements are met. Over time, if patient classification data reflect a change in nursing care requirements, the FTE and scheduling requirements may change. The total number of FTEs needed on this unit is known, but the actual number of shifts and types of personnel needed must still be determined (shown in Table 15.5). Furthermore, based on the number of allocated FTEs, managers must make decisions about the actual number of people to schedule to meet ongoing requirements within budget constraints. The number of shifts by type of personnel is calculated as follows:

- Days
  −20.8 shifts per day × 55% day shift × 75% RNs = 8.6 RN shifts
  −20.8 shifts per day × 55% day shift × 15% LPNs = 1.7 LPN shifts
  −20.8 shifts per day × 55% day shift × 10% NAs = 1.1 NA shifts

- Nights
  −20.8 shifts per day × 45% night shift × 75% RNs = 7.0 RN shifts
  −20.8 shifts per day × 45% night shift × 15% LPNs = 1.4 LPN shifts
  −20.8 shifts per day × 45% night shift × 10% NAs = 0.9 NA shifts

Different approaches can be used to achieve staffing needs, as determined in our example. One manager may decide to staff for 9 RNs on days and 7 on nights, 2 LPNs on days and 1 on nights, and 1 nursing assistant on days and nights. Another manager may staff for 8 RNs on days and 6 on nights, 2 LPNs on days and nights, and 1 nursing assistant on days and 2 on nights. These decisions should be based on a manager's understanding of patient needs, staff availability, and organizational policy.

FTEs are likely to be filled with various combinations of full-time and part-time personnel. For example, the 21.3 RN FTEs may be made up of 22 full-time RNs or 18 full-time RNs and 7 part-time RNs, and so forth. These decisions are necessary to determine the actual number of nursing positions that will staff the unit and, in turn, meet the unit personnel budget requirements.

Nursing care requirements may vary by day of the week. Fewer nurses may

TABLE 15.5
Shift
Calculations

Staff	Days	Nights	Total
RNs	8.6	7.0	15.6
LPNs	1.7	1.4	3.1
NAs	1.1	0.9	2.1
Total shifts per day	11.4	9.4	20.8

(Continued)

APPENDIX B

Continued

be needed on the weekends because certain services for patient care testing and procedures are available only on weekdays. For example, the 145.6 nursing shifts per week (i.e., 20.8 nursing shifts per day × 7 days per week—see Figure 15.2, item 2) can be distributed so that there are fewer than 20.8 nursing shifts per day on weekends and greater numbers on weekdays (Finkler, Kovner, and Jones 2007), depending on unit operations.

If patient census on the unit changes over time, nurse staffing requirements may change too. In this case, it may be necessary to advocate for additional permanent or temporary nursing personnel (from unit or in-house staffing pools or outside agencies), decrease permanent FTE requirements, or ask unit staff to take vacation time and work fewer shifts. In both of these cases, the perspective and judgment of the nurse or unit manager are critical.

Returning to our example, if we divide the 51.6 FTEs required to staff the unit over a year by the 20.8 daily nursing shifts, we see that 2.48 FTEs are needed to fill each nursing shift for the year. This means that approximately 2.5 nursing staff must be hired full time (or a greater number must be hired if some work part time) to cover a 12-hour shift for 365 days (4,380 hours). The difference

FIGURE 15.2

Staffing Calculations for a 30-Bed Inpatient Pediatric Unit

Determine the following:

1. Nursing care hours required each day
2. Number of nursing shifts per day and per week
3. Number of nursing personnel required on day and night shifts
4. Breakdown of RN/LPN/nursing assistant staffing for day and night shifts
5. Ratio of FTEs to shifts

Solutions

1. An average daily nursing care requirement = 91,300 nursing care hours per year/365 days per year = 250 nursing care hours per day

2. 250 nursing care hours per day, with 12-hour shifts = 20.8 nursing shifts per 24-hour day (250 hours/12 hours per shift)

    20.8 nursing shifts per day × 7 days per week = 145.6 nursing shifts per week

3. Using the 55 percent/45 percent standard:

    20.8 shifts × 55 percent = 11.44 nursing shifts on days
    20.8 shifts × 45 percent = 9.36 nursing shifts on nights

4. Days: 8.58 RN shifts (11.44 × 75 percent), 1.72 LPN shifts (11.44 × 15 percent), and 1.14 nursing assistant shifts (11.44 × 10 percent)

    Nights: 7.02 RN shifts (9.36 × 75 percent), 1.40 LPN shifts (9.36 × 15 percent), and 0.94 nursing assistant shifts (9.36 × 10 percent)

5. 2.48 FTEs are required to cover one shift for the entire year (e.g., 28.4 nurse FTEs are required to staff 11.44 nursing shifts during days, 23.2 nurse FTEs are required to staff 9.36 nursing shifts during nights, etc.). This means 2.48 full-time nurses must be hired to cover one 12-hour shift, 365 days of the year.

between hours paid to 2.48 FTEs (5,158 hours = 2.48 × 2,080 hours) and patient care hours required (4,380) takes into account the personnel needed to cover for staff days off, sick time, holidays, vacations, and so forth (Finkler, Kovner, and Jones 2007).

Finally, in our example, 8.58 RN shifts (21.3 RN FTEs) are required to cover days, and 7.02 RN shifts (17.4 RN FTEs) are required to cover nights, with a census of 25 patients. This yields an average workload of approximately 2.9 patients per RN for the day shift and 3.6 patients per RN for the night shift.

HUMAN RESOURCES BUDGETING AND EMPLOYEE PRODUCTIVITY

Eileen F. Hamby, DBA

Learning Objectives

After completing this chapter, the reader should be able to

- discuss the purposes and components of the labor budget,
- translate the labor budget into human resources requirements,
- determine staffing levels based on productivity standards,
- identify staffing requirements based on patient acuity levels,
- analyze employee productivity based on benchmarking,
- list the challenges in managing the labor budget,
- compare and contrast the benefits and barriers to outsourcing services, and
- explain the impact of mergers and other organizational changes on managing human resources.

Introduction

Budgeting for human resources (HR) is an important consideration when addressing the human capital needs of any organization. Because the healthcare industry is a service industry and requires people to perform the major portion of its business, the cost of the HR component usually accounts for its largest expense. Paying for appropriate manpower can be a conundrum, especially in light of the hyperturbulence in the industry and ongoing changes in reimbursement. The constant search for the perfect third-party-payer system will undoubtedly cause continued stress within the healthcare industry and the population that it serves. Healthcare organizations must weigh the financial aspect of HR carefully and ensure that they can afford the people whom they hire or engage in service. HR needs differ from one organization to the next, depending on the vision, mission, goals, and objectives of the organization. The number and type of people needed in a given situation are dependent on many factors, including the skill level of the workers, the workers' familiarity with the organization, the standards the organization sets for productivity, and regulatory and accreditation requirements.

This chapter examines factors that link budgeting with human resources management (HRM) and link HRM budgeting with productivity. The components of the labor budget are enumerated, and the use of standard and nonstandard labor practices is considered from a financial standpoint.

Linking Budgeting with Human Resources Management

If an organization employs the number of staff its managers think is ideal; hires only the best candidates; and provides comprehensive benefits, high raises, and superb incentive programs, the organization will not be able to afford anything else to run its business. The total cost of HR comprises the majority of most organizations' expenses; therefore, managers must be careful not to overspend in this area.

A budget puts the financial status of the organization into perspective, as it allows a view into projected revenues and expenses over the period of a fiscal year. This process ensures that the organization has more revenues than expenses. To plan HR activities without looking at their financial impact on the organization is negligent and is difficult to do even for the most profitable of businesses. The type and quantity of HR activities must be determined based on the fiscal priorities and allowance of the organization.

The Labor Budget

The labor budget, also known as the salary budget, consists of the expenses allocated for salary, wages, benefits, and other employee costs. The revenue portion of the budget is influenced by the human component. Skillful, efficient employees can usually help the facility produce more revenue. On the other hand, workers who do not perform well and who are not motivated may impede revenue growth. Using a past history of productivity and activity measures, most organizations can predict both revenue and labor costs fairly accurately. The purpose of the labor budget is to predict the following:

- Required staffing levels based on volume projections and productivity measures
- Projected expenses related to regular, overtime, and overall productive hours
- Nonproductive hour expenses related to paid time off, including vacation, sick, holiday, personal, and education and other training hours
- Expenses for benefits, including payroll taxes, insurance, and other benefits provided to employees
- Total salary, wage, and benefits costs

Healthcare organizations should develop flexible budgets—that is, budgets that include revenues that are dependent on volume and expenses that fluctuate with volume. Each organization needs to prepare a budget to determine its financial break-even point and the profits it needs to remain viable.

Labor Budget Terminology
A standard labor budget terminology exists, and some of these terms are defined in this section. Table 16.1 lists the most common terms used in a healthcare setting.

Salaried employees (exempt) are paid a fixed amount of income regardless of how many hours worked in a period of time. *Wage earners* (nonexempt), on the other hand, are paid per each hour worked and receive overtime pay for any hours put in over the standard 40 hours per week. Hours worked are regarded as productive hours, including time spent for nonbillable work (down time) such as attending meetings, making phone calls, writing correspondence and documenting patient care or incidents, and doing other nonrevenue-producing but work-related activities. Nonproductive hours are those that constitute time paid to the employee even when work is not produced, or in the case of nonrevenue-producing departments, days paid for but not worked. The paid hours of a full-time equivalent (FTE) consist of both productive and nonproductive hours. The amount of care a patient needs based on the degree or difficulty of illness—acuity level—must be monitored continuously to determine the required amount of FTEs.

Components of the Expense Side of the Labor Budget
The components of the expense side of the labor budget are listed in Figure 16.1 in the order in which they normally appear on a budget spreadsheet.

The cost of payroll taxes includes the employer contribution to Social Security and Medicare taxes, which amount to 6.2 percent and 1.45 percent, respectively, of an employee's gross wages. Social Security has a wage cap beyond which it no longer taxes the employer or employee during the remainder of the calendar year. Medicare has no wage cap. Federal unemployment tax is 6.2 percent of the first $7,000 of each employee's gross wages (IRS 2007). Workers' Compensation insurance, also part of the employer's responsibility, is paid at a predetermined rate for specific employee classifications. An experience-modification rating modifies this amount by up to 50 percent less and up to 300 percent more, depending on the amount and severity of employee injuries. Employee benefits, including the employer share of Medicare and Social Security, often range between 25 percent and 35 percent of total salary. In recent years, the cost of healthcare insurance has dramatically increased. Other benefits may include pension, child day care, elder

TABLE 16.1
Labor Budget
Terminology

Term	Definition
Acuity level	This is the level of caregiving difficulty that determines staffing needs (for example, because intensive care patients are sicker, higher staffing levels are needed).
Down time	These are hours spent at work that are important to the job role but do not generate revenue (for example, a respiratory therapist documenting a patient treatment is time considered "down time"; this is not billable, but it is still important for patient care).
Full-time equivalent	This is the equivalent hours of one full-time person—normally 40 hours per week. This may consist of one, two, or more employees whose working hours combined equal the hours that one full-time employee normally puts in.
Labor (salary) budget	This includes all expenses associated with salaries, wages, and benefits.
Nonproductive hours	These are hours paid but not worked, including paid time off, vacation, sick, holiday, education, and personal.
Productive hours	These are hours actually worked, including down time.
Salaried employee (or exempt employee)	This is any employee who is exempt from overtime law and whose paycheck is not dependent on hours worked.
Wage-earning employee (or nonexempt employee)	This is an employee who is not exempt from overtime law and who receives payment based on hours worked and overtime pay for time worked after 40 hours.

FIGURE 16.1
Worksheet for
Expense Side
of the Labor
Budget

Line Item	Jan	Feb	Mar	Apr	May	June	July	Aug	Sept	Oct	Nov	Dec	Total
Regular hours													
Overtime hours													
Total productive hours													
Total productive FTEs													
Holiday hours													
Vacation hours													
Personal hours													
Sick time hours													
Off-site education hours													
Total nonproductive hours													
Total nonproductive FTEs													
Total hours													
Total FTEs													
Average hourly rate													
Average overtime rate													
Total salaries and wages													
Payroll taxes, insurance, and benefits													
Total salaries, wages, and benefits													

care, life insurance, tuition reimbursement, and travel and education. These benefits all add to the expense side of the labor budget.

Following is a step-by-step illustration of how these expense components are considered when developing a labor budget:

1. A physical therapy manager determines, through a trend analysis and new program volume projection, that next year's total volume for the department will be 100,000 procedures. In this department, all of the therapists are wage earners and are paid by the hour. No overtime is allowed. To calculate the number of total hours needed to cover the projected number of procedures, knowledge of how long it takes to perform one procedure, including both productive and nonproductive hours required, is necessary. Normally, the previous year's productivity standards are used as the basis for this calculation. If the average procedure takes one-half hour, then the productivity standard is 0.50 total hours per procedure:

$$100,000 \text{ procedures} \times 0.50 \text{ total hours/procedure} = 50,000 \text{ total hours.}$$

2. The number of FTE personnel needed to perform the projected work is calculated. Based on one FTE working 40 hours per week, a year's calculation would be 2,080 hours:

$$50,000 \text{ total hours} \div 2,080 \text{ hours/FTE} = 24.04 \text{ total FTEs.}$$

3. For each FTE in the department, the following nonproductive hours will be assumed:

Vacation—80   Personal—16
Holiday—48   Education—24
Sick—80

These nonproductive hours total 248 per FTE. Therefore,

$$24.04 \text{ FTEs} \times 248 \text{ nonproductive hours/FTE} = 5,962 \text{ nonproductive hours.}$$

4. Based on 2,080 hours per year, the number of nonproductive FTEs is calculated as follows:

$$5,962 \text{ nonproductive hours} \div 2,080 \text{ total hours/FTE} = 2.87 \text{ nonproductive FTEs.}$$

5. Because the total hours are 50,000 and the nonproductive hours are 5,962, the total productive hours are calculated as such:

$$50,000 \text{ total hours} - 5,962 \text{ nonproductive hours} = 44,038 \text{ total productive hours.}$$

6. Given that there are 2,080 total hours in a year, the calculation is as follows:

$$44{,}038 \text{ total productive hours} \div 2{,}080 \text{ total hours/year} =$$
$$21.17 \text{ productive FTEs.}$$

7. Because no overtime is permitted in the department, total productive hours equal to total regular hours.

8. The average wage rate of $25 per hour is then multiplied by the 50,000 total hours:

$$\$25.00/\text{hour} \times 50{,}000 \text{ total hours} = \$1{,}250{,}000 \text{ total wages.}$$

9. Given that the average payroll taxes, insurance, and benefits make up 30 percent of wages, the calculation is as follows:

$$\$1{,}250{,}000 \times 30\% = \$375{,}000 \text{ payroll taxes, insurance, and benefits.}$$

10. To calculate the total salaries, wages, and benefits, add the total wages and the payroll taxes, insurance, and benefits:

$$\$1{,}250{,}000 + \$375{,}000 = \$1{,}625{,}000 \text{ total salaries,}$$
$$\text{wages, and benefits.}$$

For 24.04 FTEs, the physical therapy department must budget $1,625,000 for total salaries, wages, and benefits based on an average hourly rate of $25, and 30 percent must be attributed to taxes, insurance, and benefits.

Linking Human Resources Budgeting to Employee Productivity

HR budgeting cannot be discussed without examining worker productivity. Productivity is a critical determinant of a healthcare system's performance, and it may be defined as the physical inputs used (including labor, capital, and supplies) to achieve a given level of outcomes (Bailey et al. 1997). Productivity is the measure of how long it takes to perform a unit of service and how well it is done. The quality aspect of productivity distinguishes it from efficiency. Budgeted staffing requirements are dependent on productivity of the workers.

Managers need flexibility to make changes when warranted, but productivity standards should be set and adhered to, following the best practices in patient care and nonpatient care areas. Projecting profit is difficult without productivity standards in place.

An employee who can perform 30 procedures when the average is 15 is efficient but not productive, because the speed in which the employee is performing is likely compromising the quality of the work. However, the manager must assess whether the average of 15 is actually productive. In this assessment, managers sometimes use the average as a base and benchmark against that number. For the next budget quarter, the manager may set a goal of 16 procedures per day per employee and may then increase the number of procedures incrementally until it appears that quality may be negatively affected if any additional procedures are performed. When comparing employee productivity, the manager must compare employees who perform similar tasks or compare employees with themselves.

Inefficiencies cost the organization money. Managers can often identify inefficiencies in their areas by walking around and observing, by asking employees what is inefficient, and by evaluating budget metrics. In healthcare, the following are areas of inefficiencies that add expense to the organization:

1. *Unclear work policies and procedures.* Workplace rules are not adhered to because they are either not enforced or vague; for example, employees arrive for work on time, but they leave immediately to get coffee or take an extra few minutes at break time or at lunch. Twenty minutes of waste per day × 500 employees is equivalent to more than 20 FTEs worth of employees per day not working.

2. *Lack of productivity standards, or lack of monitoring of these standards.* Some organizations use hours per unit of service to set budget figures, but they do not share this information with their employees. Others do communicate the rules but fail to monitor them, so no repercussions exist for nonadherence.

3. *Inefficient use of time.* Some healthcare workers only view the service side of what they do, not the business end. They do not value time nor equate it to revenues gained or lost. For example, many clinicians write their patient notes at the end of the day, instead of at the time they are treating the patient or directly after. Some employees hold personal conversations throughout the day, instead of work.

4. *Poor work layout.* In some departments, employees have to walk down the hall for supplies, which wastes time and effort.

5. *Poor training.* Many errors are made because of poor training. Insufficient or inadequate training also causes workers to perform slower than the standard because they do not have a good grasp of what they are doing.

6. *Poor system.* Often, work processes are not evaluated to ensure that they flow in the best possible manner. This can cause employees to turn a three-step process into a five-step process.

Managing employees so that they work productively is a difficult task. Each department or functional service area should perform an audit of itself to identify areas in which waste or lack of efficiency exists. *Multiskilling,* also known as cross-training, is a viable method of managing productivity, especially during times of seasonal fluctuations of volume (Hamby 1995). Nursing throughput, productivity, and resource utilization should all be monitored on a unit level. Although national benchmarks are helpful, variances among similar nursing units in the same facilities should identify internal best practices, and internal benchmarks should be created (Leeth 2004). Skill mix should be identified for productivity and resource utilization. Assistive personnel, also called extenders, can be used where labor shortages and cost restrictions surface (Leeth 2004). Hospitals are required by the Joint Commission to establish staffing effectiveness standards and to measure their HR indicators. Long-term care and assistive living facilities are required to also use these types of metrics. Data should be collected for both direct and indirect caregivers (Mooney 2004).

The Joint Commission developed the ORYX performance improvement initiative in 1997, and it continues to perform upgrades each year. It integrates the performance metrics with outcomes data. These performance metrics are added, deleted, or modified according to their relevance for certain diagnoses and improvement initiatives. New or upcoming projects include the Surgical Care Improvement Project, the Critical Care Measure Set, and Children's Asthma Care Measures (see www.jointcommission.org/AccreditationPrograms/Hospitals/ORYX/). With ORYX, productivity is linked with performance and patient outcomes. Change in the productivity standard of the physical therapy department used in the earlier example can make a significant difference in the amount of total FTEs the department needs. This in turn affects the total salaries, wages, and benefits needed to be budgeted. For example, if the productivity standard is 0.4 instead of 0.5 hours per unit of service, the total hours required is 40,000 (instead of 50,000); the total FTEs is 19.23 (instead of 24.04); and the total cost of salaries, wages, and benefits is $1,300,000 (instead of $1,625,000).

This cost savings demonstrates that productivity plays a major role in the profits of the organization, a fact that makes productivity a key area to consider when budgeting. Additionally, if the reimbursement received does not cover labor and nonlabor costs, then the manager may need to reassess the services being offered.

Acuity Levels' Impact on Staffing Needs

Patient acuity is the degree of severity of illness on a given day. Traditionally, nurse staffing has been based on hours per patient day. To predict staffing levels accurately, the patient's severity variance on different hospital days must be recognized, and the staffing levels must be adjusted appropriately (Lacovara 1999). The Resource Utilization Group Classification System (RUGS) used in long-term-care facilities is based on the premise that different case-mix groups of residents in nursing homes have different acuity levels, which in turn vary treatment costs. A lengthy assessment form called the Minimum Data Set is used to assess and categorize nursing home residents into 1 of 44 RUGS categories. Reimbursement is based on these RUGS categories (Adams-Wendling 2003). Kane (2004) suggests that staffing in nursing homes should be based on both the clinical and social challenges present in the job.

Providing nursing care in the intensive care unit (ICU) is quite different from providing it in a traditional medical-surgical unit. ICU patients are sicker and normally need more nursing hours per patient day of care; sicker patients in a medical-surgical unit also need an increased number of nursing hours per patient day. Each unit must be analyzed for the type and severity of patients that they treat, and nursing workloads must be adjusted according to this assessment. The same acuity assessment and staffing adjustment are needed for other healthcare professionals. The work intensity—procedures per patient day—for respiratory therapists who work in the ICU and step-down units varies from that for therapists who work on the orthopedic surgical unit. Likewise, an inpatient physical therapist (PT) who treats stroke patients needs more one-on-one time with the patient than the PT who treats orthopedic patients. Patients with comorbidities—those with multiple medical problems—also need more treatment time, requiring additional staffing. These variations in patient care needs add expenses to the budget. Under current models of reimbursement, these additional expenses are not always recouped.

For inpatients in any setting, a daily patient classification system must be in place so that the required nursing hours can be correlated based on the intensity of care needed. Applied late in the afternoon, a patient classification system has proven to be a good predictor of need for the next day and allows nursing leaders to allocate their resources more appropriately (Flagle 2002). Information technology or a computerized system that captures census data, care hours, patient acuity, and patient activities is invaluable in formulating staffing ratios (Walsh 2003). Carter (2004) suggests that a system that considers patient acuity, the level of staff needed to handle activities not related to volume, and patient volumes is invaluable in making staffing decisions. Physician offices have traditionally chosen units of service as a guideline for staffing. Modification of traditional levels of staffing should be adjusted to account for the requirements of new technology (Marco 2004).

Other HR Practices Related to the Labor Budget

Nonstandard Staffing

Nonstandard staffing involves the hiring of employees on a temporary or contingency basis. These employees include per diem staff, temporary agency staff, temporary pool staff, and other contingency workers. Using nonstandard employment in healthcare presents advantages and disadvantages. On the positive side, the organization meets the current need for staffing and the patients are taken care of. In addition, the organization does not need to provide benefits to these staff. During slow times, these employees do not show up at work, preventing the organization from incurring additional labor expenses. The greatest advantage is that atypical employment allows managers to better match working time to business activity at different times of the day (Rothwell 1995).

On the negative side, however, nonstandard employees are usually very expensive. In the case of a registered nurse, the organization often pays much more than the average hourly expense of a permanent employee, especially on holidays. Quite often, nonstandard staff members are less psychologically committed to the organization, which can lead to problems of motivation, communication, confidentiality, and turnover (Brewster 1995). Because of the nonpermanent nature of their jobs, these staff members tend to not adhere to high-quality service standards (Brewster 1995). According to the Joint Commission (2007), nonstandard employees should attend to their work with the same detailed orientation as do permanent full-time employees. Additionally, to be in compliance with Joint Commission standards, organizations must ensure that temporary clinical staff must prove competency in the procedures they are hired to perform before they are allowed to give that service. These additional requirements drive up the staffing cost per hour. The labor cost per unit of service for both permanent and nonstandard staff for each affected functional service area must first be determined and accounted for in the budget.

Outsourcing

Outsourcing, which in healthcare has also been called contract management, is the use of services offered and performed by companies outside of the organization. The reasons for outsourcing include the following (Lanser 2003):

- Accessing expertise or capability in a given area
- Obtaining sufficient personnel in the needed area
- Accessing better technology for advanced applications
- Controlling costs
- Gaining a competitive advantage through specialization and economies of scale

According to *Modern Healthcare's* 2007 Outsourcing Survey, the number of healthcare organizations that received on-site management on a contract or outsourced basis continues to rise. In the healthcare industry, laundry services is the most outsourced area, followed by housekeeping, clinical/diagnostic equipment maintenance, and food services. Other frequently outsourced services include rehabilitation services, foreign language translation services, and emergency department physician services. Among the benefits is higher patient satisfaction with the services. Quality and performance, and speed and accuracy, are just as important as controlling costs (DerGurahian 2007). Approximately 75 percent of hospitals outsource at least one function (Moon 2003). Some of these functions include human resources, business office administration, radiology, surgery, case management, revenue cycle management, real estate management, and information technology. In fact, the top 20 outsourcing firms earned $4.4 billion in gross revenue in 2006, which was an astonishing 37.5 percent increase over 2005 numbers (DerGurahian 2007).

Outsourcing human resources may include one or all HR functions. A healthcare organization can also use employee leasing. With *employee leasing*, the organization remains responsible for the day-to-day supervision of the employees, the hiring and firing of employees, and most of the regular HR functions. The exception is that the employees are leased from the leasing company. Even the owner of the company can lease himself or herself from the leasing company. With employee leasing, the organization pays the leasing company for the salaries, wages, and benefits of the employees, plus all taxes and insurances related to the use of those employees. The organization then pays the leasing company one lump sum once a week or another agreed-upon time frame. Organizations normally can get better benefits for reduced costs because of economies of scale. Also, they can usually get better Workers' Compensation rates.

Outsourcing companies are becoming more creative and offering more nontraditional contract services to better accommodate the healthcare industry's needs. Key to the success of outsourcing is choosing a company whose organizational culture is aligned with that of the partner organization and whose outcomes focus is similar as well. The organization that will be contracting with an outsourcing company needs to set up a performance evaluation system in advance of signing the contract. The outsourcing company must be able to seamlessly integrate into the fabric of its partner organization (Lanser 2003). Lawler, Ulrich, and Fitz-enz (2004) analyzed the impact of outsourcing business processes, in particular the HR department, on the budget of both large and small organizations. The authors give examples of how major companies, such as Prudential and Bank of America, outsource the HR department, including its management function and benefits component. From a budgetary viewpoint, these companies have achieved substantial cost savings. These savings come from the fact that outsourcing firms have many customers and are able to pass on the benefits of economies of scale. For healthcare organizations and systems with many employees, business process outsourcing may be the wave of the future.

Using Labor Budget Metrics for Measurement

The success of the HR function can be measured using metrics that can be benchmarked against performance of similar organizations and against performance of the organization itself. This benchmarking provides information that can help in decisions regarding whether to outsource, change certain processes within the organization, or use temporary staffing. Each healthcare facility must decide which metrics are applicable to its own needs and must gather data for the purpose of comparisons. Workload measurement and unit costing are pertinent metrics.

Lawler, Ulrich, and Fitz-enz (2004) discuss commonly used HR and organizational metrics. The metrics for the HR department include accession rate, cost per employee hired, time to fill jobs, benefits claims response time, training hours produced, number of employees trained, HR expense per employee, and HR FTE ratio. The metrics for the organization include revenue per employee, human capital, value-added human capital, return on investment, compensation versus operating expense, healthcare costs, training cost as a percentage of payroll, voluntary separation rate, and contingent versus regular employees. From the chief executive and chief financial officers' viewpoints of healthcare facilities, budgetary metrics are imperative so that comparisons can be made on a regular basis against other facilities within the same healthcare system, peer facilities outside the system, and within the facility. Healthcare institutions must use metrics for both the revenue and the expense sides of human resources. The analysis of key budgetary metrics, along with reporting of the variances, is usually performed monthly in most healthcare institutions. This is done so that organizations can make necessary adjustments to be in compliance with or to adjust their budgets. Figure 16.2 presents a labor budget metrics variance worksheet with key metrics.

Actual versus budgeted amounts for the predetermined metrics are calculated and then compared. A variance of 5 percent or more in either direction requires an explanation. If the variance is positive, then the manager would like to know why so that the good result can be repeated. Alternately, if the variance is negative, then the manager would want to figure out the reason so that corrective action can be taken. Organizations that do not evaluate metrics can find themselves in a financially poor situation, which could have been foreseen. Using metrics promotes financial responsibility and accountability within the organization.

Other metrics that may be of interest to healthcare facilities are not purely financial, but they are imperative to the success of the organization. These measures relate to improving overall business performance that also includes clinical and operational performance. Ultimately, it is the combination of using best practices and continual measurement that will enable an

FIGURE 16.2
Worksheet
for Labor
Budget
Metrics
Variance

Month _____

Description	Budget	Actual	Percentage Variance	Reason
Units of service				
Total productive hours				
Total productive FTEs				
Total nonproductive hours				
Total nonproductive FTEs				
Total hours				
Total FTEs				
Average productivity/ unit of service				
Revenue/unit of service				
Revenue per FTE				
Average hourly rate				
Average hourly rate/ unit of service				
Salaries, wages, and benefits/unit of service				
Salaries, wages, and benefits/FTE				
Total net revenues				
Total labor expenses				
Total labor expenses/ total net revenues				

organization to sustain performance improvement. Evidence, with its supporting data, must be provided to ensure accountability and assess the effectiveness of the performance improvement initiatives (HFMA 2004). Cost-effective opportunities include looking at data from high-risk, high-volume, and problem-prone areas that may now be quality and performance issues, but later may become risk management issues. Risk management problems can be costly to an organization. Other types of data measured may involve areas of patient satisfaction such as patient wait time, number of facility-acquired infections, and number of readmissions within seven days. The focus should be on the outcomes.

Standardization of procedures and implementing strategies for improved clinical outcomes will provide a long-term gain for the facility. The use of integrated information systems also permits the analysis of real-time performance data (HFMA 2004).

Mergers, Acquisitions, and Strategic Alliances

With high performance and competitive advantage having become important factors in the success and viability of organizations, mergers, acquisitions, and strategic alliances have become increasingly attractive. Many organizations that once were major competitors are now strategically aligned. A merger or acquisition often results in a duplication of services, forcing the aligned institution to make decisions on which employees to keep and which to terminate. Although this decision is often difficult, it gives the organization an opportunity to retain only the best employees so that the organization can become stronger not only from operational and quality standpoints but also financially.

When the leadership of such a consolidation is focused on instilling a positive culture systemwide and when policies and procedures are in place that promote the well-being of all the stakeholders in that firm, the merged organization's value to its investors increases. To maximize net operating margin, a merged organization has to take advantage of its human capital, working to align its key personnel, nonstandard staff, and outsourcing partners.

A recent acquisition trend involves *hospitalists*. These are physicians who usually contract with a hospital to provide inpatient care when the patient's regular physician is not on staff at the hospital. Many private-practice physicians have decided not to obtain privileges at local hospitals and are leaving the inpatient care of their patients to these hospital-based physicians. Hospitalist companies are acquiring smaller practices and then contracting the physicians' services to hospitals. Outsourcing this function to hospitalist companies helps hospitals be more efficient and effective when it comes to inpatient care (Greene 2007).

Summary

This chapter extensively examines the labor budget and its components, addressing how crucial this budget is to the success and survival of an organization. Predicting future revenues and expenses is an important step in ensuring funds will be available to pay for HR expenses. An organizational budget has a relationship with HRM, and HR budgeting has a link to employee productivity. Productivity standards have to be assessed to determine staffing requirements, and even small increases in productivity can provide substantial cost savings to an organization. Acuity levels also influence staffing needs. Nonstandard staffing and outsourcing are viable alternatives to permanent, traditional staffing. This practice offers both negative and positive outcomes. Using budget metrics is necessary to measure and compare (benchmark) an organization's performance to that of itself and of peer institutions. Such measurement is a step toward promoting best practices within the organization.

Discussion Questions

1. What is a labor budget, and why is it important in human resources management?
2. What are the benefits and drawbacks of using nonstandard employees, standard employees, and outsourced staff?
3. What are some of the reasons that certain staff members may be more productive than others?
4. Define the following terms:
   - Full-time equivalent
   - Labor budget
   - Acuity level
   - Productive hours
   - Down time
5. What is meant by the term benchmarking, and why is it important in human resources management?
6. Explain why the revenue side of the budget is just as important as the cost side when it comes to determining the quantity and quality of human resources.

Experiential Exercises

Exercise   Meet with the chief financial officer of a local healthcare organization. Conduct an interview to determine what financial metrics (e.g., hours per unit of services, hours per billable test) are used for the organization's HR function. Then find out the productivity performance expectation for different job functions (e.g., 0.3 hours per outpatient procedure; 20 worked hours per 100 billable tests). Do the same thing with a similar healthcare organization. Compare and contrast the metrics used and the productivity performance expectations with the other organization. Which organization appears more productive? Why?

Case 1   Mr. Richards is the department manager for speech pathology services at ABC Hospital. The average productivity per visit at the department is 0.75 hours per procedure.

Case 1 Questions

1. Based on one FTE equaling 2,080 hours and 48,000 predicted patient procedures, how many FTEs will be needed to adequately staff the department?
2. If the department productivity changes from 0.75 to 0.70 hours per procedure, what is the new number of FTEs required to staff the department?
3. What are some of the reasons that the average productivity standard in a department changes?

Case 2 XYZ Hospital is a community hospital that is not part of a larger healthcare system. This acute care hospital has 160 beds and 348 employees. Benefits and employee pay account for 30 percent of the hospital's total salaries and wages budget. Currently, the HR function is done in-house, and the chief executive officer, Ms. Jones, is evaluating whether to keep the HR function internally or outsource it.

An outsourcing company that services several large companies in the area has approached Ms. Jones, proposing that it can perform the hospital's HR function and provide benefits to each employee for a price of 28 percent of the hospital's total salary budget. As a result, employees would get better health insurance and pension benefits because of the advantages of economies of scale obtained by the business processes of the outsourcing company.

Case 2 Question

1. What key factors should Ms. Jones address, and what benefits should be evaluated?

References

Adams-Wendling, L. 2003. "Clocking Care Hours with Workload Measurement Tools." *Nursing Management* 34 (8): 34.

Bailey, M. N., A. M. Garger, E. R. Bernddt, and D. M. Cutler. 1997. "Healthcare Productivity." *Brookings Papers on Economic Activity* 143–203.

Brewster, C. 1995. "HRM: The European Dimension." In *Human Resource Management: A Critical Text*, edited by J. Storey. London: International Thompson Publishing.

Carter, M. 2004. "The ABCs of Staffing Decisions." *Nursing Management* 35 (6): 16.

DerGurahian, J. 2007. "Emphasis on Innovation." *Modern Healthcare* 37 (39): 28–30.

Flagle, C. 2002. "Some Origins of Operations Research in the Health Services." *Operations Research* 50 (1): 52–62.

Greene, J. 2007. "Hospitalist Business Enters New Stage." *Modern Healthcare* 37 (15): 33–34.

Hamby, E. 1995. "The Use of the Multiskilled Practitioner to Manage Care." *Orthopedic Physical Therapy Clinics of North America* 4 (3): 335–50.

Healthcare Financial Management Association (HFMA). 2004. "Key Strategies for Sustained Performance Improvement." *HFM Magazine* 58 (11): 1–11.

Internal Revenue Service (IRS). 2007. "Circular E." Washington, DC: IRS.

Joint Commission. 2007. [Online information; retrieved 3/08.] www.jointcommission. org/AccreditationPrograms/Hospitals/ORYX/.

Kane, R. 2004. "Commentary: Nursing Home Staffing—More Is Necessary but Not Necessarily." *Health Services Research* 38 (2): 251.

Lacovara, J. E. 1999. "Does Your Acuity System Come Up Short?" *Nursing Management* 30 (6): 40A–43A.

Lanser, E. 2003. "Core Competencies of Successful Outsourcing." *Healthcare Executive* 18 (4): 52.

Lawler, E. E., D. Ulrich, and J. Fitz-enz. 2004. *Human Resources Business Process Outsourcing: Transforming How HR Gets Its Work Done.* San Francisco: Jossey-Bass.

Leeth, L. 2004. "Are You Fiscally Fit?" *Nursing Management* 35 (4): 42–49.

Marco, A. 2004. "The Virtual Patient Encounter—Units of Service in the Electronic Age." *Physician Executive* 30 (3): 32.

Moon, S. 2003. "Out With the Old." *Modern Healthcare* 33 (35): 28.

Mooney, M. 2004. "Stay Current with Staffing Effectiveness Standards." *Nursing Management* 35 (2): 14.

Rothwell, S. 1995. "Human Resource Planning." *Human Resource Management: A Critical Text,* edited by J. Storey. London: International Thompson Publishing.

Walsh, E. 2003. "Get Real with Workload Measurement." *Nursing Management* 34 (2): 38–42.

CREATING CUSTOMER-FOCUSED HEALTHCARE ORGANIZATIONS THROUGH HUMAN RESOURCES

Myron D. Fottler, PhD, and Robert C. Ford, PhD

Learning Objectives

After completing this chapter, the reader should be able to

- describe the significance of customer service in the highly competitive healthcare market,
- distinguish healthcare organizations that exhibit high levels of customer service from those that do not,
- explain the role of human resources management practices in enhancing customer service, and
- discuss six specific human resources strategies that can enhance customer service.

Introduction

The problem with human resources management (HRM) thinking is that it addresses only 50 percent of the "people equation," focusing on internal customers to the exclusion of external customers. The goal should be to link the external customer's requirement with the internal human capabilities, thereby optimizing the utility of both. Consequently, the goal of the human resources (HR) function is not to make employees happy or satisfied at work; rather, it is to make happy those employees who are making the external customers happy. Most healthcare organizations' mission proclaims, "People are our most important asset." Yet no one really believes such statements. What they really mean is, "People who are serving customers well are our most important asset. Others must either convert to serving customers well or leave."

Healthcare organizations have not traditionally been focused on the needs, wants, or desires of their patients/customers. As a result of their history and reimbursement sources, they have concentrated on meeting the expectations of their medical staff and third-party payers. The medical staff have historically had the power to decide where their patients would go for services, and their provider organizations have gone to great lengths to make them happy. Because third-party payers pay the bills, organizations have also spent considerable effort in satisfying them. This limited definition of "customer" has resulted in organizations focusing only on increasing market share, decreasing costs, and expanding revenues to retain the support of their third-party payers and on providing sophisticated technology and in-house amenities to satisfy their doctors. Meanwhile, the patient has been overlooked and underappreciated as the ultimate customer. Even the term "patient" implies a passive person who patiently waits for service from experts who know what that patient needs and who often provide it without consultation with or explanation to the patient.

This paradigm has led to an increasingly unhappy and vocal patient. One study commissioned by the Voluntary Hospitals of America and another survey published in *Fortune* magazine report the following consumer attitudinal trends toward healthcare organizations (*Alliance* 1998):

> Public trust in healthcare institutions has declined...with health plans losing more ground than physicians or hospitals. The decline in trust is especially pronounced among consumers age 40 to 59; those with higher income and education levels; and those who have recently changed, added, or selected a physician or hospital. Consumers gave hospitals only a 67 percent satisfaction rating, and compared with 31 other industries, hospitals rank 27th. This placed them just above the Internal Revenue Service and 10 percentage points below the tobacco industry.

Furthermore, 80 percent of Americans agree that hospitals have cut corners to save money, and 77 percent agree that these cuts endanger patients (Healthcare Advisory Board 1999). While these findings are from 1999, such dissatisfaction and cynicism from the public continue and are probably worse today. Currently, many consumers think that in the event that they become seriously ill, their health plan will be more concerned about saving money than providing the best medical care (National Coalition on Health Care 2008).

None of these findings is surprising given that the services paid for by private insurers and government are not likely to reflect consumer preferences for convenience and personal control (Herzlinger 1997, 95). The increasingly involved healthcare consumer (this term, or plainly "consumer," is used throughout the chapter to refer to "patient") and the newly evolved competitive market are forcing healthcare institutions to consider who their customers really are. They are starting to rethink the old paradigm of "take care of the doctors and third-party payers and all good things will follow" and follow the new paradigm of "don't forget the patient as customer" (Ford and

Fottler 2000). Today's consumers, however, have much more knowledge and access to information about the value and quality of their healthcare alternatives. They are more savvy about what they are getting for their healthcare dollar and are increasingly involved in the decisions about how those dollars are spent. Because they have many choices when it comes to insurance coverage and healthcare providers, their voice is being heard. In addition, increasingly vocal consumer groups have changed patients' mind-set from being passive consumers into active participants in their own healthcare decisions.

Regina Herzlinger (1997, 3–4) describes this new healthcare consumer as follows:

> They want what they want, they want it fast, and they want it when they want it. Well-informed, overworked, and overburdened with child and elder-care responsibilities, they are a new breed of consumer, and their demands for convenience and control have caused many American businesses to greatly enhance their quality and control their costs...the consumer revolutionaries want their healthcare system to provide them with the same kinds of convenience and mastery they have found with Home Depot, Consumer Reports, and Nordic Track, so that their health status and costs will improve even further.

An Emerging Customer Focus

Current Trends

No one is arguing that physicians and third-party payers are unimportant, but a lot of healthcare observers and insiders are echoing the same point: The patient's significant role in the success or failure of a healthcare organization has grown. Consequently, thriving healthcare organizations are increasingly viewing patients and their families as the "real customers" in the market. These providers are spending more time, money, and energy to convince these customers that the healthcare product they offer has both quality and value.

The results of this change in customer focus can be seen in a number of ways. First, third-party payers are more willing to pay for homeopathic treatments, acupuncture, and even chiropractic treatments, in spite of established medical practice resistance. Second, pharmaceutical companies now spend enormous sums on television and print ads in hopes of directly influencing consumers' use of branded drugs. Direct marketing has proven to be an effective strategy that sways doctors to prescribe certain drugs and circumvents HMO (health maintenance organization) drug guidelines. Third, hospitals have begun to offer such patient amenities as chef-prepared foods, valet parking, and comprehensive single nurse care to retain existing patients and families and to attract new consumers who are still deciding on where to seek services.

Consumers now have access to more information through provider report cards, the Internet, and other means; however, this question remains: Why should providers be more responsive to consumers now than they have been in the past? The major environmental forces that led to the increase in competition and greater provider responsiveness to consumers include excess capacity, the consumer movement, deregulation of the healthcare industry, changes to reimbursement systems, declines in occupancy rates, medical tourism, health savings accounts, and retail clinics. Such increased provider competition has resulted in greater interest in redesigning healthcare organizations to make them more customer focused.

An even more potent factor is the changing views of corporate America toward its role in healthcare cost management. After long relying on managed care companies as the defense against rising employee healthcare benefit costs, some U.S. employers are undergoing a fundamental change in their healthcare cost management strategy by turning healthcare decisions over to their employees. This idea is driven by a confluence of interacting forces, including the backlash against managed care, the popularity of 401K plans, the use of web-based information to help consumers make more informed decisions, the staggering costs of healthcare, and a growing feeling that the nation's healthcare system will not work well until patients themselves hold the purse strings (Weber 1997). The trend of allowing employees to handle their own healthcare benefits, just as they control their retirement money, adds momentum to the growing customer involvement in healthcare decisions (Winslow and Gentry 2000). Other employers have created websites to help employees make health benefit decisions and to sign up for plans. Entrepreneurs are responding to this trend by developing web-based services that would greatly reduce the need for employers to manage this information. In addition, these entrepreneurs are more creative in providing customers with new tools to navigate the healthcare system and to take health into their own hands (Winslow and Gentry 2000).

Corporations are also self-insuring in increasing numbers. This means that healthcare services are increasingly paid for by the corporation's own administrators, instead of the insurance companies. One of the significant advantages of self-insurance is that it allows greater flexibility in the health plans offered. When the employer manages healthcare plans, the employee has a significantly greater voice in how and what these plans provide. Employees or their union representatives need to only persuade their employer of the need to change their choices of healthcare provider or health plan. Thus, the growth of self-insurance leads to patients having a louder voice in making their own healthcare decisions. It also highlights the need for healthcare organizations to understand and use successful best practices of the guest-service industry to gain a competitive advantage in this new patient-as-customer environment.

Ranking and then publicizing the scores (on myriad patient-related measures) of healthcare organizations has changed the attitudes of many healthcare providers about the importance of the patient as customer. Data generated by the Healthcare Advisory Board (1999) suggest that healthcare executives are beginning to respond to the patient-as-customer movement. Interviews with 321 healthcare executives in 1998 reveal that they agree (with a response average greater than 4.0 on a 5-point scale) with each of the following statements:

1. Consumers' new predominance in the healthcare marketplace is increasingly influencing policy, strategy, operations, and investment decisions of organizations in all segments of healthcare.
2. Healthcare organizations will provide education and readily available data to encourage and empower consumers to be direct purchasers of care.
3. Healthcare organizations will develop new products, offer more choices, and provide service enhancements to respond directly to consumer preferences.
4. Healthcare organizations will increasingly invest in feedback mechanisms to ensure that they are in touch with consumer needs and are meeting customer expectations.

Furthermore, national magazines, such as the *U.S. News & World Report,* publish lists of "best hospitals," while local television and newspaper outlets rate the best physicians in their area. National and regional magazines publicize the best physicians and hospitals in the area and across the country. The U.S. Department of Health and Human Services (2008) rates skilled nursing facilities in all states and posts the information on its website. Major clinical users track clinical and satisfaction measures, and these results are publicized in newspapers and on television.

Healthcare executives have begun to expand their customer focus to meet the needs, wants, and desires of their patients, giving them a positive clinical and healthcare experience (Fottler et al. 2000; Fottler, Ford, and Heaton 2002; Pines and Gilmore 1998). In an environment where the consumer can make choices about where to seek care, it is no longer enough for a healthcare organization to just be the best medical provider at the lowest price. The organization now also needs to persuade the consumer that its facility is the most responsive to needs and can meet expectations for a total healthcare experience. The business of healthcare must transform its view of patients, from clinical material to customers with decision-making power.

Studer's Nine Principles of Service

Quint Studer, a major figure in the field of service- and customer-focused healthcare, is a former hospital chief executive officer (CEO) who turned around two different hospitals financially by focusing on enhanced customer service through human resources management. Subsequently, he set up the Studer Group, a service management consulting firm. Studer's 2004 book *Hardwiring Excellence* details nine principles of service and operational excellence, all of which relate to one or more aspects of human resources management:

1. *Principle 1: Commit to excellence.* This principle is about setting measurable service, quality, finance, growth, and HR goals and identifying the desired results for each goal. Sample HR goals are reduced turnover, reduced vacancies, and reduced agency costs.

2. *Principle 2: Measure the important things.* This principle focuses on objectively assessing the organization's current status and then tracking its progress toward the goals that have been set. Such measurement aligns leadership and employee behaviors toward achievement of goals. Under this principle, HR goals are measured and reported periodically and individuals are held responsible for results.

3. *Principle 3: Build a culture around service.* This principle connects organizational values to actions through the use of employee service teams that focus on areas such as standards of employee behavior, patient satisfaction, becoming an employer of choice, measurement, service recovery, communications, and reward and recognition. Building the culture also involves training staff on saying "key words at key times" and making discharge and post-visit phone calls.

4. *Principle 4: Create and develop leaders.* This principle addresses the fact that gains from the first three principles will not be sustained if leaders are not continuously developed. Healthcare organizations need to equip their leaders with competencies through formal training programs, coaching, support, and evaluation.

5. *Principle 5: Focus on employee satisfaction.* Satisfied employees do a better job of satisfying customers (Denove and Power 2006). Employees want to know that the organization has the right purpose, that their job is worthwhile, and that what they do makes a difference. Managers should also recognize and reward positive employee behaviors.

6. *Principle 6: Build individual accountability.* This principle focuses on how to create a sense of ownership. This process starts when employees take part in interviewing a job candidate during selection. It continues with employees helping to orient and train and being a role model for coworkers. With this principle, new employees are asked to read and sign a Performance Standards Agreement, and managers seek input from these new hires about the job and how it could be improved. Managers should also establish a process to review, recognize, and reward employee suggestions and work innovations.

7. *Principle 7: Align behavior with goals and values.* Management needs to develop an objective evaluation tool that includes a component for holding everyone responsible for results. Such evaluations should be aligned with desired behaviors. Monthly progress reports and 90-day plans can reinforce desired behaviors for both leaders and subordinates. Research has shown that employees are more satisfied with their jobs if they are evaluated by measures that are aligned with organizational mission and values that are communicated to them (Ford et al. 2006).

8. *Principle 8: Communicate at all levels.* When all employees understand what is important and what is expected, they take charge of their own development and feel more fulfilled. As a result, patients get better care and leaders are more effective. Possible tools for achieving excellent communication include a 90-day work plan, employee forums, communication boards, and storytelling.

9. *Principle 9: Recognize and reward success.* Success that is acknowledged by leaders is success that is repeated. Staff members appreciate specific feedback. Studies show that employees need three complements for every criticism to maintain a good relationship with their supervisor (Studer 2004, 232–33). Reward and recognition teams can assist leaders in identifying reward and recognition strategies that have the greatest impact. Rewards and recognition align everyone's behavior toward desired results.

Customer-Oriented Human Resources

The challenges today for healthcare organizations are building loyalty and retaining customers. Employees are a key component and a major link to long-term customer loyalty (McCarthy 1997). They are also significant internal customers whom the organization must serve.

Having loyal customers brings multiple values to the organization (Berkowitz 2006). It costs five times more to acquire a new customer than to keep an existing one. The loyal customer also delivers a greater "lifetime value" in terms of financial return to the organization. Per customer revenue growth and profits are greater with loyal customers because they already interact with the employees, understand the scheduling and billing processes, or know who to contact in the event of a problem. That is, loyal customers are more efficient to serve than customers who are less familiar with the organization.

Furthermore, loyal customers are advocates who provide referrals to the organization. They have a broader "zone of tolerance" in that they are more willing to give an organization the benefit of the doubt when a problem arises. Also, loyal customers pay a premium price to stay with the service provider (Reichheld 1996).

The healthcare service value from the patient's viewpoint can be defined by the following equation (Heskett, Sasser, and Schlesinger 1997):

$$\text{Value} = \text{Clinical quality} + \text{Service process quality} -$$
$$(\text{Price} + \text{Service acquisition cost})$$

Clinical quality is the result of the technology and the staff expertise provided by the organization. Service process quality reflects the patient's perception of the dependability, responsiveness, authority, empathy, and tangible qualities of the service. The importance of service process quality is indicated by the fact that 80 percent of medical malpractice suits have nothing to do with the actual clinical quality of the service encounter (Berkowitz 2006). A major explanation is that the patient or loved one was angered by the service process quality, independent of the clinical quality of the care provided (Heskett, Sasser, and Schlesinger 1997). Price is the out-of-pocket cost to access services. Service acquisition cost refers to how much effort the customer puts in to access the service. In sum, clinical quality, service process quality, and service acquisition cost (from the patient's perspective) are all significantly affected by how well the human resources of the organization are managed.

The HR function can proactively add strategic value by enhancing the customer service capability of the organization. This capability, in turn, may enhance retention of existing customers while attracting additional customers to build market share. To enhance customer service, two preconditions must exist. First, key decision makers must make a conscious decision to make customer service a desirable organizational focus or agenda. Second, obstacles to customer service must be removed. Such barriers include overly bureaucratic infrastructure, too many people involved in obtaining an approval, and supervisors who are threatened by subordinate initiative. Each of these needs to be addressed if the HR function is to effectively enhance customer service (Ashkenas et al. 1995).

With these preconditions in place, organizations can then build an HR infrastructure that fosters and maintains customer service ethics. Key components of this infrastructure will include the following:

- Senior leaders communicate customer service initiatives.
- Customer service role models are publicly acknowledged through multiple media.
- Evidence of customer service is explicitly applied as a criterion for hiring at all levels.
- Promotion of current staff specifically considers the employee's customer service commitment and capability.
- Development of customer service skills is included in organization-wide training initiatives.
- Senior executives model customer service concepts.

- Specific organizational, departmental, and individual goals exist for customer service measures, such as ensuring patient satisfaction and addressing customer complaints.
- Customer service success is measured at multiple levels using various methods and is then publicized.
- Economic and noneconomic rewards for achieving customer service goals are provided and publicized.

In the next section, we examine six key HRM strategies that leading or benchmark healthcare and customer-focused organizations have discovered as critical in meeting and exceeding their customers' expectations. Lessons learned by the hospitality industry from their guest-relations experience can be readily adopted by the healthcare industry as it moves from the old paradigm to the new paradigm. If the competitive market demands that healthcare providers treat patients as important, primary customers (instead of as willing bystanders to their own healthcare experience), then these principles of hospitality can make the difference.

Exemplars of customer-driven organizations such as Disney, Marriott, and Southwest Airlines know that their success is based on meeting and exceeding their guests' expectations. This means that they spend considerable time and energy identifying and measuring what their guests say are the factors behind the quality and value of the service experience. Benchmark organizations manage the entire experience to the highest degree possible so that their guests' expectations are met and even exceeded. They know that the best predictor of intention to return and satisfaction with the guest-service experience can be identified and managed. They make sure that the key drivers in their guests' decision processes become the key drivers in their organizations' decision processes. This is especially important because the service product is largely intangible.

Just as benchmark hospitality organizations know that the quality and value of the service experience are in the minds of the guests, so too must healthcare organizations recognize this simple truth. Even if a surgical tool, an x-ray machine, or some other physical component is involved in the healthcare experience, every healthcare provider knows well the significance of the intangibles. Healthcare customers expect that not only will the surgeon successfully remove the diseased organ, but the surgeon will also show empathy and concern before and after the procedure. Healthcare customers also expect the operating room and the inpatient room to be sterile, the physical surroundings to be bright and tidy, the nursing staff to be responsive, and the services to be prompt.

The New Paradigm

As we have been emphasizing, a patient's determination of the quality and value of his or her total healthcare experience depends on more than the success or failure of the medical procedure or clinical service. It is derived from a holistic perception of the experience, beginning with the admission and ending with the bill payment. In a sense, this view (negative or positive) may never end, as the nature of a provider's relationship with the patient is inherently ongoing in that the customer continues to receive direct or indirect reminders (through ads and other communications) that the organization is a high-quality provider and welcomes the patient should he or she seek to return if a need arises. As it is for famous retailers (such as Nordstrom) and all hospitality businesses, the idea of repeat customers is a critical consideration for healthcare organizations as well.

Whom the organization defines as its customers determines how it makes various decisions, a consideration that drives the new paradigm. Table 17.1 summarizes the differences between the old paradigm (focus on physicians and third-party payers) and the new paradigm (focus on the patient as customer).

Six Customer-Focused Strategies

Following is a discussion of six strategies that healthcare executives can use to respond to the new paradigm and to implement them in a healthcare environment. Examples from both the guest-service and healthcare industries are cited (Ford and Fottler 2000; Fottler, Ford, and Heaton 2002).

Strategy 1: Identify the Key Drivers of Customer Satisfaction

Successful customer service organizations learn what makes their customers happy through the customers themselves. They extensively conduct surveys to find out needs, wants, expectations, and definitions of a quality service experience. Findings from such surveys then become the basis for organizational plans, operational strategies, and other service decisions. In other words, the key drivers should be identified by the healthcare consumer, not the strategic planners sitting in their isolated offices.

A firm that runs a theme park, for example, may find through its guest research that patrons like cleanliness of the park, friendliness and helpfulness of the staff, and short waits in ride and concession lines. With this knowledge, the firm can then strategically respond, putting its effort and financial resources into keeping the park clean, training employees to be pleasant and helpful, and building enough capacity to keep the waiting lines minimal. This attention to customer drivers is especially important when the customer's intention to return hinges on his or her overall satisfaction with the park.

Similarly, a healthcare organization can survey its patients. Key patient drivers may include quality of hospital food; physician's communication skills; and the staff's courtesy, warmth, and friendliness. Once these drivers are identified and their relationship to the patient's intention to return is shown, the organization can then make improvements to each driver. Such enhancements

Human Resources Strategy	Old Paradigm (Focus on Physicians and Third-Party Payers)	New Paradigm (Focus on Patients as Customers)
1. Key drivers of patient/ customer satisfaction	Clinical effectiveness and cost efficiency	Patient/customer perceptions of quality and value
2. Patient involvement in healthcare	Limited involvement	Maximum involvement
3. Organizational culture	Provider driven	Patient/customer driven
4. Staff selection and training	Focused only on clinical skills	Focused on both clinical and patient/customer service skills
5. Employee motivation	Rewards for technical proficiency	Rewards for both technical and customer service proficiency
6. Measures of effectiveness	Costs, clinical processes, and medical outcomes	Total service experience

TABLE 17.1

A Comparison Between the Old Paradigm and the New Paradigm

may translate into providing communication training to both physicians and staff and evaluating hospital menus.

In the past, joint-replacement patients at the University of Alabama at Birmingham Health System were required to arrive early in the morning for surgery and to stay long enough to receive the service and procedure they needed. Now, these patients are able to purchase an entire package that includes a three-night stay in redesigned rooms similar to those at high-quality hotels, preadmission one day before surgery, gourmet meals served in a communal setting with other joint-replacement patients, and specially assigned nursing staff. The hospital is so pleased with its patients' reactions to this package that it is beginning to provide such an amenity to patients with other diagnoses.

All of the key drivers identified by healthcare consumers have implications on HRM practices such as employee selection, training, and performance appraisal. In turn, HR activities also have an effect on efforts to meet the patient expectations. Because good clinical outcomes alone do not make the total healthcare experience impressive, caregivers with only technical and clinical capabilities do not make a healthcare organization competitive in a market full of consumers looking to be satisfied.

Strategy 2: Encourage Customer Involvement and Participation in the Service Experience

Think of the patient as a partial employee who is responsible for coproducing the healthcare experience. Most customer service organizations are fully aware of the value and benefits of letting their customers participate in the service experience.

First, whatever customers do for themselves is one less thing that the organization has to pay someone to do for them. In other words, patients and their family can take on some tasks that employees normally perform for them. Second, customers who coproduce the service experience are more satisfied with the outcome because they cannot criticize something that they have produced and designed to suit their own tastes and needs. For example, a person who makes his or her own salad cannot complain that the salad is not exactly what he or she wanted. Third, customers involved in a process can help supervise employees. With a customer watching the moves and attitudes of the employee, the employee will tend to behave more appropriately and work more fastidiously. A loyal repeat customer can even train the employee on how to face customers or educate other customers on how to enjoy or best benefit from the service experience.

Considering an involved patient as a partial employee is a novel concept. Most physicians, employees, and organizations tend to see healthcare consumers as passive and submissive objects to whom the experts do something, instead of with whom. However, the reality today is that consumers want to get involved in their own care and are not shy about making demands and suggestions about how their care should be delivered. They are no longer passive or content with just waiting in bed as so-called experts circle them, making decisions about their life. Most healthcare employees know that, at some point, a patient has to be involved in his or her care. A surgery patient has to get up and walk after the procedure, a psychiatric patient has to attend and participate in therapy, and a person with a general illness has to tell the doctor where it hurts. However, most employees are unclear on the idea of allowing patients to coproduce the healthcare experience or to participate in their own wellness routine, even though enough studies (and discussions with hospital lawyers) have been done that repeatedly emphasize the value of the medical staff communicating and consulting with patients to enhance patient satisfaction.

Until the patient fully comprehends and agrees to the regimen of care, the best doctors and best treatment facilities in the world will not be able to help the patient prevent illness or get well. An example of how patient participation can be effective can be seen in hospices, where the family and loved ones are asked to be part of making the hospice patient comfortable and content. Another example of patient involvement is when patients are allowed to manage the administration of their own medication through the use of a pump. Often, the result of this practice is quicker healing and less discomfort for the patient and lower costs for the organization, as the patient typically uses less painkillers or another type of drug.

The Shouldice Hospital in Toronto, Canada, focuses on the repair of abdominal hernias (Herzlinger 1997, 159). Its operating procedures are the products of intense deliberation about patient comfort, convenience, and health status. Shouldice has an integrated operating system carefully designed so that each of its activities reinforces the others. The system purposely places considerable demands on the patients. Meals are served only in the dining room, and patients' rooms lack a telephone or a television. Patients even prepare themselves for surgery by shaving the area to be operated on and are expected to walk from the operating room. Staff members also discourage patients from lingering in bed and demand them to engage in aerobic exercise. This system creates higher levels of patient satisfaction because patients are empowered. It also results in lower costs and higher quality than seen in general hospitals.

Strategy 3: Develop a Customer-Focused Culture

Organizational culture is generally defined as the beliefs, values, and ways that are unique to the organization. Culture communicates to all employees what is important and what is not, what is appropriate behavior and what is not, and how to interact with others both inside and outside the organization. In other words, culture is both "the way we do things around here" and "why we are what we are."

Leaders teach and communicate the culture by what they reward, recognize, punish, and praise. They highlight points of importance and perpetuate the culture through the formal reward and recognition system and through informal stories about organizational values, heroes, and legends. A classic illustration of this point in the guest-service industry is the legend told to employees at Olive Garden restaurants. When Olive Garden was just beginning to establish a strong customer service culture and teach it to all employees, one of its restaurants encountered a portly customer named Larry. Larry wrote a letter to the president of Olive Garden to tell him of the delightful meal, the great service, and the wonderful dining experience he had. Unfortunately, according to Larry, the armchairs in the restaurant were too narrow for someone his size, making him uncomfortable. Larry suggested that Olive Garden do something to better accommodate people like him. Olive Garden's president immediately responded by ordering two chairs for each restaurant that did not have arms (now known throughout the chain as "Larry chairs") to accommodate heavier guests. This one letter and a simple suggestion gave Olive Garden not only an opportunity to better serve its customers but also an inspiring story that can be told to new employees to illustrate how dedicated the company is in providing exceptional customer service. Legends strongly communicate the cultural value of customer service.

In healthcare organizations, telling stories of legends and heroes helps to explain the new paradigm of a service culture that the patient expects. Under the old paradigm, staff told only stories about how the hospital had responded to or accommodated a physician's or an HMO's needs, wants, and demands. The shift to the new paradigm, however, necessitates the creation or recollection of stories, legends, and heroes that extol an employee who provided effective patient care that enhanced a patient's overall satisfaction with the healthcare experience. For example, in one nursing home, the legend is about a nurse's aide. The aide one day discovered that an elderly resident, who had no interest in eating anything, had a passion for peanut butter milkshakes. The aide went out of her way, on her own time, to make such a concoction so that the resident would eat something. A top manager told this story in an employee gathering and recognized this person with a customer satisfaction award. This story and the subsequent satisfaction from the organization, employee, and resident had an enormous impact on defining the culture in this nursing home: Do whatever it takes to achieve patient satisfaction.

A strong culture with the "right" values can reinforce customer service. More and more healthcare executives are seeking ways to identify job candidates whose values are similar to those of the organization. Irvine Medical Center in California uses testing and interviews to evaluate employee–hospital congruence on values such as service orientation, proactiveness, and teamwork (Eubanks 1991). The medical center has found that selecting employees who share its core values has greatly reinforced its corporate culture. These hiring practices have achieved better results than the "chit-chat" interviews and reference checks that previously were the norm. Research indicates that nurses whose values are congruent with those of their employing hospitals tend to remain in their organizations longer (Vandenberghe 1991).

Culture building should not start and end at the new-employee orientation; cultural values have to be reinforced. One appropriate venue for doing this is the staff retreat. One of the objectives of a retreat should be to build a customer service culture, leading employees to discuss questions such as who are our customers, what do they want, what values does the organization need to adopt to deliver what customers want, and what human resources practices will nurture those values? (*Hospitals* 1991). Neutral outside facilitators can help staff participants differentiate between their individual and institutional values and to reconcile the two when necessary.

The stronger the culture, the less necessary it is to rely on typical bureaucratic control mechanisms such as policies, procedures, and managerial directives. Because so much of the healthcare experience happens in the encounter between the patient and staff, healthcare organizations must be able to depend on staff to do the right things (i.e., exceed expectations). Culture is critically important in ensuring that these right things happen, guiding employees even when their supervisors are not nearby.

Unlike a manufacturing organization in which the production process is fairly predictable, the process of providing a healthcare experience is subject to incredible variation—that is, as many different things can happen as there are different types of people. Because defining all the possibilities is impossible, the healthcare organization must rely on its employees to understand what is expected and deliver that expectation to the customer every time. The more uncertain the task, the more employees must depend on corporate values rather than on managerial instructions, formal policies, and established procedures to guide their behavior (Davidoff and Uttal 1989).

The HR department adds considerable value to the organization when it helps develop a customer-focused corporate culture. This entails enhancing each employee's understanding of and valuing what healthcare consumers want and need (both from a clinical and team service standpoint). This effort facilitates the organization's reactive responses to short-term market demands and enhances the organization's capability to proactively track future market directions and thus provide appropriate services (Cespedes 1995). Initial research on the HR practices that have the greatest influence on creating customer-focused cultures suggests the value of the following practices (Brockbank 1999):

- Provide a free flow of information through customer focus groups, videotapes or DVDs, audiotapes or CDs, in-house visits, and employee involvement in market research.
- Implement a comprehensive communication program that emphasizes the importance of organizational unity to win the hearts and minds of external customers.
- Ensure that measurement, rewards, training, and promotions reinforce the importance of customer focus.
- Design organizational structures and physical settings that facilitate teamwork around customer requirements.
- "Walk the walk" and "talk the talk" of customer service.

If the HR function is a strategic partner in the organization, its personnel must become highly knowledgeable about external customers. According to the HR competency study at the University of Michigan, an HR professional's knowledge base must include an understanding of competitors, customers, marketing, and sales (Brockbank, Ulrich, and James 1997). Lack of integration between marketing activities and HR practices is a major contribution to the suboptimization of organizational marketing (Ballantyne, Christopher, and Payne 1995).

The healthcare industry often does not invest in what it claims to value. Although it says that customer satisfaction and employee retention are the most important aspects of its business, the industry often fails to invest adequately in either (*Modern Healthcare* 1998). Instead, healthcare's to-do lists focus on such areas as upgrading technology, collaborating with others to build networks, diversifying business lines, and reengineering business and clerical services. In contrast, patients care most about responsiveness, information about their case, pain management, and positive attitudes from physicians and other caregivers (Studer and Boylan 2000). An obvious disconnect exists, and as a result the actions of healthcare executives indicate that they do not give high priority to the major concerns of their customers. However, both employees and healthcare consumers judge leaders not on what they say but on what they do, and what they do is focus on other organizational priorities, not on customers.

Culture begins at the top; thus, a commitment to customer service should start at the executive level. The behaviors continually shown by senior management are more important than the slogans and communications they generate. The CEO and senior management must "walk the talk" of customer service if that message is to be believed throughout the organization (Denove and Power 2006). Reinforcement of the customer-focused culture also requires appropriate employee selection and training as discussed in the next strategy.

Strategy 4: Find, Hire, and Train Competent and Caring Employees

A service business is, by definition, one that is based on people rather than on products. A gap exists between the expected service quality and the delivered service quality when staff are insufficient in numbers, poorly trained, or poorly motivated. Findings of Gallup polls of service workers suggest great cause for concern. Gallup has reported that 55 percent of service workers in its database have no enthusiasm for their work, and one in five of these workers is so unenthused and negative that he or she poisons the workplace. Gallup refers to these workers as "not engaged" (*USA Today* 2001). More recent data indicate that 59 percent of employees were "not engaged" and 14 percent were "actively disengaged" (*Gallup Management Journal* 2006).

Nonclinical staff who interact with patients or their families fulfill two critical roles: (1) as impression managers and (2) as gatekeepers. As *impression managers,* support employees must recognize that they are the organization to the customer-patient. As *gatekeepers,* they play a key role in implementing service delivery standards. When service employees work with a generally positive work attitude, the customers they serve report high satisfaction levels. Customers are highly satisfied as well when employees deliver high-quality service, and vice versa (Schneider and Bowen 1995). The guest-service literature suggests that only a certain percentage of people really care about giving high-quality service. In the book *Positively Outrageous Service,* author Scott Gross (1991) calls employees who like to provide great service "lovers." These employees give customers a feel-good level of service—that is, it feels good because the employee connects with the customer even for a brief period of time. Such a service encounter makes the customer feel that something is special and memorable about the experience.

The challenge for healthcare executives is to recruit employees who love to give great service, continually train all employees in guest-service principles, and provide positive incentives to maintain and improve on these principles. Gross (1991, 159) estimates that people who love to serve represent only one in ten of the available workforce. He states that these 10 percent cannot get enough of their customers; 5 percent of workers, however, want to be left alone; and 85 percent have a prevalent mind-set of "take 'em or leave 'em." If Gross's percentages are accurate, he raises two major challenges for healthcare executives. First, they need to develop a process that will systematically recruit and select those 10 percent who are truly committed to providing excellent service. Second, they must work even harder to teach their other employees how to provide the same quality of service that the "lovers" give naturally. In other words, the successful service organizations know how to "select the best and train the rest."

Guest-service organizations like Disney, Marriott, and Southwest Airlines know this lesson well. They spend countless dollars recruiting, selecting, and training their guest-contact employees to provide excellent customer service. They know that the impact of their service is created at the moment of truth when the customer has an encounter with the employee. Ensuring that the guest-contact employee is effective in providing an excellent service experience is vital for both meeting expectations and influencing the intent to return or use the service again. The important point to remember is that outstanding guest-service organizations know that the people they put in front of their guests must not only be well trained in the necessary job skills but must also have the personality, disposition, and willingness to provide a high-quality service experience.

Healthcare organizations that follow the old paradigm tend to select employees based on experience and clinical credentials only, overlooking the applicants' lack of customer service skills. Clinical skills are a definite requisite for caregivers and cannot be undermined; however, those organizations that seek to move into the new customer paradigm must also give consideration to, or develop ways to identify, potential employees who have an innate understanding of how to treat their patients as guests. Both Irvine Medical Center in California and Lutheran General Hospital in Illinois use testing and structured interviews to analyze a job applicant's fit with institutional values such as service orientation and servanthood (Eubanks 1991). In addition, some hospitals and healthcare systems offer courses or seminars in guest relations. Such an initiative is only the beginning of the movement toward the new paradigm. The willingness of the senior management in these organizations to sponsor such training is a strong statement of the value they place on this critical customer-orientation part of the healthcare employee's total responsibility.

The emergency department (ED) of INOVA Fairfax Hospital in Virginia initiated customer service training in 1994 (Mayer and Cates 2004). All

ED staff involved in patient contact (i.e., physicians, nurses, technicians, registration personnel, core secretaries, social workers, radiology technicians, and respiratory therapists) are required to attend an eight-hour customer service training program. The program covers basic customer service principles; teaches how to recognize patients and customers; points out service-industry benchmarking leaders; gives tips on how to recognize and manage stress, how to strengthen communication and negotiation skills, and how to be more empowered and be customer-service proactive; and discusses service transitions, service fail-safes, change management, and customer-service core competencies. Customer-service updates are offered three times a year, and attendance to these updates is mandatory. Modules on conflict resolution, advanced communication skills, and assertiveness techniques, among others, are offered in these updates.

Initial results of INOVA's efforts showed that all 14 key quality characteristics identified in the organization's customer satisfaction survey increased during the one-year study period (May 1, 1994 to April 30, 1995) (Mayer and Cates 2004). The most dramatic improvements were in the likelihood of customers returning, overall customer satisfaction, and physician and nurse skills. In addition, patient complaints declined by more than 70 percent, and patient compliments increased by more than 100 percent. The clear implication of this data is that customer service training offers a competitive market advantage to healthcare institutions.

Customer service courses in healthcare may explore the following areas:

- Standard operating procedures for interacting and handling problems
- Team orientation
- Training and use of multiskilled health practitioners
- Flexibility in addressing concerns
- Communicating
- Responsibility for customers
- Results of focus groups
- Exchange of information across organizational units
- Greeting and making eye contact
- Calling customers by name
- Responding to requests and concerns

An organization's reputation can aid its recruitment efforts. As authors Benjamin Schneider and David Bowen (1995, 115) note, employers who have a positive image in the community and a satisfied and motivated workforce have a deep applicant pool from which they can fish out the best. These "employers of choice" are good neighbors to the community and have established their reputation for hiring and developing people for the long term. Their mentality, according to Len Berry (1995), is to "recruit rather than save on those who leave." In other words, hold out employee selection for the better applicants and then invest in their growth and development; keep the challenged but motivated staff in their current jobs, and offer them future opportunities with the organization. Hiring the right people, training them, and empowering them to do the right things are critical to creating the "customer advocates" who will recruit other highly capable employees and customers (Denove and Power 2006).

Selling a healthcare employment opportunity is like selling a healthcare experience. If the company has a reputation for offering high-quality jobs and career opportunities, it will attract high-quality applicants and build a pool of people who prefer to work for that company rather than for the competition. As mentioned earlier, Quint Studer took over a hospital that suffered from high turnover and low staff morale. Within three years, Studer's strategy of emphasizing customer service by focusing on employee selection, training, and rewards had reduced turnover by 67 percent and, according to employee satisfaction surveys, tripled the level of employee morale (Studer and Boylan 2000). The hospital went on to become the "employer of choice" for northwest Florida.

Successful service companies that top the J. D. Power customer satisfaction surveys recruit for values and personality rather than technical skills alone; empower employees to act on their own; pay above market rate if necessary; attract career-minded individuals who care about the long-term satisfaction of their customers; promote from within; provide career ladders for everyone; and offer creative employee benefits such as telecommuting, flexible work schedule, and job sharing (Denove and Power 2006).

Strategy 5: Train and Motivate Staff to Provide Excellent Customer Service

In the guest-service industry, the normal practice is to recognize and reward employees not only for their technical excellence but also for their ability to deliver guest satisfaction. In other words, a delicious, one-of-a-kind gourmet meal will not make a guest happy if it is served by someone unpleasant and insulting to the guest. Similarly, a nonturbulent, quiet plane ride will not count as an excellent trip if the flight attendant is rude to the passengers. Because the customer service aspect of the total job performance is so important, managers of guest-service organizations are evaluated on the manner with which the service was provided in addition to the quality of all the components that went into that service. These managers spend countless hours motivating their employees to be both technically proficient and guest-focused.

There is also a demonstrated statistical relationship between happy employees and happy customers in the guest-service industry (Ford and Heaton 2000). If the employees are having a fun, enjoyable time of serving guests, they will positively influence the experience of the guests they are serving. This is a fundamental philosophy of CEO Herb Kellerman of Southwest Airlines. Managers in guest-service organizations know the importance of keeping their employees upbeat, happy, and positive so that they not only deliver the product in the way they were trained but do so in a way that promotes an exceptional service.

Traditionally, healthcare managers measured and reinforced healthcare services according to the definition of "excellent" service by other providers and accreditation agencies. Managers and their organizations were evaluated only on aggregate statistical measures or Joint Commission accreditation standards, which typically assessed the organization's structure, processes, or clinical outcomes. In other words, "high quality" meant a hospital that has a below-average mortality rate, or a surgeon who has a high survival rate for heart transplants, or an HMO that has a large percentage of female patients receiving mammograms. Thus, the reward and reinforcement mechanisms were focused on these provider-dominated measures of success. In the new paradigm, managers, staff, and organizations must be measured and rewarded on the extent to which they provide customer satisfaction. Because "what gets measured gets managed," the motivation and reward systems must include measures of customer satisfaction as well as employee attitudes to ensure that the managers spend the necessary time and effort on these vital aspects of customer service.

Strategy 6: Measure and Hold Staff Responsible for All Aspects of the Service Experience

Excellent service organizations, like Marriott, Disney, Nordstrom, and Southwest Airlines, send out questionnaires, interview departing guests, and pay people to sample the guest-service experience provided by the organization. These are highly systemic investigations that yield the necessary data for understanding and assessing customer perception of the quality and value of the service experience.

Asking the customer directly is especially important in healthcare for three reasons. First, the healthcare service is an intangible product that is consumed at the moment it is produced. Only the person who has undergone the experience has a complete understanding of it. Second, each healthcare consumer is unique not only in character and background but also in the way he or she experiences the service, which depends on various internal and external factors. Each consumer can deliver a personalized account of any problems that arose during the service and can give a suggestion on how to remedy and prevent such problems. Third, managers equipped with first-hand feedback can better design measures for what is important to the customer and subsequently oversee them more effectively; as the popular saying goes, "what gets measured gets managed."

Unfortunately, today, most dimensions of customer satisfaction in healthcare are neither measured nor managed, and patients' perceptions of convenience, comfort, and service quality are ignored. The healthcare equivalent of surveys of consumer perception, like the Zagat's survey of restaurants and the J. D. Power surveys of automobiles, have yet to appear (Herzlinger 1997, 94). Furthermore, accreditation of hospitals and industry-developed ratings of HMOs do not appear to be highly correlated with independent surveys of user satisfaction (*Consumer Reports* 1996). Many healthcare organizations (hospitals, healthcare systems, even physician practices), however, use measurement techniques to understand their customers' perception of the service experience. They send out questionnaires to patients after receiving care at their facility to identify areas that were satisfactory and those that were flawed or that impeded the desired level of service. More and more, the industry is realizing the consequences of failing their customers twice—once if the service is poor and twice if the problem is not determined and corrected immediately. Learning and responding to mistakes early are equally important in the pursuit of the new customer-focus paradigm.

Other measurement tactics include mystery shoppers, comment cards, focus groups, and other creative surveys. The Campbell Health System in Texas reinforces its patient satisfaction data by using mystery shoppers who report the details of the service encounters. Managers then share the feedback in a way that is meaningful and motivating for the staff (Millstead 1999). Healthcare organizations can measure and reward superior service by establishing a baseline of patient satisfaction in every unit and then continually sampling patient attitudes. This approach can help to identify both problems and opportunities. Salick Healthcare, which operates outpatient cancer centers in many states, has meticulously maintained patient records from which it has worked up detailed practice guidelines to standardize and refine the treatment of numerous types of cancer (Bianco 1998). Salick has been able to achieve better clinical outcomes, higher levels of customer satisfaction, and lower costs of care.

The key HR task is to link customer expectations and satisfaction back to the factors that are measured in the organization's performance appraisal system. This will undoubtedly mean significant differences in the criteria for different positions. Success in meeting customer expectations should also be reinforced through economic and noneconomic rewards. An increasing number of companies (e.g., Federal Express, Best Buy, various restaurants) use internal and external "customer approved" measures as sources of employee performance appraisal information. Examples are answering a telephone within four rings or responding to an e-mail within one day. Managers establish customer service measures and employee goals that are connected to company goals. Achievement of these customer service goals is often linked to compensation through incentive programs. The aim of including customer service measures in performance reviews is to produce more objective evaluations, more effective employees, more satisfied customers, and better financial performance.

Organizations also have internal customers—people who work in the facility who can provide feedback on anyone inside the organization with whom they work and/or on whose work outputs they depend. Healthcare executives who rely on the HR department for employee selection and training services can conduct an internal customer evaluation on that department. For both administrative and developmental purposes, internal customers can provide extremely useful feedback about the value added by an employee or a team of employees. Both internal and external customers should be included in the performance appraisal processes. By surveying external customers for employee performance appraisals, organizations can produce more objective evaluations, more effective employees, more satisfied customers, and better organizational outcomes (Radcliff 2002). Customer input into the appraisal process focuses the employee on what he or she can do to better meet customer needs, how customers view their performance, and what skills the employee needs to focus on improving (Jacobson 2005).

To measure service performance, an organization must remember that customer expectations are a key factor in customer perception of the ultimate level of performance. To build customer loyalty and commitment, expectations must be exceeded (Lee 2003). Note that each customer contact point (e.g., reception, admission, pharmacy) is critical to the customer's overall satisfaction with the entire service and the customer's willingness to return or recommend the organization. Therefore, at each contact point (or moment of truth), four questions must be asked:

1. How important was "x" in terms of your overall satisfaction with the organization?
2. How well did "x" meet your expectations?
3. Would you return if you need similar services in the future?
4. Would you recommend our organization to a friend or family member? Why or why not?

Answers to such questions should be fed back to both managers and staff in those contact points where the customer service encounter occurred. Such data should constitute a major factor in individual performance appraisals for both staff and managers. They can also be used to identify areas where additional staff training may be necessary. Finally, merit salary increases should be related, in part, to these data.

In sum, excellent service providers do the following (Denove and Power 2006, 232):

- Collect the right information from customers.
- Properly analyze the information and forward the analysis to those who are in a position to use it.
- Properly act on the information in terms of performance evaluations and merit salary increases.

Summary

Patients and healthcare consumers today are assertive. They are proactive in their search for convenient, cost-effective, high-quality, and customer-focused healthcare. The healthcare system is now more responsive to these demands, and the growth of medical savings accounts should enhance this trend (Goodman and Musgrave 1992).

Achieving competitive advantage in this hypercompetitive market requires developing organizational capabilities that are difficult for competitors to duplicate in the short run. Capabilities represent integrating and coordinating mechanisms that bring together resources and competencies that are superior to those of competitors (Henderson and Cockburn 1994). When implemented as a total system, the six HR strategies presented in this chapter represent one such integrative and coordinating mechanism for achieving competitive advantage through increased customer satisfaction. These strategies are derived from the best practices of the guest-service industry and have been developed and modified over many years to be applicable to the needs of the healthcare field.

Some may argue that because healthcare deals with more serious issues of life, death, and health status, healthcare consumers are not as interested in the amenities of service delivery as are customers of guest-services organizations. However, no data can support this claim, and patients who have received excellent clinical and customer care will argue otherwise. These six strategies are indivisible, and not one is more important than the other. They must be linked together and aligned to enable the organization to achieve the level of service excellence demanded by healthcare consumers today (Ford et al. 2006). That is what healthcare organizations must do under the new customer-focused paradigm.

Implementing these strategies (from identification of key drivers to measurement of employee performance) requires a champion (preferably from senior management) who will identify benchmark service organizations, cross organizational boundaries, and make true customer service the highest value in the organization. Following the strategies takes considerable time (several years) and effort, and success is not guaranteed. Most healthcare organizations have made progress toward putting some of these strategies into practice; however, we do not know of any that have been successful with all strategies.

If these strategies can be successfully implemented, they would provide capabilities that can become a core competency of the organization (Prahalad and Hamel 1990). In such a case, the core competency is the collective learning about how to coordinate diverse operational skills and integrate multiple activities toward enhancing customer satisfaction. Because the process of implementing the principles requires a long-term commitment, the principles will be extremely difficult for a competitor to emulate as a short-term fix.

Discussion Questions

1. Why is customer service important to healthcare organizations? What are the negative implications of failing to address this issue?
2. Think about your own experience or that of a family member in receiving healthcare services. To what degree was the healthcare provider customer-oriented? Why? What lessons can you derive from that experience that will help enhance your customer service orientation?
3. Describe one HR practice that can enhance customer service in healthcare.

How will you implement it, and what problems do you anticipate? If successfully implemented, what positive outcomes will you expect, and why?

4. If you were the CEO of a healthcare organization that is not customer-oriented, how will you change the culture? What are the potential obstacles, and how will you overcome them? Provide a step-by-step plan for reforming your culture.

Experiential Exercises

Case 1   Robert Casey received his master's in health administration from a major healthcare management program ten years ago. Through a series of increasingly responsible positions in various healthcare organizations, Robert was eventually appointed as the vice president for human resources at a university medical center where he had been employed for the past six months. Soon after his appointment, the CEO stepped down and was replaced by a new CEO, who is committed to making the medical center "not only the best in clinical outcomes but also the best in customer service in the region."

Robert has been asked to prepare a plan for moving the medical center in the next three years from the 40th percentile in patient satisfaction (as measured by the Gallup Organization) to the 90th percentile.

Robert asked your professor for advice on how human resources at the medical center can contribute to this objective. Your professor, in turn, asked your student group to prepare a recommendation. Your recommendation should include some element of cultural change in the organization, given that building a customer-oriented culture is more likely to be sustained.

Case Questions

1. What HR components will you suggest, and why?
2. How will you go about implementing changes in the components you chose? Why?
3. How will you monitor progress in achieving the new CEO's goal, and what will you be prepared to do if progress is inadequate?

Exercise 1 Form a group of three to five students in your class. Each student in each group should share with the group one example of poor customer service. Then the group will question that student concerning possible sources of the poor service experience. (Sources may range from lack of top management commitment to inadequate training of staff to inadequate staffing to failure to measure customer satisfaction to negative staff attitudes.) Each group should identify one or more managerial prescriptions for addressing each source. All groups should give a report to the class about (1) any commonalities they find concerning the sources of poor customer service and (2) their prescription for addressing these problems.

Exercise 2 Consider Quint Studer's nine principles of customer service (discussed in this chapter). Give examples of how your own service encounters (in healthcare or outside healthcare) illustrate any three of these principles. For each of the three principles, indicate which HR activities that you believe are most important for implementing that principle and why.

References

Alliance. 1998. "Consumer Attitudes." *Alliance* (May–June): 11.

Ashkenas, R., D. Ulrich, T. Jick, and S. Kerr. 1995. *The Boundaryless Organization: Breaking the Chains of Corporate Structures.* San Francisco: Jossey-Bass.

Ballantyne, D., M. Christopher, and A. Payne. 1995. "Improving the Quality of Service Marketing." *Journal of Marketing Management* 11 (1): 7–24.

Berkowitz, E. N. 2006. *Essentials of Health Care Marketing,* 2nd Edition, 200–06. Sudbury, MA: Jones and Bartlett Publishers.

Berry, L. L. 1995. *On Great Service: A Framework for Action,* 171. New York: Free Press.

Bianco, A. 1998. "Bernie Salnik's Business in Cancer." *Business Week* (June 22): 76–84.

Brockbank, W. 1999. "If HR Were Strategically Proactive: Present and Future Directions in HR's Contribution to Competitive Advantage." *Human Resource Management* 38 (4): 337–52.

Brockbank, W., D. Ulrich, and C. James. 1997. "Trends in Human Resource Competencies." Presented at the Third Conference on Human Resources Competencies, University of Michigan School of Business, Ann Arbor.

Cespedes, F. 1995. *Concurrent Marketing: Integrating Product, Sales, and Service.* Boston: Harvard Business School Press.

Consumer Reports. 1996. "How Good Is Your Health Plan?" *Consumer Reports* 61 (8): 34–35.

Davidoff, W., and B. Uttal. 1989. *Total Customer Service,* 96–97. New York: Harper.

Denove, C., and J. D. Power. 2006. *Satisfaction.* New York: Penguin Group.

Eubanks, P. 1991. "Hospitals Probe Applicant Values for Organizational Fit." *Hospitals* 65 (20): 36–38.

Ford, R. C., and M. D. Fottler. 2000. "Creating Customer-Focused Healthcare Organizations." *Healthcare Management Review* 25 (4): 18–33.

Ford, R. C., and C. P. Heaton. 2000. *Managing the Guest Experience in Hospitality.* Albany, NY: Delmar.

Ford, R. C., S. A. Sivo, M. D. Fottler, D. Dickson, K. Bradley, and L. Johnson. 2006. "Aligning Internal Organizational Factors with a Service Excellence Mission: An Exploratory Investigation in Health Care." *Health Care Management Review* 31 (4): 259–69.

Fottler, M. D., R. C. Ford, V. Roberts, and E. Ford. 2000. "Creating a Healing Environment: The Importance of the Service Setting on the New Customer-Oriented Healthcare System." *Journal of Healthcare Management* 45 (2): 91–106.

Fottler, M. D., R. C. Ford, and C. P. Heaton. 2002. *Achieving Service Excellence: Strategies for Healthcare.* Chicago: Health Administration Press.

Gallup Management Journal. 2006. "Gallup Study: Feeling Good Matters in the Workplace." [Online article; retrieved 3/8/08.] http://gmj.gallup.com/content/20770Gallup-Study-Feeling-Good-Matters-in-the.aspx?verysi.

Goodman, J., and G. Musgrave. 1992. *Patient Power.* Washington, DC: Cato Institute.

Gross, T. S. 1991. *Positively Outrageous Service.* New York: Warner Books.

Healthcare Advisory Board. 1999. *Hardwiring for Service Excellence: Breakthrough Improvements in Patient Satisfaction.* Washington, DC: Healthcare Advisory Board.

Henderson, R., and I. Cockburn. 1994. "Measuring Competence." *Strategic Management Journal* 15 (1): 63–84.

Herzlinger, R. 1997. *Market Driven Healthcare: Who Wins in the Transformation of America's Largest Service Industry.* Reading, MA: Addison-Wesley.

Heskett, J. L., W. E. Sasser, and L. A. Schlesinger. 1997. *The Service Profit Chain.* New York: Free Press.

Hospitals. 1991. "Retreats Advance Corporate Culture." *Hospitals* 65 (18): 58.

Jacobson, L. 2005. "Ask the Customer." *Incentive* 179 (8): 8–12.

Lee, F. 2003. "Stop Measuring Patient Satisfaction." *Marketing Health Services* 23 (2): 33–37.

Mayer, T., and, R. J. Cates. 2004. *Leadership for Great Customer Service: Satisfied Patients, Satisfied Employees.* Chicago: Health Administration Press.

McCarthy, D. C. 1997. *The Loyalty Link.* New York: John Wiley and Sons.

Millstead, J. B. 1999. "Satisfying Your Customers: Mystery Shopping in Your Organization." *Healthcare Executive* 14 (3): 66–67.

Modern Healthcare. 1998. "Put Up or Shut Up: Study Finds Execs Not Investing in What They Claim to Value." *Modern Healthcare* 11 (28): 42.

National Coalition on Health Care. 2008. "News Worthy Trends: Increasing Concerns about Health Care." [Online article; retrieved 3/3/08.] www.nchc.org/materials/ articles/index.shtml.

Pines, B. J., and J. H. Gilmore. 1998. "Welcome to the Experience Economy." *Harvard Business Review* 78 (4): 97–105.

Prahalad, C. K., and G. Hamel. 1990. "The Core Competence of the Corporation." *Harvard Business Review* 68 (1): 78–90.

Radcliff, D. L. 2002. "A New Paradigm of Feedback." *Executive Excellence* 19 (4): 20–26.

Reichheld, F. F. 1996. *The Loyalty Effect,* 40–49. Boston: Harvard Business School Press.

Schneider, B., and D. E. Bowen. 1995. *Winning the Service Game.* Boston: Harvard Business School Press.

Studer, Q. 2004. *Hardwiring Excellence.* Gulf Breeze, FL: Fire Starter Publishing.

Studer, Q., and G. Boylan. 2000. "Turning Customer Satisfaction into Bottom-Line Results." Presentation at the Baptist Healthcare Leadership Institute, July 8–9, Pensacola, Florida.

U.S. Department of Health and Human Services. 2008. "Nursing Homes Certification and Compliance." [Online information; retrieved 3/3/08.] www.cms.hhs.gov/certificationandcompliance/12_NHsasp.

USA Today. 2001. (May 10): 2A.

Vandenberghe, C. 1991. "Organizational Culture, Person-Culture Fit, and Turnover: A Replication in the Healthcare Industry." *Journal of Organizational Behavior* 20: 175–84.

Weber, D. 1997. "The Empowered Consumer." *Healthcare Forum Journal* (September/ October): 28.

Winslow, R., and C. Gentry. 2000. "Medical Vouchers: Healthcare Trend—Give Workers Money, Let Them Buy a Plan." *Wall Street Journal* (February 8): A1, A12.

PRESENT TRENDS THAT AFFECT THE FUTURE OF HUMAN RESOURCES MANAGEMENT AND THE HEALTHCARE WORKFORCE

Bruce J. Fried, PhD, and Myron D. Fottler, PhD

Learning Objectives

After completing this chapter, the reader should be able to

- enumerate and discuss the trends that are occurring in the healthcare marketplace, and
- list and explain the challenges in healthcare human resources management.

Introduction

Healthcare human resources management (HRM) operates within a complex external environment. Therefore, when we consider the future of healthcare HRM and the healthcare workforce, we must take into consideration the trends that are specific to the healthcare industry and its workforce, the concerns that affect HRM as a whole, and the changes that will have an impact on human resources (HR) functions in the future. These three sets of issues are overlapping and interrelated.

Ten Healthcare Trends

Of all industries, the healthcare industry can easily be considered the most dynamic and, at least in some respects, the most unpredictable. This unpredictability is natural in that healthcare is about people and hence absorbs the changes that happen in all areas of society, including politics, the economy, immigration, and popular culture. The ten key trends that are expected to cause major changes in the healthcare industry, and consequently on its workforce, are examined in this section and summarized in Figure 18.1.

Technological Innovation

One area that is not yet clearly understood but is geared to make an impact on healthcare is genetics. The Human Genome Project reached a turning point in April 2003 when the full human genome sequence was completed. As research continues about the hereditary and genetic factors associated with disease, more details concerning the treatment and management of disease will emerge, raising the question, what kind of education, training, and specialization do physicians and other caregivers need?

Genetic counseling will continue to grow as a field, but how will this profession change as a result of discovery and technological advances? What new types of personnel will be required as the field of human genetics comes out of the laboratory and into the clinical setting? Advances in genetic diagnosis and treatment likely will require a broad range of professionals in medical genetics, gene therapy, organ transplantation, and pharmacogenomics, among others. Demand for personnel in these areas will increase, and demand will continue for researchers in gene sequencing, biotechnology, functional genomics, proteomics, and microbial genetics.

The point here is that not only will personnel in genetics and research be in greater demand but also that jobs will be created in these areas.

Other emerging technologies, including imaging, information technology, and telemedicine, are also poised to make an impact on the healthcare workforce, similarly generating new types of positions and specializations. More unpredictable than the types of jobs that may emerge is the impact of these changes on the structure and functioning of healthcare organizations.

FIGURE 18.1
Ten Healthcare Trends

1. Technological innovation
2. Consumer mind-set of patients
3. Focus on quality and evidence-based medicine
4. Security and privacy
5. New healthcare professionals
6. Information technology and decision support systems
7. Globalization
8. Demographic changes (aging, diversity)
9. Prevention and disease management
10. Patient safety

Will current organizational charts be viewed as simplistic and obsolete as new types of relationships form across organizational boundaries and as new organizational forms develop? Will current models of supervision become archaic in the advent of new information technologies and innovations?

Information technology has changed the face of HR through the increasing impact of human resources information systems (HRIS). Since HR affects the entire workforce, the impact of HRIS can be dramatic in terms of lowering administrative costs, increasing productivity, speeding up response times, enhancing decision making, and improving customer service. These impacts are achieved by automating routine HR functions. The most frequent uses of HRIS include automating payroll processing, maintaining employee records, and administering benefits programs (*Human Resource Department Management Report* 2004).

One of the major HRIS trends today is *self-service*. This involves Internet-based systems that allow managers to access employee records for administrative purposes and enable employees at all levels to change personal information or benefits. The self-service system then reduces paperwork and offers greater convenience to both managers and employees. Also, more and more managers are using software to recruit, screen, and pretest job applicants online before interviewing and hiring them. Software for training and promotion purposes are also being used (Snell, Stueber, and Lepak 2007).

Consumer Mind-Set of Patients

With the increased availability of medical and health information on the Internet come consumers who are more healthcare literate and savvy. This trend is leading to a healthcare environment that is driven by consumers. In the future, consumers will likely have possession of their own healthcare record and perhaps maintain their health information through a personal website. As consumers assume a larger share of their own healthcare costs, we may see customized health benefit plans designed to meet the person's unique needs. Consequently, the healthcare workforce will need to be more attuned to consumer demands and concerns, and healthcare organizations have to improve the manner by which patients participate in their own medical decision making. See Chapter 17 for a discussion on consumer-driven healthcare.

Focus on Quality and Evidence-Based Medicine

Business pressures and the movement toward evidence-based medicine will force healthcare organizations to set quality and clinical outcomes goals, work toward achieving them, monitor them, and publicize the results. Organizations will need clinicians and teams to work together on quality improvement initiatives, and those who are trained in quality improvement methodologies will be more in demand.

Total quality management (TQM) is a set of principles and practices whose core ideas include understanding customer needs, doing things right the first time, and striving for continuous improvement. Criteria for the Malcolm Baldridge National Quality Award have provided the impetus for organizations to rethink their approach to managing their human resources. Each year, the Baldrige Award is given to an organization in each of these five areas: manufacturing, service, small business, education, and healthcare (*Quality* 2004). However, TQM programs have not been a panacea for improving productivity and responding to customer needs. In many cases, managers viewed quality as a quick fix and became disillusioned when results did not come easily.

Recently, many organizations (both in and out of healthcare) have adopted Six Sigma, a more systematic approach to quality that requires major changes in philosophy and HR programs. Six Sigma is a statistical method of translating a customer's needs into separate tasks and defining the best way to perform each task in concert with others. By examining the optimum process, Six Sigma can have a powerful effect on the quality of products, the enhancement of customer service, and the development of employees. Unlike other quality tools, Six Sigma allows process mistakes and medical errors to be caught before they happen (Pande, Newman, and Cavanagh 2000). This system has also helped HR departments to shift their focus from administrative activities to strategic planning (Gubman 2004).

Security and Privacy

Concerns over the security and privacy of medical records, heralded in large part by the Health Insurance Portability and Accountability Act (HIPAA) of 1996, will shift focus, as patient records become accessible and shareable through electronic means (e.g., website, personal digital assistant, e-mail). Information technology specialists who understand the technological, legal, and ethical imperatives involved in healthcare information privacy will be highly sought after.

Maintenance and storage of personnel files are another issue in this area. Employee files contain critical personal information, including performance appraisals, salary history, and disciplinary actions. Easy accessibility to medical and personnel records, identity theft, and other technology-driven security breaches will plague healthcare managers and necessitate new policies and standards. Generally, HR managers and supervisors recognize the importance of discretion in handling all types of employee information. Also, HIPAA and its Privacy Rule protect the use and disclosure of medical information, and the Electronic Communications Privacy Act (ECPA) of 1986 protects private electronic communications, although the ECPA offers limited protection for e-mail use (a discussion of which is beyond the scope of this chapter). One recent survey of 400 HR professionals found that 54 percent of respondents work for organizations that have written privacy policies that safeguard employee data (Bohlander and Snell 2007).

Employer challenges to privacy rights in the workplace have sparked a heated debate over the extent to which fundamental rights previously thought untouchable may be lessened through the employment relationship. Employers defend their intrusion into employee privacy by noting their legitimate interest in some of the personal affairs of employees, particularly those that may directly affect productivity, workplace safety, and motivation or morale (Chieh and Kleiner 2003). Examples are drug use, criminal activity, and coworker dating. Court decisions generally attempt to balance an employee's legitimate expectation of privacy against the employer's need to supervise and control the efficient operation of the organization.

New Healthcare Professionals
Advances in technology and changes in the way disease is treated and managed will bring about the possible reeducation and retraining of existing professionals and the birth of new healthcare professionals. New employees, as always, will need to be trained and their competencies will need to be assessed, and managers will have to determine these professionals' role and place within the organization. Existing professions will evolve in both predictable and unforeseen ways.

Information Technology and Decision Support Systems
Information technology has increasingly touched all aspects of healthcare. The era of the manual, paper medical record is ending and moving toward the age of paperless systems. Use of decision support systems will be more prevalent, helping clinicians and teams to effectively use new diagnostic, surgical, clinical, and medical devices and new pharmaceuticals. Information technology literacy will be a core competency among healthcare personnel, enabling them to match the technological savvy of healthcare consumers.

Globalization
The emergence of illnesses and health-related concerns that took root in other countries (e.g., HIV/AIDS, SARS, foot-and-mouth disease, mad cow disease) and the ongoing threat of biological and chemical terrorism signal the effects of globalization on healthcare. This trend will lead to the disintegration of the fine line between traditional medicine and public health, requiring the healthcare workforce of all hospitals and healthcare systems to be trained in areas such as disaster management and community surveillance. Public health workers, physicians, and other caregivers will need to work together to respond to new strains of diseases and to develop new methods of treatment. These groups will require training in and acculturation to this collaborative imperative.

In the United States, some consumers are going abroad to receive health services. Known as *medical tourism,* this phenomenon is driven by the high costs of healthcare and the limited availability of certain products and services in the United States. To respond to this trend, some healthcare organizations in this country are partnering with foreign healthcare institutions through a process of *mutual patient referrals*. Expected to be widely adopted in the future, mutual patient referral initiatives will need to be staffed. The HR department will play a role not only in staffing but also in evaluating such initiatives.

Demographic Changes

The aging of the population is a predictable change that will affect society overall and healthcare in particular. The demographic projections are very clear: By 2011, the number of U.S. residents in the over-65 age bracket will be 40 million; by 2019, this number will grow to 50 million. The over-80 population will also see rapid growth: By 2020, the number of octogenarians will reach 7 million (U.S. Census Bureau 2004).

Such rapid increases in the number of senior citizens have profound implications on the types and volume of services demanded and on the competencies required of healthcare professionals. Employers are concerned that older workers' retirement will mean the loss of these employees' expertise, a loss that will be difficult to replace. Consequently, employers are making a real effort to attract and retain older workers, particularly those who have taken early retirement, and many of these workers are responding positively to such initiatives. AARP reports that 68 percent of workers between the ages of 50 and 70 years plan to work in retirement, either full-time or part-time (Bohlander and Snell 2007). The healthcare costs for older workers are higher than that for younger employees, but such costs are more than offset by the minimized need (and costs) for recruitment, turnover, training, and transitions (Hall 2005).

By 2050, the ratio of the nonwhite to white population in the United States will be 1 to 3 (see Chapter 6 for this changing racial profile). The growth in diversity will demand cultural competency and sensitivity from the healthcare workforce. Healthcare organizations may meet this demand through retraining their staff on diversity issues, recruiting members of underrepresented or minority groups to be part of the caregiving staff and/or management team, and incorporating cultural competence education into the staff orientation and training curriculum.

Prevention and Disease Management

The aging of the population will mean not only more demand for healthcare services but also more emphasis on geriatrics and its various subfields such as chronic disease management and home health care. The concept of disease prevention, although not new, continues to regain momentum as healthcare consumers take more charge of their bodies and learn alternatives to traditional medicine. Healthcare organizations are heeding these cues, providing more preventive services and boosting their current disease management programs. New professions will likely emerge to meet this trend, and again the onus falls on healthcare organizations to provide training to current caregivers and to recruit employees who are skilled and knowledgeable in these concepts.

Patient Safety

As we learn more about medical errors and their causes, changes will likely be required in healthcare processes and information technology. Such changes affect HR practices in that staff will need to be trained in communicating outcomes (adverse or otherwise) to patients and their family, reporting incidences of errors to management, managing conflicts that arise, and other tasks within the purview of the staff's responsibilities. Training in the use and application of medical technology and in the dissemination and sharing of patient health information using electronic means is an appropriate response to this trend.

Also, healthcare organizations have to create a culture in which staff are not penalized for reporting errors or ostracized for committing mistakes. Such a culture encourages improvement in staff performance and morale, which then leads to fewer medical errors and higher quality. Performance evaluation criteria should include a patient safety component as well.

SHRM's Survey Results

In 2004, the Society for Human Resource Management (SHRM) conducted a survey of HR executives. That survey revealed ten trends in the workplace that respondents believed would affect the future of HRM. The order in which these developments are presented here corresponds to the level of importance given to them by the survey respondents (see Figure 18.2).

In 2006, SHRM updated this study to include six additional trends (Schramm 2006):

1. Increased demand for work–life balance
2. New attitudes toward aging and retirement as baby boomers reach retirement age
3. Growth in the number of individuals and families without health insurance
4. More incidents of identity theft
5. Work intensification as employers strive for higher productivity with fewer employees
6. Vulnerability of existing technology to attack or disaster

FIGURE 18.2

Developments
and Practices
Inside and
Outside
Healthcare

2004 SHRM Study

1. Rise in healthcare costs

2. Focus on domestic safety and security

3. Use of technology to communicate with employees

4. Legal compliance

5. Use of technology to perform transactional HR functions

6. Global-market issues

7. Retirement and labor shortages

8. E-learning

9. Export of U.S. jobs to developing countries

10. Changing definition of family

2006 SHRM Update

1. Increased demand for work–life balance

2. New attitudes toward aging and retirement

3. Growth in the number of uninsured

4. Growth of identity theft

5. Work intensification

6. Vulnerability of technology to attack or disaster

SOURCE: SHRM (2004); Schramm (2006)

Rise in Healthcare Costs

The rise in healthcare costs has multiple effects not only on individual healthcare organizations but also on the U.S. economy. First, it stifles economic
growth: The more expensive healthcare services get, the less able people are
to afford them and the less willing the government and third-party payers will
be to reimburse. Second, it causes greater tension between employers and employees, as organizations are forced to shift their healthcare costs to employees, which results in higher insurance premiums and higher copays. Third, it
fuels strike actions from employees who get frustrated with the employer's attempts to cut down on organizational costs.

Focus on Domestic Safety and Security

The threat of terrorism is pushing employers to devote substantial resources to
ensuring employee safety and security and to training employees on disaster

management. Security policies are being revised and tightened, and multiple units of organizations, including HR, are involved in this process.

Use of Technology to Communicate with Employees
Developments in information and communication technology have changed the manner in which employers communicate with employees. This trend has brought out other issues, such as ensuring the privacy of the information being communicated, the need for employees to learn to use the new communication methods, and the concern over security of such communication tools.

Legal Compliance
Legal requirements, particularly state-level legislation, concerning employment will continue to become increasingly complex and unpredictable. The globalization of the economy has resulted in the need for employers to be knowledgeable about the legal implications of recruiting and hiring employees from other countries. The emergence of the European Union places particular demands on human resources, as European countries' employment requirements in such areas as privacy, pension, and discrimination differ from those observed in the United States.

Use of Technology to Perform Transactional HR Functions
HR departments face pressures to bring value to the organization and to provide HR services in an efficient and effective manner. One approach to hitting this imperative is to use technology for a variety of functions, including training, evaluating compensation and benefits, and managing performance.

Global-Market Issues
Global insecurity and conflict are affecting all aspects of the economy, particularly businesses with an international presence. Organizations, especially healthcare systems, are establishing tight security measures to protect their interests. They are also coping with the economic downturn brought on by the war in Iraq and by homeland security initiatives. The oil market, which is deeply affected by the disturbance within oil-producing countries, is causing significant fluctuations in prices as well. These global issues directly and indirectly influence the supply of healthcare workers as well.

Retirement and Labor Shortages
The aging of the population is ushering the retirement of older healthcare professionals and is consequently contributing to labor shortages. Healthcare organizations situated in locales with a high proportion of older workers may need to assess new approaches to retirement, including phased retirement.

E-Learning

Training and skills development will continue to be an important part of organizational strategies. However, training programs will increasingly be required to demonstrate their value, in terms of improving the performance of employees and showing a return on investment. Use of more efficient computer-based training modalities will continue to be popular.

Export of U.S. Jobs to Developing Countries

The debate continues over the appropriateness of offshoring jobs, especially white-collar jobs, which once seemed immune from globalization. Whether the practice of exporting jobs for the purpose of cutting costs will in any way abate is uncertain, although security concerns may place some limits on this practice.

Changing Definition of Family

Debates over same-sex marriage and providing benefits to domestic partners will likely continue, even as the number of companies that offer such benefits rises. An annual survey by *Business & Legal Reports* states that the percentage of companies that provide domestic-partner benefits to exempt and nonexempt workers increased from 13 percent in 2003 to 19 percent in 2005 (Human Rights Campaign Foundation 2008). Eleven percent of plant employers provided such benefits (up from 8 percent in 2003), and 7,768 companies made this benefit available in 2005 (Human Rights Campaign Foundation 2008).

Six Overall Challenges in Human Resources Management

Recently, SHRM examined and categorized various HR literatures to identify current and emerging HRM challenges and issues (Schwind 2007). The top ten were talent management, cultural transformation, managing change, leadership development, HR technology, work–life programs, diversity, healthcare cost management, globalization, and ethical leadership.

Table 18.1 shows the connection between the HR trends and the HR management challenges identified by SHRM through its survey and study. Each trend identified in the 2006 survey update involves implications that must be addressed by both the HR department personnel and line managers (Schramm 2006; Schwind 2007). Three of these trends (see trends 1, 3, and 7 in Table 18.1) will specifically affect healthcare, not just the general U.S. workplace. All organizations inside and outside healthcare are forced to confront the cost dilemma and the uninsured status of many residents in the United States. Whether these issues will be addressed in the 2008 presidential election and whether politically acceptable solutions will be implemented in subsequent years remain to be seen.

HR Trends	HRM Issues/Challenges
1. Rising healthcare costs	• HR technology • Management of healthcare costs • Globalization • Ethical leadership
2. Increased outsourcing of jobs to other countries	• Cultural transformation • Change management • Diversity • Globalization • Ethical leadership
3. Threat of high healthcare costs to U.S. economic competitiveness	• HR technology • Management of healthcare costs • Globalization • Cultural transformation • Ethical leadership
4. Increased demand for work–life balance	• Talent management • Cultural transformation • Change management • Work–life programs
5. Retirement of large numbers of baby boomers	• Talent management • Change management • Leadership development • Work–life programs
6. New attitudes toward aging and retirement	• Cultural transformation • Change management • Work–life programs
7. Rise in number of uninsured individuals and families	• Change management • HR technology • Management of healthcare costs • Ethical leadership
8. Increase in identity theft	• HR technology • Ethical leadership
9. Work intensification through increased productivity	• Cultural transformation • Change management • Leadership development • Ethical leadership
10. Vulnerability of technology to attack or disaster	• Change management • HR technology • Ethical leadership

TABLE 18.1

The Connections Between HR Trends and HRM Challenges

Table 18.2 shows the overall and specific HRM challenges of healthcare organizations today. These factors extend beyond "people issues" and require the development of a skilled and flexible workforce as well as a professional HR function. Overriding the overall challenges is the need to measure the effectiveness of HRM in achieving human resources goals and objectives (again, what gets measured gets managed). Benchmarking of HR functions is crucial. It requires that the levels of performance be determined on a wide range of HR areas, including employee commitment, turnover and retention, productivity, cost containment, diversity, job satisfaction, and compliance with legal regulations. In addition, the organization may benchmark its own outcomes against those of its competitors in areas such as cost effectiveness, market share, customer satisfaction, clinical quality, technology, profitability, and reputation in the community. Obviously, the HR department can more directly influence employee outcomes than organizational outcomes, given that the latter are affected by various external and non-HR factors. Nevertheless, determining where an organization stands on both employee and organizational outcomes relative to its competitors is a necessary prerequisite to maximizing the impact of the HR function.

Human Resources and Strategic Management

Human resources represent the single most important cost in most healthcare organizations. How effectively the organization uses and integrates its human resources with its strategy can have a dramatic effect on its ability to compete and survive in a hypercompetitive environment. The goal is to develop the organization's human resources so that its skill, knowledge, and distinctive capability exceed those of its competitors. Obviously, the specifics depend on the nature of the organization and its market. By assessing external factors, the organization can exploit environmental opportunities and neutralize threats.

Human resources management should also be responsive to the market. HR functions should be focused on producing staff who are ready, willing, and able to respond to customer needs and wants in terms of quality, innovation, variety, and service excellence. As seen in Table 18.2, such goals are not easy to achieve in light of environmental challenges such as rapid change, workforce diversity, and skill shortages. Shortages, in particular, represent a severe challenge because a typical healthcare organization does not educate and graduate healthcare professionals, so it is dependent on educational institutions to produce appropriately trained graduates.

In addition, the integration of HR and strategy does not occur in a static internal environment. The organization faces continual pressure from external stakeholders to restructure, outsource, downsize, and modify its

TABLE 18.2
General and Specific HRM Challenges

Specific Challenges	General Challenges						
	Integrating HR and Strategy	Using Technology	Enhancing Productivity	Containing Costs	Managing Diversity	Complying with Legal Standards
Environmental						
1. Rapid change	X	X			X	
2. The Internet revolution	X	X	X			
3. Workforce diversity	X	X	X			X
4. Evolving work and family roles	X	X	X			
5. Skill shortages	X	X	X	X		

(Continued)

TABLE 18.2
Continued

Specific Challenges	Integrating HR and Strategy	General Challenges				
		Using Technology	Enhancing Productivity	Containing Costs	Managing Diversity	Complying with Legal Standards
Organizational						
1. Competitive position	X	X	X	X	X	
2. Organizational restructuring	X	X	X			
3. Organizational culture	X	X	X	X		
4. Outsourcing and downsizing	X	X	X			
5. Optimal recruitment and retention	X	X	X	X	X	X
6. Design of compensation systems	X	X	X			
7. Ethical behavior	X	X				X
8. Employee empowerment	X	X	X			
9. Benchmarking of the HR functions	X	X	X	X	X	X

culture. While integration of HR and strategy can enhance organizational performance in the long run, many short-term pressures can impede this integration in the real world.

Nevertheless, benefits of such integration include the following (Gomez-Mejia, Balkin, and Cardy 2004, 21–22):

- Encouragement of proactive rather than reactive behavior
- Explicit communication of organizational goals to all stakeholders
- Stimulation of cultural thinking and examination of assumptions
- Identification of gaps between the current situation and the future vision
- Participation of line managers
- Identification of HR constraints and opportunities
- Creation of a common bond

Using Technology

Advancements in information technology have enabled healthcare organizations to take advantage of the information explosion. With myriad electronic and Internet-based networks, unlimited amounts of information can be stored, retrieved, and used in a variety of ways. Even in healthcare, which has a long tradition of "hands-on" service, the web is transforming the way organizational goals are accomplished. Computer-mediated connections are giving rise to a new generation of virtual workers, who work from home or wherever the work takes them.

The implications of information technology for managing human resources are enormous. Because it allows coordination of activities with individuals and groups outside the organization, information technology can:

- lower administrative costs, increase productivity, speed response times, improve decision making, and enhance service;
- support efforts to link and leverage the organization's human resources to achieve competitive advantage;
- enhance service and employee empowerment (through remote access to HR databases that can support HR decisions and increase the ability to connect with other parts of the organization); and
- expand the scope and function of the HR department because it enables the provision of training through e-learning or distance learning.

Technology has changed the speed with which HR communicates with employees. HR can draft a company memo and, within minutes, e-mail it to all employees. Also, many organizations have created intranet sites that provide employees with a variety of information. Lastly, technology can assist in benchmarking the HR function against that of similar organizations. Such a comparison reveals which areas of the HR function are strong and weak and what HR experiences can be benchmarks.

As beneficial as it is, technology also presents a number of concerns, including employee privacy and intellectual property rights. Confidentiality of employee data is a growing concern, and employer liability in the event of security breaches is still unclear (SHRM 2004).

Enhancing Productivity

Obviously, the Internet can enhance employee and organizational productivity—defined as quantity and quality of output divided by input. Other factors also enhance productivity as noted in Table 18.2, including flexibility in job design to accommodate different family patterns; organizational restructuring, outsourcing, and downsizing; optimal recruitment and retention policies; encouragement of a high-productivity culture; design of a compensation system to enhance motivation; employee empowerment; and benchmarking HR organizational processes and outcomes against those of other organizations. These and other factors have been discussed throughout this book.

The challenge is to find the appropriate mix of tactics that will enhance productivity without reducing organizational commitment, loyalty, and retention. Many healthcare organizations recognize that employees are more likely to choose an employer and to stay if they perceive the environment offers a high quality of work life. A perception that the workplace is great is positively related to high job satisfaction, low absenteeism, and low turnover, and these traits in turn are related to good customer service. An exclusive focus on quantitative/accounting measures of productivity to the exclusion of HR considerations can reduce an organization's employee commitment, loyalty, and retention.

New investments in technology have rapidly increased the productivity of American workers over the past decade. However, investments in faster computers and other technologies are beginning to level off. Thus, additional and continued productivity will have to be the result of developing knowledge and ability, improving work environments, and providing enhanced employee motivation. This makes the role of human resources management all the more crucial in the future (Miller 2005).

Containing Costs

Employees, managed care, and government insurance programs (i.e., Medicare and Medicaid) have all put pressures on healthcare organizations to lower costs and to improve efficiency. In response, organizations have tried a number of approaches, including restructuring, downsizing, outsourcing, and employee leasing. Each method has had a direct impact on HR policies and practices.

Each approach presents significant potential downsides, particularly in terms of reducing employee attachment to the organization. In well-managed healthcare organizations, accounting considerations focused on short-term data should never have priority over longer-term HR considerations. Labor costs can be controlled through a compensation system that uses innovative reward structures to control labor costs and reward staff for behaviors that relate to achieving strategic goals. In addition, costs may also be contained by some combination of the following HR tactics:

- Select better candidates, which will lead to the likelihood that they will stay and perform better.
- Train employees to make them more efficient and productive.
- Structure work to reduce time and resources needed to deliver quality services (i.e., decentralization).
- Empower employees through reducing direct supervision and increasing the span of control.
- Reinforce cultural values that emphasize service and efficiency.
- Create economic incentives for employees to enhance their health status and economize their use of healthcare services.

Managing Diversity

Nearly 90 percent of the growth in the U.S. workforce from 1995 through 2005 involved women; immigrants; and people of African American, Hispanic, or Asian heritage (U.S. Census Bureau 2005). In the past, the typical U.S. worker was a white male and a member of a single-earner household. Fewer than 20 percent of today's employees fit that "typical" description. In March 2005, an estimated 10.9 percent (or 30 million) of the U.S. population was foreign born, and this percentage is rising as a result of high rates of international immigration (U.S. Census Bureau 2005).

A diverse workforce is becoming the norm in American businesses. Healthcare consumers and employees alike have become and will continue to become more diverse. Specific diversity challenges include the following (Gomez-Mejia, Balkin, and Cardy 2004, 120–53):

- Linking affirmative action programs to employee diversity so that the two systems support one another
- Identifying how each of the HR functions can contribute to the successful management of diversity
- Reducing potential conflicts among employees that cause cultural clashes and misunderstandings
- Developing a profile of employee groups who are less likely to be well represented in higher-level positions, and creating policies targeted to their needs
- Implementing HR systems that assist the organization in managing diversity

To accommodate the changing demographic trends, many healthcare organizations have increased their efforts to recruit and train a more diverse workforce through providing more internships to members of minority groups, flexible work-schedule options for women and older workers, phased-retirement options for older workers, diversity training programs, a culture of mutual respect, access to higher-level positions, and an environment that respects and is sensitive to different cultural beliefs.

Among the most important impediments to managing employee diversity are prejudice, resistance to change, group cohesiveness, segmented communication networks, resentment of perceived favoritism to minorities, and competition for opportunities. Managing diversity requires awareness and sensitivity to all of these factors.

Complying with Legal Standards

Much of the growth of the HR function in the past four decades is attributable to its crucial role in keeping the organization out of legal trouble. Most healthcare organizations are concerned about potential liability resulting from HR decisions that may violate laws or regulatory guidelines set by federal, state, and local governments and legislators. These laws and regulations are continually interpreted and reinterpreted in cases brought before government agencies, state and federal courts, and the U.S. Supreme Court.

We live in a highly litigious society, and this fact shows no sign of letting up. In fact, federal lawsuits that charge violation of human resources legislation have increased faster than any other area of civil litigation—up by 125 percent since 1991 (Bernardin 2007). In 2005, 24 percent of judgments against companies were for $1 million or more, compared with only 7 percent in 1994.

A healthcare organization's HRM depends significantly on its ability to deal with government legislation and regulation. This requires keeping track of the external legal environment and developing internal systems to ensure compliance and to minimize legal challenges. Establishing formal policies and internal administrative channels to address sensitive legal issues (e.g., sexual harassment) can help to reduce claims.

Healthcare managers need to understand legal issues that affect how they manage their staff because many of their decisions are constrained to some extent by laws. They should be particularly sensitive to legal issues when making decisions about whom to hire or promote, how to compensate, what benefits to offer or not offer, how to accommodate dependents, and how and when to terminate.

Legal compliance in HR practices has become more complex as a result of new employment laws, regulatory guidelines, and court decisions that interpret existing laws. Examples of newer employment laws are the Americans with Disabilities Act and the Family and Medical Leave Act. Court decisions relate to issues such as worker safety and sexual harassment. All of these changes have made HR decisions more difficult and risky and have increased the cost of making poor decisions. HR managers can advise and consult with departmental managers about the legal aspects of personnel decisions. Obviously, legal compliance is not the only priority in employment decisions but should be heavily considered along with other work-related factors such as timeliness, service quality, and productivity. Well-managed healthcare organizations go well beyond legal compliance in managing their human resources; they attempt to consistently practice the golden rule—do unto others as you would have them do unto you.

Summary

This chapter examines the present and future trends in the business and healthcare industries to determine the effects they will have on healthcare HRM. Six overall challenges are also identified, with the overriding challenge being how to best integrate strategic management and human resources management so that the HR function becomes a full partner in the pursuit of the organization's objectives.

Strategic human resources management requires that each HR function be aligned both horizontally and vertically. Horizontal alignment occurs when each HR function reinforces and supports other HR functions. For example, it would make no sense to recruit the best people and then fail to offer them opportunities for growth and advancement. Vertical alignment, on the other hand, occurs when each HR function reinforces and supports one or more strategic goals or objectives. For example, it would make no sense to have a strategic goal of providing the highest-quality service and then compensate staff below the market or provide little or no training. The result of that would be mediocre staff, high turnover, and dissatisfied patients.

Continually monitoring and evaluating the organization's programs are critical. This can be done using a variety of HR indicators, such as absenteeism, turnover, employee attitude survey data, time to fill positions, and customer satisfaction data. Benchmarking such indicators against those of other organizations that provide similar services provides an external validation of organizational strengths and weaknesses. Such data should then be used to implement a cycle of continuous improvement.

Discussion Questions

1. Which of the specific environmental and organizational HR challenges identified in this chapter will be most important in healthcare in the next 20 years? Use your own experience in your answer.

2. Most HR executives in healthcare do not have a major responsibility for achieving top management priorities such as improving productivity, quality of care, cost containment, customer

service, and financial performance. What do you think are some of the reasons for this gap? Outline several ways that an HR department can align its practices with the strategic goals of the organization.

3. What are the pros and cons of a more diverse workforce? Are more diverse healthcare organizations better able to compete because of their diversity? Why?

Experiential Exercise

Case For the past 20 years, Metropolitan Hospital celebrated the fact that 50 percent of its new hires in management positions had been women. The hospital assumed that with such a practice, women would eventually represent 50 percent of their top management executives (vice presidential level and above). But something unexpected happened. Five years ago, the hospital became concerned that its diversity program was not producing results. Instead of seeing an increase in the number of women in executive positions, the organization was observing a decline. Talented female managers were leaving, draining the pool of capable people.

To address this problem, the hospital founded the Task Force on Retention and Advancement of Women in Executive Positions. This task force aimed to pinpoint the reasons that female executives were leaving. The task force conducted a massive information-gathering initiative, interviewing women in all position levels and women who left. The team uncovered three main areas of concern through the interviews: (1) limited opportunity for advancement, (2) lack of mentoring and networking, and (3) existing work and family issues.

In response to these findings, Metropolitan Hospital retooled the workplace, renewing its commitment to flexible work arrangements, reduced workloads, and flex time. The hospital also developed plans for company-sponsored networking and formal career planning for its women employees. Since these initiatives were implemented, the results have been positive. Retention of women employees at all levels has risen, and turnover rates of those in management positions (just below the executive level) have been lower for women than for men. In addition, the hospital promoted the highest percentage (41 percent) of women as new executives in its history.

Metropolitan Hospital is now basking in its new reputation as a woman-friendly employer. This gives the organization external recognition in the marketplace, which helps with recruiting efforts, and enhances their reputation in the community.

Case Questions

1. How and why did the problems at Metropolitan Hospital occur in the first place?
2. How did the changes address the underlying problems?
3. What managerial actions are required to successfully implement a diversity program?

References

Bernardin, H. J. 2007. *Human Resources Management: An Experiential Approach,* 11. New York: McGraw-Hill.

Bohlander, G., and S. Snell. 2007. *Managing Human Resources.* Mason, OH: Thomson-South Western.

Chieh, C. M., and B. H. Kleiner. 2003. "How Organizations Manage the Issue of Employee Privacy Today." *Managerial Research News* 2 (4): 82–90.

Gomez-Mejia, L. R., D. B. Balkin, and R. L. Cardy. 2004. *Managing Human Resources,* 4th Edition. Upper Saddle River, NJ: Prentice-Hall.

Gubman, E. 2004. "HR Strategy and Planning: From Birth to Business Results." *Human Resources Planning* 27 (1): 13–21.

Hall, K. G. 2005. "Age Old Dilemma." *Fort Worth Star Telegram* (March 7): C3–C4.

Human Resource Department Management Report. 2004. "How HR Managers Use Technology Applications to Control Department Costs." *Human Resource Department Management Report,* Number 4–5.

Human Rights Campaign Foundation. 2008. "Domestic Partner Benefits Up, Signing Bonuses Down in 2005." [Online article; retrieved 3/7/08.] http:// benefitslink.com/ links/20050126-033749.html.

Miller, K. L. 2005. "Economy Out of Steam—A Dip in U.S. Productivity Provoke Anxious Questions." *Newsweek International* (February 21): 34.

Pande, P. S., R. P. Newman, and R. R. Cavanagh. 2000. *The Six Sigma Way.* New York: McGraw-Hill.

Quality. 2004. "Nonprofits Aim to Apply for the Baldrige Award." *Quality* 43 (1): 11–13.

Schramm, J. 2006. *SHRM Workplace Forecast.* Alexandria, VA: Society for Human Resources Management.

Schwind, K. M. 2007. *The Future of Human Resources Management: Emerging HRM Needs and Tools.* Alexandria, VA: Society for Human Resources Management.

Snell, S. A., D. Stueber, and D. P. Lepak. 2007. "Virtual HR Departments: Getting Out of the Middle." *Human Resource Management in Virtual Organizations,* edited by R. L. Heneman and D. B. Greenberger. Columbus, OH: Information Age Publishing.

Society for Human Resource Management (SHRM). 2004. *Workplace Forecast: A Strategic Outlook, 2004–2005.* Alexandria, VA: SHRM.

U.S. Census Bureau. 2004. *Aging in the United States: Past, Present, and Future.* [Online information; retrieved 12/24/04.] www.census.gov/ipc/prod/97agewc.pdf.

———. 2005. *Profile of the Foreign Born Population in the U.S. Current Population.* Reports 23–206 Extrapolation. Washington, DC: U.S. Census Bureau.

REDUCTION IN FORCE AT SIERRA VETERANS AFFAIRS MEDICAL CENTER

Sarah Huth and Sara Hofstetter

Background

One windy morning, as Paul Marquez pulled into the parking lot of Sierra Veterans Affairs Medical Center (SVAMC), he was struck by the sound of the American flag flapping overhead. As he entered the double doors to the facility, his eyes fixated on the brass plaque that hung in the hallway. The plaque bears the mission of the Department of Veterans Affairs (VA): "To care for him who shall have borne the battle and for his widow and his orphan." That day, more than any other, Mr. Marquez found himself deep in thought. He chose to work at the VA because of its worthy mission, but now he was unsure how to best carry out this mission in light of his current predicament.

Mr. Marquez was assistant chief of the Human Resource and Management Service (HRMS) department at SVAMC. The year before, in 1996, he was charged with overseeing the strategic reduction of the facility's workforce—a move ordered by SVAMC's executive leadership team (ELT) in response to budget constraints. That morning, Mr. Marquez was due to meet with the ELT to discuss the final stages of the reduction in force (RIF).

Located in a mid-sized metropolitan area, SVAMC operates 215 beds and employs between 1,300 and 1,400 personnel. A major referral medical center, SVAMC serves the community in conjunction with the VA's nursing home care units and its Community-Based Outpatient Clinics. Also, the medical center is affiliated with the medical, pharmacy, and nursing schools in the area.

The RIF Order

Mr. Marquez received the RIF order memo from the medical center director of SVAMC. The RIF had been approved by VA headquarters in Washington, DC, and was cleared by the director of the Veterans Integrated

Service Network (VISN) for the region. The memo laid out the following reasons for the RIF:

1. The need to redistribute resources in the VISN in conjunction with the strategic plan to close certain inpatient services that will enable the enhancement of outpatient services
2. An anticipated non-growth budget from the federal government that would result in an actual reduction in purchasing power of approximately 6 percent over two years
3. The need to address issues related to supervisor–employee ratios, reorganize internal functions in a more efficient manner, and abolish positions in excess of VA's needs and/or contrary to its mission

SVAMC was experiencing a shrinking reserve. In fiscal year (FY) 1995, the amount of this reserve was $4.5 million, but in FY 1996 it was down to less than $200,000. Because of this, a $7 million shortfall was predicted over the next two years and no additional funds were expected to be allocated from the VISN. Table C1.1 lays out the action plan for the RIF, a proposal expected to create a savings of more than $5 million by 1997.

The RIF order at SVAMC came at a time of widespread transformation of the Veterans Health Administration (VHA) as a whole. (See the organizational chart in Figure C1.1 to understand how SVAMC fits into the national structure of the VA.) From 1994 through 1999, the VHA was led by visionary Under Secretary for Health Dr. Kenneth Kizer. Dr. Kizer decentralized the VHA into VISNs, giving local-level control to network directors and individual medical center leaders. Also, at this time the VA faced fiscal constraints as the government worked to balance the federal budget. Because the VA budget

TABLE C1.1 Proposal to Meet Budgetary Needs by Implementing the RIF

Action	Full-Time Equivalent Employees	Salary Savings	All Other Savings/Costs	Net Savings
Reorganization	58.8	$1,488,170	$27,596	$1,515,766
Cut MD/PhD/DSS*	9.9	$1,227,484	$(85,857)	$1,141,627
Consolidate 7W/ 8S inpatient units	22.0	$995,094	$(325,000)	$670,094
Close HBHC**	6.5	$260,000	$(91,000)	$169,000
Contract dialysis service	9.8	$555,000	$(109,000)	$446,000
Miscellaneous	2.0	$266,000	$1,114,000	$1,380,000
Total	109.0	$4,791,748	$530,000	$5,322,487

*Decision support system; **Hospital-based home care

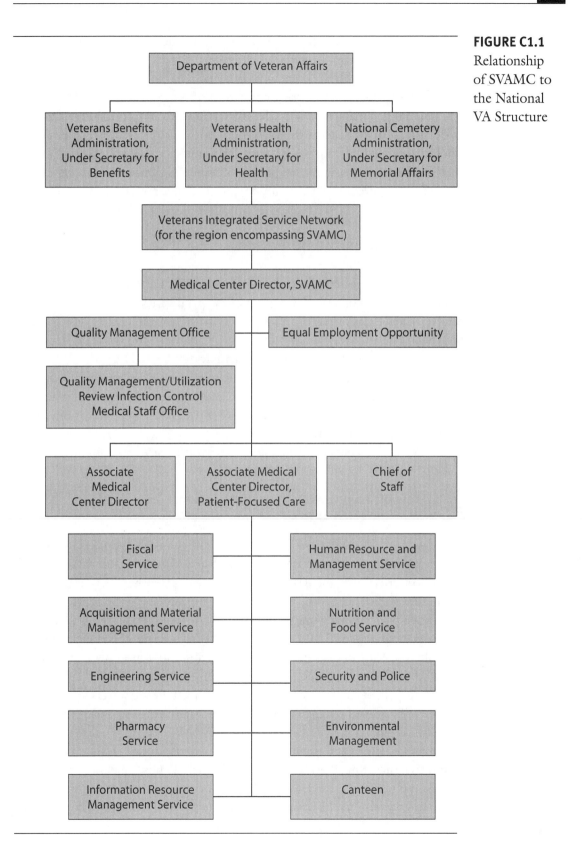

FIGURE C1.1

Relationship of SVAMC to the National VA Structure

is subject to the annual appropriations process conducted by Congress, it was vulnerable to fluctuations from year to year.

As with healthcare systems in other sectors, the VHA was undergoing a shift from inpatient to outpatient care. From a personnel standpoint, this shift eliminated many inpatient clinical positions. In addition, during this time a document referred to as the Farsetta Report was released, which evaluated inefficiencies within the VA system. This report catalyzed the systemwide elimination of all assistant chief positions in the VA, which made it possible for the agency to provide a greater number of health services at lower cost.

Process and Implementation

The RIF process included the identification of 109 full-time equivalent (FTE) employees, who composed 8 percent of the total FTEs at SVAMC, to be separated. Employees of the VHA fall under one of two categories: Title 5 (General Schedule and Wage Grade) and Title 38 (Nurses and Physicians); employees in both categories would be vulnerable to the RIF. Of the 109 FTEs identified for reduction, 68 held clinical positions and 41 performed administrative functions. Forty to 50 of these employees were expected to actually lose their jobs, while the rest would leave through attrition, early retirement, or reassignment within the VHA.

Various management measures were put in place to minimize the impact of the RIF, including the following:

• Instituting a hiring freeze on vacant positions
• Moving projected "RIFees" to nonvulnerable positions
• Awarding buyouts to other vulnerable employees

Consistent with the VA's national policy, SVAMC informed employees that those affected by the RIF could be transferred to other VA facilities within commuting distance. Also, when deemed appropriate, early retirement and severance pay options would be offered. The maximum amount allotted for severance pay was $25,000 per employee. To alleviate effects on employee morale, the HRMS department began distributing a monthly newsletter to keep all employees updated on the impending staff cuts.

As part of the RIF process, the VA national headquarters and the U.S. Office of Personnel Management (OPM) mandated the establishment of a career transition assistance plan (CTAP) at SVAMC. CTAP would provide career services aimed at lessening the impact of a job loss as a result of downsizing or restructuring. These services would include tips, guidance, or training in resumé writing, interviewing, financial planning, and dealing with creditors. In addition, OPM offered the interagency CTAP to provide displaced employees a special selection priority with other federal agencies in the event vacancies arose. RIF-affected employees at SVAMC were allowed to take a percentage of work time to participate in career transition programs.

Figure C1.2 provides a chronological timeline of the specific functions required to complete the RIF. The process could not begin earlier than January 27, 1997, after VA headquarters completed its update and entry of salary schedules into the Personnel and Accounting Integrated Data (PAID) system.

FIGURE C1.2   RIF Timeline

Early 1996	Employees began receiving information on the RIF and Title 38 staffing adjustments. HRMS offered briefings on these processes for each service.
January 15, 1996	HRMS committed extensive staff time to verify the accuracy of all PAID criteria for every employee who would be entered into the RIF Runner.
September 5, 1996	The medical center director held a town hall meeting with employees to present the final proposed reorganization.
January 4, 1997	This was the end of the pay period. To ensure that the PAID data received from VA headquarters remained accurate, all Title 5 personnel changes (e.g., appointments, changes to lower grade, reassignments) were frozen. Restrictions were also made to Title 38 personnel changes so that resources could be dedicated to conducting the RIF.
January 27–31, 1997	PAID data were downloaded into the RIF Runner program, and all necessary adjustments were made, including manually inputting all employee performance information for the last three years and deleting all Title 38 personnel data. The RIF Runner program was also tested to ensure the accuracy of the data and the proper functioning of the software. During this period, meetings were held with members of the ELT to identify vacant positions that were available for displaced employees.
February 3–7, 1997	All employees affected by the RIF were identified. For each individual, it was determined whether he or she should be placed in another position or separated completely from the system. This step was the actual bump/retreat process.
February 10–14, 1997	RIF letters were issued to all employees who were projected to be released from their positions by change to lower grade, reassignment, or separation. All RIF letters were issued on the same day during this week.
March 31, 1997– April 4, 1997	All temporary employees displaced by permanent staff were issued separation notices.
April 14–18, 1997	All RIF actions took effect during this week.

ELT: executive leadership team; HRMS: human resource and management service; PAID: personnel and accounting integrated data; RIF: reduction in force

FIGURE C1.3

Employee
Information
and Criteria
Verified by
HRMS

TYPE OF APPPOINTMENT: There are appointments in the competitive service and in the excepted service. Appointments in the competitive service are commonly known as Title 5, and those in the excepted service are usually referred to as Title 38. The excepted service also includes all Veterans Readjustment Appointment (VRA) employees and all employees appointed under a Schedule Authority.

POSITION OF RECORD: Official pay plan, job title, series and grade, and position description number. This information is found on the Notification of Personnel Action (SF-50) and on the official position description (PD).

TEMPORARY ASSIGNMENT: If an employee is currently on detail, temporary promotion, or temporary reassignment, it will be noted here.

WORK SCHEDULE: Full time is regularly scheduled 40 hours per week. Part time is regularly scheduled hours fewer than 40 hours per week. Intermittent is non-regularly scheduled work.

TENURE GROUP: There are three categories for tenure: I, II, and III.

COMPETITIVE SERVICE	EXCEPTED SERVICE
Career (Group I) Career employee not serving a probationary period.	Permanent (Group I) Appointment carries no restriction or condition.
Career Conditional (Group II) Employee usually having less than 3 years of continuous service; or a career employee serving a probationary period.	Conditional (Group II) Serving a trial period.
Non-Status/Non-Temporary (Group III) Term appointments made for more than 1 year, but not more than 4.	Indefinite (Group III) Indefinite but does not lead to permanent; or appointment with time limit of more than 1 year; or more than 1 year of current, continuous temporary employment.
Temporary (Group 0) Current appointment is for 1 year or less.	Temporary (Group 0) Appointment made for 1 year or less and has less than 1 year of continuous employment.

This system in turn provided information for the RIF Runner, a software designed to generate a list of employees and designate them for reassignment or separation based on objective criteria. HRMS verified every piece of employee information and criteria on the PAID system before they were fed into the RIF Runner (see Figure C1.3). Employees who were downgraded or laid off as a result of the RIF process were given the opportunity to challenge and appeal the decision.

SUBGROUP: There are 3 levels of preference: AD, A, and B.

AD: Preference eligible who has a compensable service-connected disability rated at 30% or more.

A: All other preference eligibles not included in group AD.

B: Employees not eligible for veterans preference. Some retired military personnel may be included in this group, depending on the conditions of retirement and the rank at the time of retirement.

CREDITABLE MILITARY SERVICE: Prior military service will be noted here.

RETIRED MILITARY: In receipt of uniformed service retired pay.

SERVICE COMPUTATION DATE (MONTH, DAY, YEAR): A date, either actual or constructed, that reflects creditable civilian and uniformed service. For individuals without any prior creditable service, the service computation date will normally be the date they entered on duty.

PERFORMANCE RATINGS: Annual performance ratings add additional years to the service computation date based on an average of three ratings. If a hard copy of a performance appraisal for a specific year at SVAMC is not on file in your Official Personnel Folder, an "05B" appears along with the rating obtained from another system of VA records. Hard copies of the actual performance appraisal must be located if at all possible. If during a performance rating period, there is no record on file of your performance rating, please provide a hard copy of the missing information. If fewer than three annual ratings were received during the last four years, an assumed rating of "Fully Successful" will be given. The amount of credit received for each rating is:

> Outstanding = 20 years of service
> Highly Successful = 16 years of service
> Fully Successful = 12 years of service

ADJUSTED SERVICE COMPUTATION DATE: The service computation date is adjusted based on the average years of credit for performance. This is the date used to determine retention standing in a reduction in force.

SOURCE: Apapted from U.S. Department of Veterans Affairs. "Running a Reduction in Force (RIF): Verification of RIF Essential Employee Data." Washington, DC: VA.

Unexpected News

As the RIF process advanced, Mr. Marquez spent countless hours responding to questions about job security. Many employees were unwilling to accept the prolonged uncertainty and began seeking jobs outside the VA system. As assistant chief of HRMS, Mr. Marquez had the responsibility to mitigate both employee concerns about their livelihood and management concerns about ensuring that the RIF met its cost-savings goals. In the midst of all this, he checked his mailbox and found a disconcerting memo from the chief of HRMS.

The memo notified him that he, too, was affected by the current RIF. According to the memo, the action was in response to budget constraints and not a reflection of his job performance, for which he had consistently received "Highly Successful" ratings. The memo went on to offer him a position as Supervisory Employee Relations Specialist at a lower pay grade, and it warned him that failure to accept the offer within six weeks would mean that he would be separated from the VA at that time. A phone number was included in this correspondence, directing him to contact a RIF specialist if necessary. The specialist would review information on personnel retention, applicable rules and regulations, and appeal/grievance procedures.

The Outcome

One year after the RIF process began, SVAMC attained its budget goals. As mentioned earlier, initially 109 FTEs were identified to be separated. However, only a total of eight employees were actually separated at the conclusion of the RIF. Many were reorganized to fill other positions within SVAMC or were relocated to nearby VA facilities. A significant number voluntarily left for other employment, particularly those with the most marketable skills. As for Mr. Marquez, he opted to accept the lower position with a decreased pay grade.

Years later, the effects of the RIF were still apparent. A series of turnovers occurred among members of the ELT, hindering the ability of leadership to build trust throughout the organization. Longstanding employees still speculate as to whether another RIF may be on the horizon.

For a brief definition of the VA terms used in this case, see Figure C1.4.

Discussion Questions

1. In evaluating the series of events that unfolded during the RIF process, do you think the RIF was successful? Why or why not?
2. Would you have chosen a RIF as the best way to solve SVAMC's impending budget problems? In hindsight, what alternative courses of action could have been pursued?
3. Assuming he had no other choice than to follow the directive to carry out the RIF, what additional steps could Mr. Marquez have taken to lessen the impact of the RIF on employees? What actions can SVAMC leadership undertake now to heal the wounds caused by the RIF?
4. What are the advantages and disadvantages of using the RIF Runner software to identify employees to be targeted for the RIF?
5. From a personnel standpoint, what repercussions may arise at SVAMC as a result of the layoffs?

Bumping and retreating. Displacement of a lower-grade employee who has less service by another employee qualified for that position.

Buyout. A separation incentive for an employee to voluntarily leave his or her position. A maximum payment of $25,000 may be offered.

Department of Veterans Affairs (VA). The federal agency responsible for operating nationwide programs for healthcare, financial assistance, and burial benefits for U.S. veterans. The VA is the second largest department of the 15 cabinets in the U.S. government.

Reduction in force (RIF). A coordinated method used to release employees from their jobs for reasons other than disciplinary. RIF refers to layoffs, demotions, relocation, or any other significant employee-removal action.

Veterans Affairs Medical Center (VAMC). A major healthcare facility operated by the VA (such as the SVAMC in this case). A VAMC is located in every state and offers a variety of services, including primary care, inpatient care, long-term care, psychiatric care, and rehabilitation.

Veterans Health Administration (VHA). One of the three branches of the VA, the VHA operates the largest integrated health system in the United States. It consists of several types of healthcare facilities, including approximately 155 VAMCs nationwide, that provide a continuum of health services to veterans.

Veterans Integrated Service Network (VISN). One of multiple regional organizations of VHA facilities that provides the structure for planning, budgeting, and service delivery within its respective geographic area.

MANAGEMENT CHALLENGES OF A CUSTOMER SERVICE CENTER

Andy Garrard and Heather Grant

Background

Wells Medicine is a public, not-for-profit health system that comprised an 800-bed academic medical center, a children's hospital, and several community hospitals that together earn more than $2 billion in annual revenues. The main campus, located in a busy metropolitan area, is ranked as one of the top hospitals in the United States, attracting patients from around the globe. Wells Medicine is a nationally recognized leader in clinical services, research, innovation, and teaching, all of which are components of the system's vision.

The healthcare system attracts employees from many geographic areas, ranging from the local, poor, inner city to other states and countries. It recruits talent from local universities, community colleges, trade schools, high schools, and placement agencies. Especially because Wells Medicine is one of the largest employers in its financially challenged location, the city and county governments are great supporters, providing job placement and development programs.

Wells Medicine's radiology department prides itself on employing internationally renowned physician faculty and using the latest technology to provide the highest-quality care. Annually, the department performs more than 400,000 exams and generates $200 million in revenue. In addition, the department has consistently been ranked one of the top radiology programs in the United States. To run this 166,000-square-foot department, 1,000 full-time employees are required.

Imaging Customer Service Center

The radiology department recently established the Imaging Customer Service Center (ICSC) to provide a central location in which patients and physicians can request and receive duplications of radiology images. Other services offered include image duplication for employed physicians and patients, stat orders typically for inpatients, and troubleshooting when something is wrong with an image order. The ICSC is located at the bottom level of Wells

Medicine's main inpatient tower and has been open for one year. Patients and physicians can fill out an order form either directly at the center or online, and images can be picked up in person or by a third party or can be mailed to an individual or a doctor. Customer groups that obtain services at the ICSC include patients, patient-designated representatives, physicians, and physician offices; each of these groups can be internal or external to the system.

Outside image processing is a service that the ICSC offers to patients who request from the system's prestigious radiologists a secondary interpretation or reading of their results. Outside reads generate substantial revenue, in the form of professional fees, for the physician practice owned by Wells Medicine. Figure C2.1 highlights the growth in outside-read transactions processed at the ICSC, versus at hospitals within the system; order volume has more than doubled in the first year of ICSC operation.

The process of duplicating an image consists of three primary actions: order entry, order processing, and order delivery. ICSC employees are expected to perform all three functions within the center and provide excellent customer service, given that the ICSC is the first thing that inpatients see when they enter the radiology department. For convenience, the ICSC is open 24 hours a day, 7 days a week, 365 days a year.

FIGURE C2.1
Growth
in Outside
Image Orders

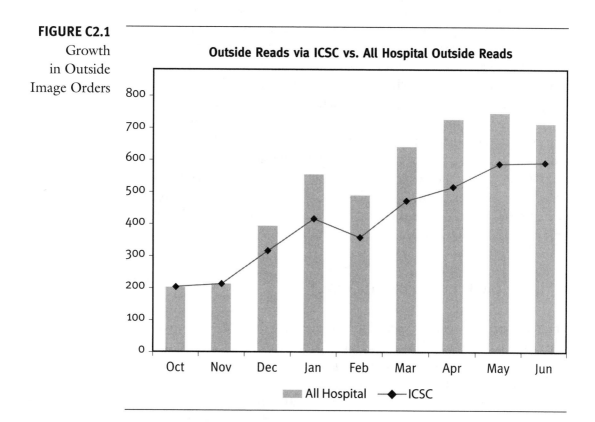

The initial goal of the ICSC was to implement the following strategic initiatives:

- Create a single point of contact for radiology patients
- Cross-train radiology employees
- Reduce film costs
- Transform the role of film clerks into an information technology (IT) role; doing so aligns these workers with the department's overall business focus

For cross-trained employees to have the ability to work at any station, the original layout of the ICSC was designed with a one-size-fits-all mentality. With this mentality, all workstations are supposed to be cross-functional and multipurpose. Unfortunately, however, technology limitations made this concept almost impossible. The current workstations are not truly multipurpose, forcing employees to constantly shift stations and wait for the appropriately equipped station to open up. The other part of the cross-training goal is for employees to stay current in the imaging field and be able to help any coworker at any time. To do this, employees must rotate roles.

Perhaps most important was the goal to have every employee always present his or her best face to the customer. Unfortunately, the ICSC ran into unforeseen time constraints and opened for business prematurely. This rapid start left gaps in the development of policies and procedures, training, and support that have impeded efficient, customer-focused staffing.

The Situation

As the administrator of the radiology department, Robert Walker just finished a meeting with the interim committee that manages daily operations in the department in the absence of a full-time administrator of operations. The former administrator of operations left six months ago to pursue opportunities at one of Wells Medicine's facilities abroad. The interim committee was then formed to ensure that operations, billing, and customer service in the radiology department continue to function smoothly until a replacement administrator can be hired.

During the meeting, Meg Johnston, manager of diagnostic radiology and leader of the interim committee, discussed the progress of moving film storage off-site and outsourcing film management. Although that project is moving along well, several other issues needed to be resolved that involve the supervision and performance of the ICSC staff. Ms. Johnston is responsible for the ICSC as a leader of the interim committee. Also, she is among the internal and external candidates applying for the administrator of operations position, and she, along with another internal applicant, is a front-runner for the job. While the department is functioning well under the interim committee, Mr. Walker knows that the vacant position needs to be filled shortly. At the meeting, Ms. Johnston reported that she has just learned that the current policies and procedures at ICSC are not HIPAA compliant and thus need to be addressed immediately. The internal auditor is scheduled to come to the department in the next couple of weeks, and the situation has to be handled proactively to avoid any formal violations. However, Ms. Johnston has neither the time nor the personnel needed to effectively revise and then implement the policies and processes. Beyond that, she is not sure exactly which HIPAA regulations are being violated.

Normally when such a case arises, she turns to Frank Thompson, the day-shift supervisor of the ICSC, but Mr. Thompson came to her just last week to admit that he does not like managing people—an unfortunate fact given that he supervises ten line employees. Ms. Johnston also consulted with the evening supervisor, Sarah Boyd, an employee of 35 years, to help with implementation. However, Ms. Boyd does not have many direct reports, as she has transferred most of them to other supervisors without her supervisor's consent. Ms. Boyd does not process orders nor manage people, yet she is on the payroll. Although Ms. Boyd has been a good employee in the past, she is not currently adding value to the ICSC team. Wells Medicine's policy is for management to make an honest effort in finding the best fit for an employee's capability before considering letting the employee go. The hospital also frowns on discharging employees who have put in many years of service. Now, Ms. Johnston does not know where to turn, and all of this is happening while she is trying to put her best foot forward as she vies for the administrator of operations position.

The other item Ms. Johnston noted at the meeting concerns the off-site move of the entire film vault operations. This move means that current film vault clerks, supervisors, and physical space are being reviewed for how they can best be used in the organization, if they are to continue at all. The assessment involves 20 employees across three shifts. Outsourcing film management is a real money saver for the radiology department, especially as it has moved to primarily digital imaging; the only service of the department that is not yet digital is mammography. However, monitoring the outsourcing project is taking a lot of Ms. Johnston's time to ensure that it is moving ahead according to plan.

Some ICSC clerks are concerned that the amount of work is continuing to grow, given that more modalities are removing film from their services, resulting in more customers for the ICSC. Also, now that the film vault operations will be outsourced, requests for pulling images will most likely flow through the ICSC. This makes staff feel that they are underpaid, overworked, undertrained, and understaffed. Ms. Johnston and Mr. Walker, however, do not agree with this mind-set. They believe the ICSC has great potential, providing employment to individuals who would otherwise lose their jobs with the decline in film imaging and increase in digital imaging.

These are the challenges that Ms. Johnston has to tackle in a short time frame. Although she has a good handle on the outsourcing project, she is going to need professional help in improving staff morale and compensation and in revising and implementing policies and procedures.

The Handover

Mr. Walker, the administrator of radiology, appoints Ms. Johnston as the new administrator of operations for the department. While elated about her promotion, she is still anxious about what to do for the ICSC, and her bid for the job and other duties kept her too busy to complete the revisions to the ICSC policies and procedures or to attend to the issues of staff morale and compensation.

Initial ICSC Assessment

Ms. Mary Pilcher, the interim manager for the ICSC, begins her assessment of the center by walking up to the window and seeing how long it takes for someone to acknowledge and greet a customer. She is amazed that it takes nearly 90 seconds for anyone to look up and say hello, but she decides to keep her observation to herself until she has gained the staff's trust. Once the staff are aware of her presence, she introduces herself and lets them know that she is there to support their work and provide what they need. She asks to come into the unit to get a feel for what they do on a regular basis.

One of the first things that Ms. Pilcher notices is that the unit is cluttered and the layout is poorly designed, making the space feel smaller and less efficient. The staff's personal belongings are strewn everywhere, and paperwork is piled up on all surfaces. Desks are small and seemingly temporary, and they are positioned so that staff's backs face the oncoming customers. Although workstations were initially designed to be multipurpose, they are not functioning as such because staff training and equipment have not been standardized. Ms. Pilcher realizes that the ICSC caters to many patients and physicians daily, and the current environment does not present a professional image—one that provides excellent service to customers. Without proper training, supervision, and support, the staff are marginally proficient and the workflow is horribly inefficient. She wants to think about these issues first before she brings in a company that can redesign the layout and provide better furniture and equipment.

Ms. Pilcher moves on to watching the staff work, with the staff's permission. One clerk gets very frustrated with the system as she processes an order, and she confesses that she really does not know what she is doing because she has never been trained. Ms. Pilcher then remembers from her conversation with Ms. Johnston that the day supervisor, Mr. Thompson, does not like to work with people, and that may explain why the day staff have not been trained. She also notices a general lack of communication and poor attitude among staff. Several clerks, who have worked on both day and night shifts, informed her that they are uncomfortable fulfilling their job tasks and, on the whole, are frustrated with the constant changes and lack of training and managerial support. She acknowledges these concerns and spends a few more minutes taking note of the physical space as well as the employee morale.

After returning to her office, Ms. Pilcher writes down the following observations and questions about the ICSC:

- Who is supporting this team? Mr. Thompson never seems to be on the unit, nor is Ms. Boyd, the night supervisor. Who is watching out for the staff?
- Many desk-help requests to the IT unit remain open, and some requests were completed or closed without communication from IT.
- What training have staff received? No documentation supports what actual training has been provided. A skills assessment matched with job requirements may need to occur.
- Who is supposed to work on the day shift, evening shift, and night shift? The day shift seems to have more than enough people—five are currently working. The staffing plan for the ICSC calls for three to four on the day shift and two on the evening and night shifts.
- What can be done to make the work environment look and feel more professional? Orders are left everywhere and are difficult to find. Outside images fill up the cabinets and are not being purged. Work is left in process and not handed over at shift change. Personal items are visible by customers. The whole place needs organization!
- What technology problems crop up regularly? The equipment gets backed up or goes down frequently. Some workstations can do outside reads, and some can do image duplications, but only certain stations can actually print film. No equipment is labeled that indicates what machine can do what. What is the process flow? Who fixes technology malfunctions?
- Where is the policy and procedure manual? It is nowhere to be found. Staff say that Ms. Johnston may have it.
- What is the order management process? Who makes sure that orders get done and get done well? The cross-training philosophy does not match the chaotic environment, leading to work not getting done efficiently. There is gross variation in order processing time.

Process Review

Over the next few days, Ms. Pilcher spends more time learning the processes at ICSC, which provides outside image processing, image duplication, stat order fulfillment, and troubleshooting. However, tracking occurs only for outside image orders, which are logged manually into a logbook: The clerk indicates what the images are, when they were received, and who received them. Beside this process, no other work orders are tracked.

Outside Imaging

Ms. Pilcher notices that for outside image orders, the original images are stored on the unit, although the policy states that once scanned into the hospital's system the images are to be picked up by or returned to the originating party. The clerks inform her that rarely does a doctor or a patient come to pick up the original images. Looking into the policy further, Ms. Pilcher discovers that very little process is defined for outside imaging and for all other services at ICSC. It is, therefore, not surprising that the average time to complete an outside image order varies significantly, ranging from five minutes to more than one hour.

During one of Ms. Pilcher's rounds, she overhears a clerk taking an outside image order from a physician. The doctor has walked several blocks through tunnels to reach the ICSC, which is located in the main inpatient tower. Although the doctor is really glad that the service is available, he asks if there is a better way to send film to the ICSC for third-party reading. Unfortunately, the ICSC only has one site, and no tubes run across the Wells Medicine campus into the center. As Figure C2.2 illustrates, physicians are the second highest users of ICSC services. Accordingly, in an effort to improve customer satisfaction, Ms. Pilcher wants to explore the possibility of providing better access through installing a second center in another part of the campus, creating drop locations, or using a clerk as a campus runner. Logistical challenges are associated with each of these options, but she wants to ensure that customer needs are met in the best way possible.

Image Duplication

Image duplication is a simple process that presents two main problems: lost orders and unreadable CDs. Because of disorganization, sometimes a clerk cannot find the original duplication order or the completed paperwork; Ms. Pilcher thinks that an order management system can alleviate this issue. The unreadable CD problem appears to be caused by the incompatibility of ICSC computers with various software, an issue that the IT unit can fix. Both problems put the radiology department at risk for customer complaints or even a medical malpractice lawsuit. If an order is lost, confirming that an order has been received, is in process, or has been completed is impossible.

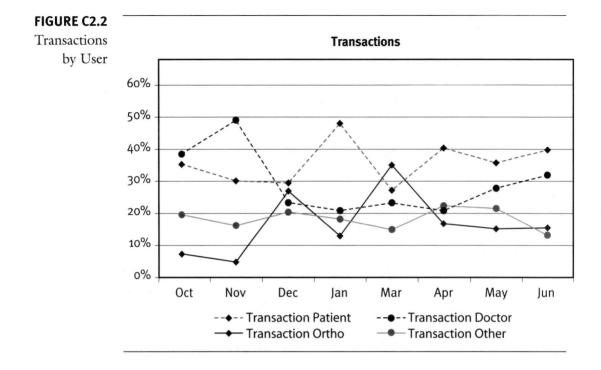

If a CD cannot be read because of technical difficulties, the customers are frustrated. Although image duplication demands minimal technical skills, it requires those who perform the process to be adequately trained because it is most prone to error. Errors at this stage can then lead to other clinical consequences.

Another problem with image duplication at the ICSC is that not all workstations can print images. This leads to lag time, when a clerk has to wait for a properly equipped workstation to become available so that an image can be printed. The average time to print an image is between 15 minutes and 20 minutes.

Work handoff is also troubling at the ICSC. Orders that are in process at the end of a shift are not handed off to the next batch of clerks. Sometimes, these orders are stored in clerks' personal lockers, giving no one else access in case of an emergency. As a result, patients or physicians who need the films or CDs for an appointment or surgery may not get them in time. Ms. Pilcher is aware that this lack of handoff procedure goes against the standards of the Joint Commission's National Patient Safety Goals. Per her observation, distrust among staff is obvious, and it is significantly affecting the work and must be addressed.

Stat and Troubleshooting

Stat and troubleshooting orders constitute a fair amount of the workload at ICSC. Stat orders are those that need to be completed quickly. Because these orders demand immediacy and preciseness, staff who fulfill them have to be technically proficient and appropriately trained. Troubleshooting usually arises when outside images cannot be scanned into the system. This technical difficulty can potentially delay surgery or another medical procedure and in turn introduce health risks to the patient or lower the quality of care. For troubleshooting, an employee who has superb technical skills and technology know-how is needed. Ms. Pilcher does not know who at the ICSC performs these highly technical duties or who coordinates them to ensure that they are completed correctly and in a timely manner.

Other Operational Issues

According to staff, Ms. Johnston keeps the books along with the policy and procedure manual. The staff also explain that a customer can request as many copies of the images on CDs for free but film costs $5.00 per sheet. Customers have to pay for the images first, and to pay they have to go to patient accounting services, which is located on another floor. Ms. Pilcher thinks that this setup is inconvenient for customers, as they come to the ICSC first, are then told to go somewhere else to pay, and have to return to the ICSC just to retrieve their order. Although a customer relations representative for the department is just across the hall from the ICSC, she decides that this system has to be improved.

As Ms. Johnston informed her, practices at the ICSC are noncompliant with HIPAA regulations. Currently, clerks receive and fill orders and give out images without asking customers to show identification or paperwork that verifies identity, without notifying customers of their HIPAA rights, and without requiring signature for the order and release of images. Ms. Pilcher knows that such violations have to stop immediately and all other issues have to be prioritized and handled appropriately. Which problem should be tackled first? What improvement will have the greatest impact? Which problem poses the biggest risk?

Next on her list is understanding and dealing with human resources issues.

Personnel Review

Over the week, Ms. Pilcher receives both good and bad news about ICSC staff. Several e-mails and phone calls have come in about the good work of two clerks—one on the day shift and one on the evening shift. These two exemplify the kind of customer service that Ms. Pilcher wants to instill in the ICSC. Both clerks went an extra mile to calm and comfort patients and their families, ensuring that orders were completed properly and on time.

On the other hand, a complaint from a physician about another clerk has reached her as well. The physician arrived with a stat order for a patient in preoperative surgery. The clerk refused to enter the order because the physician had not filled out an online order form. In fact, the clerk said, "no form, no images" and then flashed a smile. Although the clerk was only trying to follow procedures, he did not handle the situation in a customer-friendly manner. Plus, this specific clerk is technically astute and is the best technician at the ICSC. Thus, he needs to be approached with care. This complaint emphasizes to Ms. Pilcher the following points:

- ICSC staff need better customer service training to enable them to deal with difficult or conflicted interactions.
- Where was Mr. Thompson when the problem occurred? He is responsible for ensuring not only the quality and availability of the service but also supporting the people who provide that service.

Digging further, Ms. Pilcher reviews performance evaluations that were completed in the last fiscal year. The files contain some inconsistencies between actual performance and reviewed performance. Mr. Thompson's evaluations of the day staff appear to be subjective. For example, a clerk was rated a "4" for excellent performance, yet that clerk received several disciplinary actions during that same review year. Another clerk was rated a "3" for above-average performance, yet she was always on time, was given no disciplinary actions, and consistently received customer compliments.

During one of her rounds, Ms. Pilcher issues a warning to some staff for having a verbal dispute while customers are waiting at the window. To her amazement, the cause of the dispute is a simple disagreement about the air conditioning temperature on the unit. On another round, she finds a clerk in the back of the room with his shirt off. When asked, the clerk replies, "I feel hot." With these incidents, Ms. Pilcher starts to doubt her willingness to continue being the interim manager for the ICSC. However, they indicate deeper problems among the staff that must be addressed, including the following:

- *A generational clash.* The staff is made up of an equal number of older and young people. This creates a clash in the culture, as both parties have different ways of working that each insists is the proper approach. This also contributes to distrust.
- *Overstaffing.* The day shift is staffed by too many people, and there is not enough work to keep everybody occupied.
- *Poorly designed processes.* Staff follow steps that are inefficient and that they do not agree with nor understand. These processes cause frustrations, rework, poor quality, delays, errors, and blame. Most important, they lead to staff feeling inadequate, unappreciated, overworked, and resentful.
- *Lack of supervision.* Management on both the night and day shifts is nonexistent. Although two people are assigned to these posts, neither of

them can provide leadership, support, guidance, education, encouragement, expertise, information, improvement, advocacy, or model behavior. With a lack of ongoing supervision, it is no wonder there is a lack of training.

Information Technology Review

The next element for review is the IT support function. The ICSC depends on the IT unit to resolve technical issues and provide technical assistance. However, a significant number of IT requests (or tickets) submitted to the help desk are still open, waiting to be resolved. Although new tickets have been opened, the IT staff have no information about the status of these requests. Ms. Johnston acknowledges the presence of these issues and directs Ms. Pilcher to the IT director, Peter Hammond, who knows about them.

Mr. Hammond apologizes profusely to Ms. Pilcher for the miscommunication of information. According to him, the IT staff have resolved some of the open requests and informed Mr. Thompson. Also, IT staff are working hard to reconcile the other requests, but currently everyone on the unit is focusing on getting the digital imaging system (i.e., picture archiving and communication system or PACS) up and running. Without PACS, the radiologists cannot read images, and that will bring the entire medical center to a grinding halt. Mr. Hammond promises Ms. Pilcher that his staff will continue to work on open ICSC requests and will inform the unit once the work is finished. Ms. Pilcher then informs the ICSC clerks of her conversation with Mr. Hammond and his promise to deliver a resolution to the technical issues.

Ms. Pilcher understands that the PACS is more important, but she is concerned that the ICSC cannot provide critical services without the proper technology either. She also recognizes that the communication between the two departments and the level of support from IT leave much to be desired. She discusses her concerns with Ms. Johnston, who acknowledges these problems but does not give recommendations.

The Ultimatum

Mr. Walker, the administrator of the radiology department, has been meeting about the ICSC's performance with both Ms. Johnston and Mr. Hammond, both of whom have the same level of authority over their respective business units within the department. Mr. Hammond is vying to become manager of the ICSC because he views it as an IT unit. Although he recognizes that IT gives it a low level of support, he is confident that if it comes under his control more attention will be paid to the equipment and technology, enabling them to run smoothly. He has been successful at creating a "real IT department" in radiology over a short period of time. On the other hand, Ms. Johnston, as the former leader of the ICSC interim committee, has a larger stake on the unit and wants to see the unit succeed. She sees the successful turnaround of ICSC as an opportunity to garner a quick win in her new role. Neither of these two managers, however, has a full picture of the current challenges and the future implications at ICSC.

After a final, heated meeting between Mr. Walker, Ms. Johnston, and Mr. Hammond, Ms. Johnston is given the chance to prove she can turn the ICSC around in 60 days. Mr. Walker thinks that a lot of progress has been made at the ICSC and that Ms. Johnston now has the resources available to get it on the right track. Ms. Johnston arranges to meet with Ms. Pilcher to discuss her findings and to outline an action plan. Ms. Johnston relays the ultimatum she was given: Fix the ICSC in 60 days, or surrender its management to the IT director.

Discussion Questions

1. Prioritize the multiple challenges in this case. What will you address first, and how will you address it?
2. What are the underlying causes of the issues discussed?
3. What resources will you need to meet the 60-day turnaround target?
4. What are the key human resource and management issues, and how do they relate to the process and IT problems?
5. Who needs to be involved in developing and implementing solutions?

PERFORMANCE FEEDBACK NOW AND THEN

Lee Ellis, Dawn Morrow, and Adia Bradley

Introduction

Kristen Turtle closes the reminder on her calendar. She has 15 more minutes until a 90-day performance review of Leslie Kopalski, her newest direct report. Ms. Turtle has been director of marketing at Englewood Hospital for almost a year, and this is the first time she has supervised an employee who is not meeting expectations. She pushes the papers around her desk as she thinks about how to handle the meeting. She remembers her first hospital position ten years ago, right after she graduated.

Background

Ten years ago, Ms. Turtle just started her first job as a manager at Bayside Healthcare, the same system where only a year earlier she had completed her administrative fellowship under the chief operating officer. As a fellow, she formed great working relationships with many of the hospital's administrators, including her new boss, Jessie Morris, director of public affairs. During her fellowship, Ms. Turtle worked on several projects for Ms. Morris and thought of her as a mentor. After several months under her, however, Ms. Turtle realized that Ms. Morris was not as easy to work for as she had expected.

During the hiring process, Ms. Turtle was told that she would contribute to several public relations projects for Bayside Healthcare's outpatient clinics and that she would be directly responsible for two, large, revenue-generating projects in the emergency department each year. This type of work was what she had always wanted to do, and she was excited to get started on these projects right away. However, after her first month on the job, Ms. Turtle had not been informed of what the first project in the emergency department would be, nor had Ms. Morris posted the required formal work plan on the hospital's online project-management system.

Several months later, Corey Powers, a former manager in Bayside Healthcare's physician practice, was hired as Ms. Turtle's counterpart. Mr. Powers's job description was the same, with responsibility for two large, revenue-generating projects per year based in the outpatient clinics. He was excited to start his new position, but he was also experiencing a tense working relationship with Ms. Morris. In his first week on the job, Ms. Morris sat down with her two new managers to discuss her expectations. She said she would be sending them work daily and expected the work to be completed quickly. She would closely monitor their performance until they were able to win her trust. She wanted them to type minutes for any meetings they attended without her. They both asked when they would get the details of their first major projects, the primary focus of their position, but Ms. Morris brushed them off, promising that she would inform them later.

Two weeks passed, and Ms. Turtle and Mr. Powers grew more frustrated with their jobs. Their work plans were still not entered in the project management system, and they were only working on small projects assigned daily by Ms. Morris. Moreover, their offices had not been completed, forcing both of them to move from desk to desk wherever space was available. They finally decided to set up a meeting with Ms. Morris to discuss their frustrations. They developed an agenda for the meeting that included a discussion of the work they completed; proposals for their first projects; and a list of things they required to effectively perform their jobs, including a consistent work space. They framed the meeting as a time to develop a structured work plan, as they were unsure of their current role expectations. Unfortunately, the meeting did not go as smoothly as planned. Ms. Morris felt attacked and was defensive. Although they talked through their agenda items, they did not reach solutions on any issue. Everyone left the meeting feeling uneasy and suspicious.

The next day, Ms. Morris scolded Mr. Powers for the previous day's events, saying that he and Ms. Turtle needed to learn their place. He walked away flabbergasted and found Ms. Turtle to tell her about the encounter. She was still on a six-month probation period, during which she could be fired with few questions asked. He, however, had served the system for four years and could not be terminated as easily. Nonetheless, he called his former boss and explained his situation. The boss offered him an open position, and he turned in his resignation, only one month after he began.

Ms. Turtle was now left alone and had few options except to do as she was told to survive her probationary period. Ms. Morris finally posted a work plan for her, but the plan and its expected results were vague. Ms. Morris continued to assign daily tasks, but they all had unrealistic deadlines. Although Ms. Turtle presented several proposals for her first project, Ms. Morris continued to dismiss her.

More weeks passed and Ms. Turtle learned from a close colleague that Ms. Morris had made a disparaging comment about her during a meeting attended by many service line managers. Apparently, Ms. Morris said, "Well, that was a mistake" in reference to having hired Ms. Turtle. Also, the colleague reported that the grapevine was abuzz with talk that Ms. Morris had been making derisive comments around the hospital about Ms. Turtle.

Ms. Turtle was furious about this news and was worried about its impact on her reputation. Not knowing what to do, she decided to leverage the relationships she had developed during her time as the fellow to save her reputation. She set up meetings with several vice presidents and even her former boss, the COO, to discuss the situation. These meetings did not prove especially helpful, but she felt vindicated and avenged in some ways.

Ms. Turtle grew increasingly bitter about Ms. Morris's unrealistic demands, especially the requirement to provide minutes for any meeting that she attended alone. Ms. Morris had access to Ms. Turtle's calendar and carefully monitored it, sending her reminders about when she should send the minutes. Ms. Turtle finally quit scheduling meetings on her electronic calendar, opting instead to stop by someone's office if she needed to meet or to call for an appointment and jot down a reminder on her paper calendar. If her boss wanted to play games, then she could play too.

Two weeks before her six-month review, Ms. Turtle received a meeting request from Ms. Morris and Bruce Belding, vice president of outpatient services. She expected that this meeting would not be good news, so she prepared a rebuttal the night before. As expected, Ms. Turtle was informed that her employment with the hospital was not working out and she could either be fired and given 30-days severance pay or resign, effective immediately. The reasons cited included (1) insubordination that negatively affected teamwork and customer service and (2) failure to provide quality and quantity of work expected. Ms. Turtle resigned and left immediately.

Current Situation

Ms. Turtle was devastated by that experience, but she moved on. Right after her termination, she went to work for a competing hospital, where she stayed for several years. Although the sting of that first job has faded, she can still remember it and does not want her new direct report, Ms. Kopalski, to have the same experience. Ms. Turtle wishes now that she had given Ms. Kopalski consistent feedback throughout the past six months instead of waiting until now, her formal review date.

Ms. Kopalski is a recent graduate of a top-tier master of health administration (MHA) program. Six months ago, she accepted a position with Englewood Hospital, a private, secular, not-for-profit system that consists of a medical school, five hospitals, and a large ambulatory care facility. The system is consistently ranked among the top 25 hospitals in the United States, and it is world-renowned in oncology and cardiology. Before attending graduate school, Ms. Kopalski was a healthcare consultant in a small firm, where she was responsible for strategic planning projects with hospital clients. At that firm, she was a consistently good performer and worked her way up from analyst to contract manager. After earning her MHA, she wanted to apply the skill sets she had obtained in a different healthcare setting, so she applied for a position as a marketing manager for Englewood Hospital's outpatient clinics.

In preparation for Ms. Kopalski's performance evaluation, Ms. Turtle reviewed the job description she had given Ms. Kopalski when she joined the team (see Figure C3.1).

FIGURE C3.1
Job Description

Job Overview

- Responsible for managing development of the strategic marketing plan for the orthopedic, cardiology, and endocrinology clinics.
- Required to perform market analyses and develop strategies to increase the number of patients who receive services at these three clinics.

Supervisor: Reports to director of marketing for Outpatient Services

Direct reports: Three research analysts

Essential Job Functions

- Identify and address critical issues within each clinic pertaining to the marketing of services/service line expansion, and recommend solutions; win "buy in" from management/physician for plans.
- Lead segmentation activities for each clinic.
- Analyze emerging market opportunities, and develop justification for service line development.
- Target patient populations based on competitive strengths.
- Assess feasibility of meeting targets' needs.
- Monitor competitive environment.

Manage Resources

- Implement expansion of clinical services, and coordinate launch activities.
- Lead cross-functional groups, including Patient Satisfaction, Quality Improvement, Operations, Marketing, Communications, Legal, and Finance/Accounting.
- Recommend and implement pricing strategies and cost-reduction measures to optimize profitability.
- Establish and achieve quarterly profitability goals.

FIGURE C3.1
Continued

Deliverables Include

- Monthly report of progress on annual goals and quarterly summary statistics on clinic performance

- Semiannual report of the activities of competitive activity relating to the three service lines

- Brief reports on clinic staff and departmental meetings

- Written performance reviews for direct reports

- Other reports as requested

Core Behaviors

- Leads strategically

- Builds alignment

- Communicates directly

- Drives performance

- Collaborates

- Energizes others

- Develops people

Ms. Kopalski's Performance

On several occasions in the last six months, Ms. Turtle had been disappointed with Ms. Kopalski's performance:

- The local newspaper reported that a local hospital was launching a new service line consisting of freestanding orthopedic clinics. However, Ms. Kopalski had not mentioned this new development, even though it could have a direct impact on the outpatient clinics for which Ms. Kopalski was responsible.

- One departmental director informed Ms. Turtle that the marketing department has had no representation at 9 out of the last 12 Patient Satisfaction and General Clinic Operations meetings.

- Ms. Kopalski submitted a preliminary draft of profitability goals, but Ms. Turtle noticed several errors in the assumptions used to develop the goals. Additionally, the goals seemed shortsighted and arbitrary.

Despite these issues, Ms. Kopalski has received praise from her direct reports and colleagues, offering the following comments:

- "Leslie is smart, and a great person to work with. She does not micromanage and is always available. She gives me constructive feedback and makes me feel that I am a valued team member. She is also a team player. I remember an instance during my first month working with her when one of the clinics asked me to do a data analysis that used a software that I was unfamiliar with, and I had been working on it for hours and still couldn't figure it out. I finally went and talked to her about it, and she not only knew how to use it but also walked me through the process without ever making me feel stupid."
- "It was a pleasure having Leslie in our staff meeting today. She spoke clearly and perceptively about the issues facing our clinic. She knew the key issues we faced and the threats that we were seeing from our competitors. She advised us on clinic positioning for maximum growth and recommended several initiatives for both short-term and long-term growth, offering to develop and lead the implementation teams. We really feel like she helped us take a giant step forward."

Ms. Turtle believes that, although Ms. Kopalski has not performed up to expectations so far, she has a lot of potential. Ms. Turtle wants to retain and develop Ms. Kopalski and give her some meaningful feedback.

Discussion Questions

1. Assume that the performance review is still a few days away. How should Ms. Turtle prepare for this meeting? Personally, how should she prepare to maximize the effectiveness of the review?
2. What additional information should Ms. Turtle have gathered before the meeting?
3. What could Ms. Turtle have done to prevent the current situation with Ms. Kopalski?
4. If you were Ms. Turtle, how will you give feedback to Ms. Kopalski? Outline an agenda for the performance review, and think about how you will discuss each agenda topic.

5. What reaction do you anticipate Ms. Kopalski will have to Ms. Turtle's concerns about her performance, and how should Ms. Turtle respond to this reaction? Every story always has multiple sides, and this scenario is no exception. It is possible that Ms. Turtle's perception of Ms. Kopalski's performance only represents a portion of a bigger story. How do you expect Ms. Kopalski to talk about this situation?
6. How will Ms. Turtle determine if the performance review was successful? What outcomes should she expect?

INDEX

ABOUT THE EDITORS

Bruce J. Fried, PhD, is an associate professor and director of the Residential Master's Program in the Department of Health Policy and Administration in the School of Public Health at the University of North Carolina at Chapel Hill. He teaches in the areas of human resources management, international and comparative health systems, and globalization and health. He has written numerous journal articles, book chapters, commentaries, and book reviews. Dr. Fried is also coeditor of and contributor to *World Health Systems: Challenges and Perspectives.* Among his research interests are the impact of organizational factors and culture on quality in healthcare settings, healthcare workforce, mental health services, and global health. Dr. Fried has conducted workshops and management training courses in Eastern Europe, Asia, Latin America, and the Caribbean. He received his undergraduate degree from the State University of New York at Buffalo, his master's degree from the University of Chicago, and his doctorate from the University of North Carolina at Chapel Hill.

Myron D. Fottler, PhD, is a professor and executive director of the Health Services Administration Programs at the University of Central Florida, where he teaches courses in healthcare human resources management, service management and marketing, and dissertation research. His research addresses human resources management, service management, and strategic management issues in the healthcare industry. His publications include more than 130 journal articles and 16 books. He has been active in both the Academy of Management and the Association of University Programs in Health Administration. He also serves on several editorial review boards and is a founding coeditor of *Advances in Health Care Management,* an annual research volume published by JAI/Elsevier.

ABOUT THE CONTRIBUTORS

William Atkinson, PhD, FACHE, is president and chief executive officer of WakeMed Health & Hospitals. He has more than 20 years' experience as a hospital president and chief executive officer in rural and urban settings in several states. He earned a doctorate degree in public policy and master's degrees in public health and public policy. He is also a graduate of the Executive Management Program of Yale University. Dr. Atkinson holds adjunct faculty positions in the School of Public Health and the School of Medicine at the University of North Carolina at Chapel Hill and in the School of Public Health at the University of South Carolina, Columbia. In 2007, Dr. Atkinson was named Business Leader of the Year by *Business Leader Magazine* and was named on the Who's Who 2006 list by *Metro Magazine*. He is recognized nationally for his leadership in disaster preparedness, emergency medical services, and workforce development, among other areas. He lectures frequently on innovation diffusion in healthcare.

Adia Bradley, MHA, is a graduate of the University of North Carolina at Chapel Hill (UNC) Gillings School of Global Public Health and is currently a fourth-year medical student at the UNC School of Medicine. She earned a bachelor's degree in finance from the University of Florida.

Dolores G. Clement, DrPH, FACHE, is a tenured professor in the Department of Health Administration at Virginia Commonwealth University (VCU) and the program director of VCU's Professional MSHA Program. She holds a joint appointment in the Department of Preventive and Community Medicine in the School of Medicine at VCU. Dr. Clement earned her doctorate in health policy and administration from the University of California, Berkeley. She has investigated such areas as community health and well-being; curriculum development in allied health professions; distance learning; Medicare risk contracting with HMOs for the elderly in the areas of quality, access, and beneficiary satisfaction; patterns of diffusion; growth and survival of HMOs; and use of alternative payment strategies by various providers.

Maria A. Curran, MA, is the vice president of Human Resources and Family Care Services at Virginia Commonwealth University (VCU) Health System. She is also an adjunct faculty member of the VCU Department of Health Administration and teaches a graduate-level course that focuses on the myriad issues facing executives when managing human capital. Ms. Curran earned a master's degree from the University of Virginia and a bachelor's degree from Rollins College.

Lee Ellis, MHA, is a consultant for Deloitte Consulting. Previously, she worked in operations for the University of North Carolina at Chapel Hill (UNC) Department of Family Medicine and in event planning for the National Multiple Sclerosis Society, Eastern North Carolina Chapter. She received her bachelor's and master's degrees in health policy and administration from the UNC Gillings School of Global Public Health.

Rupert M. Evans, Sr., DHA, FACHE, is an assistant professor and associate director of the Master Healthcare Administration Program in the College of Health Professions at Governors State University. He earned his doctorate from Central Michigan University. Dr. Evans is the principal of Trepur LLC, a healthcare management and diversity consulting company and is senior vice president for the Desir Group Executive Search. He is the immediate past president of the Institute for Diversity in Health Management, a nonprofit organization that seeks to expand opportunities for ethnic minorities in the healthcare field. He has more than 25 years' experience as a healthcare executive and has written several articles, which have appeared in *Hospitals & Health Networks, Modern Healthcare,* and *Journal of Healthcare Management.* A well-known speaker on the subject of diversity in healthcare, Dr. Evans was twice named by *Modern Healthcare* as one of the top 100 "Most Powerful People in Healthcare."

Robert C. Ford, PhD, is a professor of management in the College of Business Administration at the University of Central Florida (UCF). At UCF, he is chair of the Department of Hospitality Management and associate dean for Graduate and External Programs. He has authored or coauthored more than 100 articles, books, and presentations. He has published in a wide variety of academic and practitioner journals, including the *Journal of Applied Psychology, Academy of Management Journal, Organizational Dynamics, Health Care Management Review,* and *The Academy of Management Executive.* His books include *Principles of Management, Organization Theory, Managing the Guest Experience in Hospitality, Achieving Service Excellence, Leading with a Laugh,* and *Managing Destination Marketing Organizations.* He was editor of the *Academy of Management Executive* and chair of both the Management History and Management Education and Management Development divisions of the Academy of Management. He is a Fellow and former dean of the Southern Management Association.

Andy Garrard, MHA, is a graduate of the Department of Health Policy and Administration at the University of North Carolina at Chapel Hill. Previously, he was a senior consultant specializing in supply chain and operations at IBM

Business Consulting Services. Mr. Garrard graduated with high honors from The Georgia Institute of Technology, earning a BS in industrial engineering.

Michael Gates, PhD, RN, is assistant professor in the Hahn School of Nursing and Health Science at the University of San Diego. He has a doctorate in nursing from the University of North Carolina at Chapel Hill. He began his nursing career at the University of Tennessee in Memphis after two years as a research assistant with the health policy group at the Urban Institute and after receiving his BS in applied mathematics/economics from Brown University. His research interests include diversity and the nursing workforce, and he is particularly interested in the link between the healthcare workforce and outcomes of care. His current work examines nurse labor market behaviors, migration, and employment trends.

William Gentry is director of the Community Preparedness and Disaster Management Certificate Program in the Department of Health Policy and Administration in the School of Public Health at the University of North Carolina at Chapel Hill. Mr. Gentry is also an instructor in the program and is the main representative of the program to the first-responder community. Previously, he worked for the North Carolina Division of Emergency Management for more than 15 years. In addition, he has responded to the World Trade Center disaster as part of a national overhead team, to the Red River Flood disaster in North Dakota, and to eight major East Coast hurricanes. He has run statewide operations for several tornados, floods, and ice storms, and he was deployed as the incident commander of a state incident management team to assist after Hurricane Katrina. Mr. Gentry provides consulting services to healthcare institutions for disaster planning and preparedness initiatives.

Heather Grant, MHA, is a graduate of the Department of Health Policy and Administration at the University of North Carolina at Chapel Hill. Previously, she was an office manager for a private dental office and was an intern in the marketing department of a large multispecialty medical practice. She graduated summa cum laude with a BA in business administration from the University of Kentucky. Ms. Grant is a Member of the American College of Healthcare Executives and the Healthcare Financial Management Association.

Eileen F. Hamby, DBA, is vice president of the College of Baccalaureate Studies and Management Programs at Daytona Beach College (DBC). Formerly, she was senior professor and dean of the School of Baccalaureate Studies at DBC. She was also a tenured associate professor and regional campus coordinator for the Master of Science Program in Health Services Administration at the University of Central Florida. She received a bachelor's degree in physical therapy from Hunter College and earned a master's degree in business administration and a doctorate in business administration from Nova University. Dr. Hamby is a Certified Professional in Healthcare Quality, a Diplomate in the American Board of Quality Assurance and Utilization Review Physicians, and a licensed healthcare risk manager in the state of Florida. She has served as chief executive officer of a nursing home and a hospital. In addition, she was the corecipient of the IBM Research Award from the Center for Healthcare Management for her work on patient flow management. Dr. Hamby has published many journal articles and book chapters. Her research interests include leadership, finance, human resources management, and quality management.

Sara L. Hofstetter, MHA, is a graduate of the Department of Health Policy and Administration at the University of North Carolina at Chapel Hill. She has prior experience as a member of the professional staff at the U.S. Senate Committee on Veterans Affairs. In this role, she was involved in congressional oversight of the Veterans Health Administration and making recommendations regarding federal funding levels for the Department of Veterans Affairs. She received her undergraduate degree from Princeton University.

Sarah M. Huth, MHA, is a graduate of the Department of Health Policy and Administration at the University of North Carolina at Chapel Hill. She completed her BS in healthcare administration at the University of Wisconsin, Milwaukee. As an early careerist, she has experience at a Veterans Affairs Medical Center in the areas of process and systems improvement, operations, and strategic planning.

Sharon Jahn, MS, CEBS, CMS, is benefits director for the Virginia Commonwealth University Health System. Previously, she was benefits manager for MCV Physicians, and she worked at Trigon Blue Cross/Blue Shield (now Anthem) in both the actuarial and third-party administration departments. Early in her career, she worked for the actuarial department of Life of Virginia and the Virginia Department of Medical Assistance Services (Medicaid). She received a bachelor's degree in mathematics from The College of William & Mary and a master's degree in risk management and insurance from Virginia Commonwealth University. She earned a Certified Employee Benefits Specialist designation in 2001 and a Compensation Management Specialist designation in 2004. She is currently a Fellow with the International Society of Certified Employee Benefits Specialists (ISCEBS) and is currently serving on the Board of the Richmond Chapter, ISCEBS.

Cheryl B. Jones, PhD, RN, FAAN, is an associate professor in the School of Nursing and a Research Fellow at the Cecil G. Sheps Center for Health

Services Research at the University of North Carolina at Chapel Hill. Dr. Jones has a long-standing interest in the healthcare workforce, quality of care, and the cost of care delivery. Her work on the costs of nursing turnover is cited frequently, and she has published on the nursing workforce topic in numerous peer-reviewed journals. Previously, she served as a senior health services researcher at the Agency for Healthcare Research and Quality (AHRQ), where she was involved in projects examining the nursing workforce at organizational and public policy levels. In her role at AHRQ, she collaborated with others in the public and private sectors to analyze trends in the healthcare workforce and the impacts on quality of care. Dr. Jones is also coauthor of *Financial Management for Nurse Managers and Executives,* 3rd Edition. She obtained her bachelor's degree from the University of Florida and her master's and doctoral degrees from the University of South Carolina.

John Laughlin, MBA, has been a software engineer and information technology consultant to *Fortune* 500 companies for nearly 20 years. He has a bachelor's degree in computer science from Northwest Missouri State University and an MBA from Boise State University. He is currently an independent marketing research consultant.

Donna Malvey, PhD, is an assistant professor at the University of Central Florida. She received her master's degree in health services administration from George Washington University, completed an administrative residency and post-graduate fellowship in hospital administration at the Veterans Administration Medical Center in Washington, DC, and earned her doctorate in health services administration from the University of Alabama at Birmingham. Her area of specialization is strategic management. She was the recipient of a research award from IBM's Center for Healthcare Management for her study of patient flow management. Dr. Malvey is a nationally known speaker, has published extensively in the field, has served on the editorial board of the *Journal of Health Care Management Review,* and is chair-elect of the Faculty Forum on Distance Learning of the Association of University Programs in Health Administration. She has worked as a congressional aide and served in a variety of healthcare positions, including as executive director of a national trade association that represents health professionals.

Leah Masselink is a PhD candidate in the Department of Health Policy and Administration in the School of Public Health at the University of North Carolina at Chapel Hill. Her main research interest is the globalization of healthcare and the healthcare workforce. She holds a bachelor's degree in Spanish studies from Duke University and has worked at the Duke Center for Health Policy and the Center for Clinical and Genetic Economics at Duke Clinical

Research Institute. Her dissertation research examines public discussion and policymaking surrounding recent controversies in nursing education and migration in the Philippines.

Dawn Morrow, MBA, MHA, is a graduate of the University of North Carolina at Chapel Hill Kenan-Flagler Business School and School of Public Health. She earned a BSE in civil engineering from the University of Iowa. After practicing as a roadway designer for three years, she worked in optometry as both a technician and a front-office employee. She has experience in small business operations and marketing.

George H. Pink, PhD, is an associate professor in the Department of Health Policy and Administration in the School of Public Health at the University of North Carolina at Chapel Hill (UNC). He is also a Senior Research Fellow at the Cecil G. Sheps Center for Health Services Research at UNC. Prior to receiving a doctorate in corporate finance, he spent ten years in health services management, planning, and consulting. Dr. Pink teaches courses in healthcare finance and is involved in several large research projects, including studies of hospital financial performance. In the past 20 years, he has served on boards and committees of more than 100 hospitals and other healthcare organizations. He has written more than 60 peer-reviewed articles and has made more than 200 academic presentations in ten countries.

Rita Quinton, SPHR, MPA, is an associate vice president for Organizational and Faculty Development at Daytona Beach College (DBC) and an adjunct instructor for the Bachelor's of Applied Science program at DBC. She has worked in the human resources and organizational development field for more than 17 years. She received her bachelor's degree in business and her master's in public administration from the University of Central Florida. She also directs a nationally recognized Leadership Development Institute and is completing a doctorate in business management from North Central University.

Thomas C. Ricketts, III, PhD, is a professor of health policy and administration and Deputy Director of the Cecil G. Sheps Center for Health Services Research in the University of North Carolina at Chapel Hill. In 2003, he was named director of the North Carolina Center for Health Workforce Studies, one of six such centers funded by the federal government. Dr. Ricketts has been involved in the development of regulations and legislation that guide the distribution of health human resources and policy for primary care providers. In 2004, he was appointed to a four-year term on the National Advisory Committee on Rural Health and Human Services of the U.S. Department of Health and Human Services.

Beverly L. Rubin, JD, serves as the senior vice president and deputy general counsel for Quintiles Transnational Corp. Over the years, she has held numerous positions for Quintiles, including vice president of global human resources operations. Previously, Ms. Rubin practiced law at the firm of Moore & Van Allen, in the areas of employment, healthcare, and commercial litigation. She received her undergraduate degree from the University of Virginia and her law degree from the University of North Carolina. Ms. Rubin has published and presented extensively in the areas of human resources and healthcare litigation.

Howard L. Smith, PhD, is a professor at the Anderson Schools of Management at the University of New Mexico (UNM). From 1990 to 1994, Dr. Smith served as associate dean at the Anderson Schools, and from 1994 to 2004, he was dean of both the Anderson Schools and the School of Public Administration at UNM. He has published more than 200 articles on health services, organization theory/behavior, and strategic management in journals such as the *Academy of Management Journal, Health Care Management Review,* and the *New England Journal of Medicine.* He has published six books on prospective payment, staff development, hospital competition, financial management, strategic nursing management, and reinventing medical practice. His most recent professional book is *Reinventing Medical Practice: Care Delivery that Satisfies Doctors, Patients and the Bottom-line.* He is an active consultant both nationally and internationally.

Kristie G. Stover, MBA, PhD, is an assistant professor at George Washington University. Dr. Stover received her BA in political science from Miami University, her MS in healthcare management and MBA from Marymount University, and her PhD from Virginia Commonwealth University. She is a Member of the American College of Healthcare Executives and has experience in hospital administration, particularly in research, marketing, strategic planning, and governance.

Derek van Amerongen, MD, is vice president and chief medical officer for Humana Health Plans of Ohio in Cincinnati. Previously, he was national medical director for Anthem Blue Cross/Blue Shield, was chief of obstetrics and gynecology for the Johns Hopkins Medical Services Corporation, and was a faculty member for the Johns Hopkins School of Medicine. He has written and presented extensively on managed care and women's health topics. His articles and letters have appeared in such publications as the *New England Journal of Medicine, Physician Executive,* and *Health Affairs.* His book, *Networks and the Future of Medical Practice,* won the 1998 Robert A. Henry Literary Award of the American College of Physician Executives. He received his undergraduate degree from Princeton University, his master's in medical administration from the University of Wisconsin, and his medical degree from Rush Medical College.

Kenneth R. White, RN, PhD, FACHE, is the Charles P. Cardwell, Jr. Professor and the director of the Graduate Program in Health Administration at Virginia Commonwealth University (VCU). Dr. White received his PhD in health services organization and research from VCU, his MPH from the University of Oklahoma, and his MSN from VCU. Dr. White has extensive experience in hospital administration and consulting, particularly in the areas of leadership development, governance, marketing, facility planning, and operations management. Dr. White is a Registered Nurse and a Fellow and former Governor of the American College of Healthcare Executives. He is coauthor of *The Well-Managed Healthcare Organization*, 5th and 6th editions, and *Thinking Forward: Six Strategies for Successful Organizations*. He is a contributing author in the books *Advances in Health Care Organization Theory*, *Peri-Anesthesia Nursing: A Critical Care Approach*, and *Introduction to Health Services*.